BEST EVIDENCE FOR
SPINE SURGERY
20 Cardinal Cases

BEST EVIDENCE FOR
SPINE SURGERY
20 Cardinal Cases

EDITORS

Rahul Jandial, MD, PhD
Assistant Professor
Division of Neurosurgery
City of Hope Cancer Center
Los Angeles, California

Steven R. Garfin, MD
Distinguished Professor and
   Chairman
Department of Orthopaedic Surgery
University of California San Diego
   Health System
San Diego, California

ASSOCIATE EDITORS

Christopher P. Ames, MD
Associate Professor
Department of Neurosurgery
Co-Director, Spine Center
University of California San Francisco
San Francisco, California

Henry E. Aryan, MD
Associate Clinical Professor
Department of Neurosurgery
University of California San Francisco
Sierra Pacific Orthopaedic & Spine Center
Fresno, California

Scott D. Boden, MD
Professor of Orthopaedics
Director, Emory Orthopaedics and Spine Center
Orthopaedic Surgery
Emory University
Staff Physician, Department of Orthopaedic
   Surgery
Atlanta Veterans Affairs Medical Center
Atlanta, Georgia

Mike Y. Chen, MD, PhD
Assistant Professor
Division of Neurosurgery
City of Hope Cancer Center
Los Angeles, California

Alexander R. Vaccaro, MD, PhD
Professor and Vice Chairman
Department of Orthopaedic Surgery
Thomas Jefferson University and
   The Rothman Institute
Philadelphia, Pennsylvania

ELSEVIER
SAUNDERS

1600 John F. Kennedy Blvd.
Ste 1800
Philadelphia, PA 19103-2899

BEST EVIDENCE FOR SPINE SURGERY: 20 Cardinal Cases   ISBN: 978-1-4377-1625-2
Copyright © 2012 by Saunders, an imprint of Elsevier Inc.

Notice

Knowledge and best practice in this field are constantly changing. As new research and experience broaden our understanding, changes in research methods, professional practices, or medical treatment may become necessary.

Practitioners and researchers must always rely on their own experience and knowledge in evaluating and using any information, methods, compounds, or experiments described herein. In using such information or methods they should be mindful of their own safety and the safety of others, including parties for whom they have a professional responsibility.

With respect to any drug or pharmaceutical products identified, readers are advised to check the most current information provided (i) on procedures featured or (ii) by the manufacturer of each product to be administered, to verify the recommended dose or formula, the method and duration of administration, and contraindications. It is the responsibility of practitioners, relying on their own experience and knowledge of their patients, to make diagnoses, to determine dosages and the best treatment for each individual patient, and to take all appropriate safety precautions.

To the fullest extent of the law, neither the Publisher nor the authors, contributors, or editors assume any liability for any injury and/or damage to persons or property as a matter of products liability, negligence or otherwise, or from any use or operation of any methods, products, instructions, or ideas contained in the material herein.

Library of Congress Cataloging-in-Publication Data
Best evidence for spine surgery / editors, Rahul Jandial, Steven R. Garfin ; associate editors, Christopher Ames ... [et al.]. — 1st ed.
  p. ; cm.
Includes bibliographical references and index.
ISBN 978-1-4377-1625-2 (hardcover : alk. paper)
I. Jandial, Rahul. II. Garfin, Steven R. III. Ames, Christopher P.
[DNLM: 1. Spine—surgery—Case Reports. 2. Evidence-Based Medicine—Case Reports. 3. Orthopedic Procedures—methods—Case Reports. 4. Spinal Diseases—surgery—Case Reports. WE 725]
617.5'6059—dc23   2011045627

Content Strategist: Julie Goolsby
Senior Developmental Editor: Mary Beth Murphy
Publishing Services Manager: Anne Altepeter
Project Manager: Louise King
Designer: Louis Forgione

Working together to grow
libraries in developing countries

www.elsevier.com | www.bookaid.org | www.sabre.org

ELSEVIER   BOOK AID International   Sabre Foundation

Printed in China
Last digit is the print number: 9 8 7 6 5 4 3 2 1

To my dear wife, Danielle—for countless reasons

Rahul Jandial

I continually need to thank and offer my appreciation to my wife and family, and my UCSD friends/colleagues (particularly Liz, Wendy, Yu-Po, Todd, and others) for supporting me for the extra time it takes to work at a teaching institution, teaching young, bright surgeons and colleagues/others through attending meetings, lecturing, editing/writing books, doing research, and providing complex clinical care.

Steven R. Garfin

Contributors

Frank L. Acosta, Jr., MD
Assistant Professor
Department of Neurological Surgery
Cedars-Sinai Medical Center
Los Angeles, California

Mir H. Ali, MD, PhD
Orthopaedic Spine Surgeon
OAD Orthopaedics
Warrenville, Illinois

Edward R. Anderson III, MD
Fellow, Department of Spine Surgery
William Beaumont Hospital
Royal Oak, Michigan

Paul A. Anderson, MD
Professor of Orthopedic Surgery
University of Wisconsin
Madison, Wisconsin

Paul M. Arnold, MD, FACS
Professor of Neurosurgery
Department of Neurosurgery
University of Kansas Medical Center
Kansas City, Kansas

Edward C. Benzel, MD
Chairman, Department of Neurosurgery
Center for Spine Health
Cleveland Clinic
Cleveland, Ohio

Sigurd Berven, MD
Associate Professor in Residence
Department of Orthopaedic Surgery
University of California at San Francisco
San Francisco, California

Scott D. Boden, MD
Professor of Orthopaedics
Director, Emory Orthopaedics and
    Spine Center
Orthopaedic Surgery
Emory University
Staff Physician, Department of
    Orthopaedic Surgery
Atlanta Veterans Affairs Medical Center
Atlanta, Georgia

Christopher M. Bono, MD
Associate Professor
Department of Orthopaedic Surgery
Brigham and Women's Hospital
Harvard Medical School
Boston, Massachusetts

Ali Bydon, MD
Assistant Professor of Neurosurgery
Department of Neurosurgery
Johns Hopkins University
Baltimore, Maryland

Garrick W. Cason, MD
Fellow, Department of Spine Surgery
William Beaumont Hospital
Royal Oak, Michigan

Kelli L. Crabtree, MD
School of Medicine
University of Kansas Medical Center
Kansas City, Kansas

Bradford L. Currier, MD
Professor
Department of Orthopedic Surgery
Mayo Clinic
Rochester, Minnesota

Scott D. Daffner, MD
Assistant Professor
Department of Orthopaedics
West Virginia University School
    of Medicine
Morgantown, West Virginia

Michael F. Duffy, MD
Orthopaedic Spine Surgeon
Texas Back Institute
Mansfield, Texas

Richard G. Fessler, MD, PhD
Professor of Neurological Surgery
Department of Neurological Surgery
Northwestern University
Chicago, Illinois

Michael A. Finn, MD
Assistant Professor of Neurosurgery
University of Colorado School of Medicine
Aurora, Colorado

Steven R. Garfin, MD
Distinguished Professor and Chairman
Department of Orthopaedic Surgery
University of California San Diego
    Health System
San Diego, California

Ziya L. Gokaslan, MD
Professor of Neurosurgery, Oncology, and
    Orthopaedic Surgery
Department of Neurosurgery
Johns Hopkins University
Baltimore, Maryland

Krishna Gumidyala, MD
Orthopaedic Surgeon
OptimOrthopaedics
Savannah, Georgia

Andrew C. Hecht, MD
Assistant Professor of Orthopaedic Surgery
    and Neurosurgery
Co-Chief of Spinal Surgery
Mount Sinai Hospital
Mount Sinai School of Medicine
New York, New York

Harry N. Herkowitz, MD
Chairman, Department of Orthopaedic
    Surgery
William Beaumont Hospital
Royal Oak, Michigan

Rahul Jandial, MD, PhD
Assistant Professor
Division of Neurosurgery
City of Hope Cancer Center
Los Angeles, California

Michael G. Kaiser, MD
Assistant Professor of Neurological Surgery
Department of Neurological Surgery
The Neurological Institute
Columbia University
New York, New York

Adam S. Kanter, MD
Assistant Professor of Neurological Surgery
Department of Neurological Surgery
University of Pittsburgh
Pittsburgh, Pennsylvania

Thomas J. Kesman, MD, MBA
Fellow, Orthopedic Spine Surgery
OrthoCarolina
Charlotte, North Carolina

Tyler R. Koski, MD
Assistant Professor of Neurological Surgery
Department of Neurological Surgery
Northwestern University Feinberg School
    of Medicine and Northwestern Memorial
    Hospital
Chicago, Illinois

Yu-Po Lee
Assistant Clinical Professor
Department of Orthopaedic Surgery
University of California San Diego
University of California San Diego Medical
    Center
San Diego, California

Timothy E. Link, MD
Fellow, Clinical Instructor
Division of Neurological Surgery
Barrow Neurological Institute
St. Joseph's Hospital and Medical Center
Phoenix, Arizona

Christopher E. Mandigo, MD
Instructor of Clinical Neurosurgery
Department of Neurological Surgery
Columbia University College of Physicians
    and Surgeons
New York, New York

Steven Mardjetko
Associate Professor
Department of Orthopedic Surgery
Rush University
Chicago, Illinois

Matthew B. Maserati, MD
Resident, Neurological Surgery
Department of Neurological Surgery
University of Pittsburgh
Pittsburgh, Pennsylvania

Jamal McClendon, Jr., MD
Resident, Department of Neurological Surgery
Northwestern University Feinberg School
    of Medicine and Northwestern Memorial
    Hospital
Chicago, Illinois

Paul C. McCormick, MD, MPH
Herbert and Linda Gallen Professor
    of Neurological Surgery
Neurosurgery
Columbia University College of Physicians
    and Surgeons
New York, New York

Robert A. McGuire, Jr., MD
Professor and Chairman
Department of Orthopedic Surgery and
    Rehabilitation
The University of Mississippi Medical Center
Jackson, Mississippi

Tuan V. Nguyen, MD
Trinity Neurosurgery
Trinity Medical Center
Birmingham, Alabama

Alfred T. Ogden, MD
Assistant Professor
Department of Neurological Surgery
The Neurological Institute
Columbia University
New York, New York

Stephen L. Ondra, MD
Professor of Neurological Surgery
Department of Neurological Surgery
Northwestern University Feinberg School
    of Medicine and Northwestern Memorial
    Hospital
Chicago, Illinois

Niraj Patel
Department of Orthopaedic Surgery
University of California San Diego
University of California San Diego Medical
    Center
San Diego, California

Frank M. Phillips, MD
Professor of Orthopaedic Spine Surgery
Rush University Medical Center
Midwest Orthopedics at Rush
Chicago, Illinois

Sheeraz A. Qureshi, MD, MBA
Assistant Professor of Orthopaedic Surgery
Mount Sinai Hospital
Mount Sinai School of Medicine
New York, New York

Andrew J. Schoenfeld, MD
Assistant Professor
Department of Orthopaedic Surgery
William Beaumont Army Medical Center
Texas Technical University Health Sciences
    Center
El Paso, Texas

Daniel M. Sciubba, MD
Assistant Professor of Neurosurgery,
    Oncology, and Orthopaedic Surgery
Department of Neurosurgery
Johns Hopkins University
Baltimore, Maryland

Christopher I. Shaffrey, MD
Professor of Neurological Surgery
Department of Neurological Surgery
University of Virginia
Charlottesville, Virginia

John H. Shin, MD
Instructor in Surgery (Neurosurgery)
Harvard Medical School
Attending Neurosurgeon
Massachusetts General Hospital
Boston, Massachusetts

Harvey E. Smith, MD
Assistant Clinical Professor
Department of Orthopaedic Surgery
Tufts University School of Medicine and
    New England Baptist Hospital
Boston, Massachusetts

Volker K.H. Sonntag, MD
Vice Chairman, Emeritus
Division of Neurological Surgery
Barrow Neurological Institute
St. Joseph's Hospital and Medical Center
Phoenix, Arizona

Alexander R. Vaccaro, MD, PhD
Professor and Vice Chairman
Department of Orthopaedic Surgery
Thomas Jefferson University and
    The Rothman Institute
Philadelphia, Pennsylvania

Jean-Paul Wolinsky, MD
Assistant Professor of Neurosurgery and
    Oncology
Department of Neurosurgery
Johns Hopkins University
Baltimore, Maryland

Jack E. Zigler, MD
Orthopaedic Spine Surgeon
Co-Director, Fellowship Program
Texas Back Institute
Plano, Texas

Preface

Clinical practice based on "evidence" would seem an objective both clearly defined and easily attained, but in its application to surgical decision making essential nuances are often lacking. In the construction of this text, presenting the elusive subtleties has been a priority. By selecting cases that require a synthesis of diverse surgical knowledge and technical skill, we aim to provide insights that can be extended both to the specialized case and to the general practice of spine surgery.

For pedagogical reasons, the chapters comprising this book are titled after commonly debated topics in professional meetings and grand-rounds worldwide. Accordingly, the chapters have been designed to present decision making from the available evidence regarding two competing treatment options for a single disease entity. We believe this approach is ideal for dissecting the layers of "best evidence" through which the decision making between surgeon and patient can be personalized.

For broad appeal to both developing and veteran surgeons, each chapter opens with a brief Case Presentation followed by Surgical Options and a crisply illustrated section on Fundamental Technique. A Discussion of Best Evidence provides readers with the necessary knowledge to criticize as well as defend competing surgical interventions, thereby equipping them with the best evidence. In lieu of a summary, each chapter presents a Commentary from the senior author, who shares with readers a personal synthesis of the topic.

The credibility of a text that aims to reveal the leading edge of evolving surgical practice rests almost entirely on the strength of expert voices. Undoubtedly both neurosurgery and orthopaedics fundamentally contribute to the craft of spine surgery, and the collection of senior authors presented in *Best Evidence for Spine Surgery,* in our opinion, includes many of the best.

Our hope is that this book functions to improve both the art and expertise with which you practice.

Rahul Jandial
Steven R. Garfin

Acknowledgments

I would like to recognize my administrative staff and the team at Elsevier for not only facilitating this book, but also for helping improve it.

Rahul Jandial

It has been a wonderful opportunity and experience for me to work with Rahul Jandial, MD, PhD, on this book. He is a neurosurgeon who trained at UCSD. Though I am listed as an equal as an editor, it was his concept and his diligence that brought this to fruition. My contribution was to add to the chapters and help cajole the distinguished senior faculty to participate in this book, and then review the chapters after Rahul. At UCSD I have had the opportunity and privilege to work not only with orthopaedic surgery, but with neurosurgery, residents, and faculty in a manner I learned during my fellowship with Richard Rothman, MD, PhD (orthopaedic spine surgeon) and Frederick Simeone, MD (neurosurgeon). This has carried over into my involvement at AAOS, NASS, CSRS, ISSAS, and other organizations, as well as at UCSD.

Steven R. Garfin

Contents

Chapter 1   Cervical Disk Herniation: Anterior Cervical Diskectomy and Fusion Versus Arthroplasty

Mir H. Ali, Frank M. Phillips

Cervical disk herniation is a common problem affecting approximately 1 in 1000 adults in the United States.[1] Although it typically causes radicular pain in a dermatomal distribution (radiculopathy), it can also cause motor weakness and myelopathic symptoms, such as gait difficulty, muscle spasticity, and bowel or bladder incontinence.[2] In cases of isolated cervical radiculopathy without weakness, nonoperative treatment is usually recommended in the acute phase. Physical therapy and selective nerve root (or epidural) injections can alleviate symptoms and obviate the need for surgical intervention.[3] If these treatments are not successful, surgical intervention may be considered. Surgical options include posterior laminoforaminotomy, anterior cervical diskectomy and fusion (ACDF), and cervical total disk replacement (TDR).[4]

CASE PRESENTATION

A 42-year-old man had a 3-month history of left-sided arm pain that radiated from his neck to the level of his elbow. At presentation he described constant paresthesias and subjective weakness in his upper arm with overhead activities. He initially rated the pain at 8 out of 10 on a visual analog scale (VAS). When he first developed symptoms, he was prescribed nonsteroidal antiinflammatory medications and physical therapy, which minimally decreased his pain over the subsequent 2 weeks (pain rating of 6 out of 10). Two weeks after beginning physical therapy, the patient underwent a fluoroscopically guided C5-6 epidural steroid injection that provided some symptomatic relief, but with persistence of weakness.

- PMH: Unremarkable
- PSH: Unremarkable
- Exam: The patient had normal spinal posture with 60 degrees of cervical flexion and 20 degrees of extension. Extension beyond 20 degrees produced pain in the left shoulder and the Spurling maneuver gave a positive result for both pain and numbness into the left arm. Motor examination revealed 4/5 strength in the patient's left deltoid, external rotators, and biceps; he had normal 5/5 strength in all other muscle groups tested, including the right deltoid, external rotators, and biceps. Sensation to light touch was diminished over the lateral aspect of the shoulder on the left side, but preserved in all other dermatomal distributions in the left and right upper extremities. Reflexes were normal and symmetric in all extremities. No pathologic reflexes were present. His gait was normal with no evidence of cervical myelopathy.
- Imaging: Plain radiographs demonstrated cervical spondylosis with anterior osteophytes at C4-5 and C5-6 (Figure 1-1, *A* and *B*). There was no evidence of spondylolisthesis or instability with flexion extension (Figure 1-1, *C* and *D*). Cervical magnetic resonance imaging (MRI) demonstrated central disk herniation at C4-5 and C5-6 with left greater than right foraminal stenosis (Figure 1-2). A computed tomographic (CT) scan revealed little uncovertebral spurring and mild facet arthrosis at the lower cervical levels (Figure 1-3).

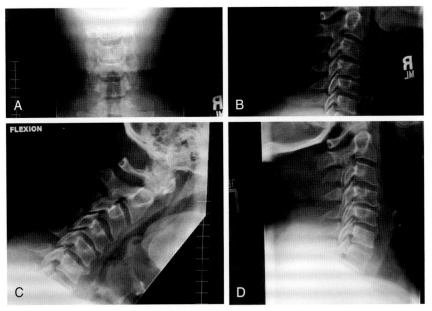

FIGURE 1-1 Plain radiographs at presentation. **A,** AP view. **B,** Lateral view. **C,** Flexion. **D,** Extension.

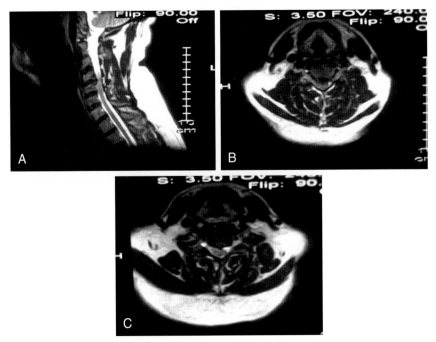

FIGURE 1-2 MRI images at presentation. **A,** T2-weighted sagittal image. **B,** T2-weighted axial image at C4-5. **C,** T2-weighted axial image at C5-6.

SURGICAL OPTIONS

Surgical indications for a herniated disk include disabling or progressive motor deficit or failure of radicular symptoms to respond to an appropriate nonoperative course of treatment. Surgical options for cervical disk herniation with indications for operative intervention include posterior laminoforaminotomy, anterior cervical diskectomy without fusion, ACDF, and cervical disk replacement. If the patient does not complain of neck pain and has only radicular symptoms, and imaging

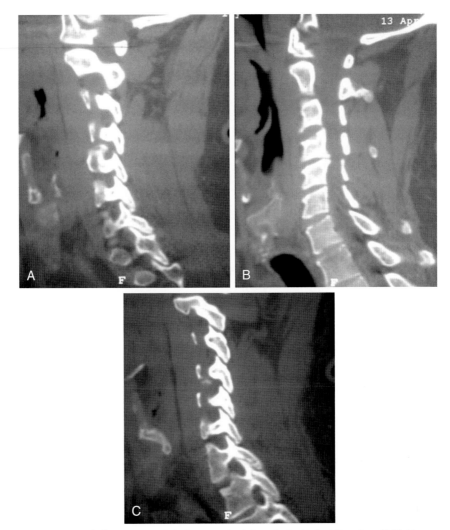

FIGURE 1-3 CT scan before surgery. **A,** Left parasagittal view. **B,** Sagittal midline view. **C,** Right parasagittal view. No significant facet disease is demonstrated.

demonstrates a "soft" disk herniation, a posterior cervical laminoforaminotomy could adequately decompress the involved nerve root if the disk is lateral and not central. This procedure avoids the need for concomitant fusion. However, in patients with radiculopathy and persistent and severe neck pain, ACDF may be preferred. In addition, in the presence of anterior spinal cord compression or localized kyphosis, ACDF is preferred. Although ACDF has been successfully performed for decades, there are concerns that fusion alters spinal kinematics and leads to accelerated degeneration of adjacent segments. Cervical TDR has been suggested as an alternative to fusion with the advantage of preserving motion at the treated level and thereby theoretically reducing the risk of adjacent-level degeneration. The indications for cervical disk replacement include radiculopathy due to disk herniation with failure of nonoperative treatment or progressive or disabling motor loss. In addition, acute myelopathy secondary to a disk herniation may be amenable to treatment with decompression and TDR (Table 1-1). In cases of advanced degenerative spondylosis, ACDF may be preferable to TDR. These would include cases showing severe loss of disk height, significant osteophyte formation, facet arthrosis, or ankylosis.

TABLE 1-1   Indications and Contraindications for Total Disk Replacement

Indications	Contraindications
Cervical radiculopathy refractory to nonoperative treatment and/or with objective motor weakness	Posterior column instability (e.g., iatrogenic or associated with trauma or rheumatoid arthritis)
Cervical myelopathy or myeloradiculopathy without retrovertebral stenosis	Retrovertebral stenosis (e.g., congenital cervical stenosis)
Isolated symptomatic cervical disk disease at one, two, or three levels	Chronic or active infection
	Ankylosing spondylitis/diffuse idiopathic skeletal hyperostosis
	Ossification of the posterior longitudinal ligament
	Symptomatic facet arthrosis
	Osteoporosis
	Axial neck pain
	Obesity

For the patient described in the case study, he had his central disk herniations at both C4-5 and C5-6, so a posterior cervical laminoforaminotomy was not a good option. The risks, benefits, and alternatives to both ACDF and cervical disk replacement were discussed. At the time of the patient's evaluation, a U.S. Food and Drug Administration (FDA) study of two-level cervical disk arthroplasties was in progress, and the patient was interested in participating in this study at the authors' institution. All appropriate consents were obtained according to study protocols, and the patient was scheduled for two-level cervical disk replacement at C4-5 and C5-6.

FUNDAMENTAL TECHNIQUE

The surgical technique for cervical disk replacement is largely based on traditional ACDF techniques.[5-7] The neck should be positioned in a neutral posture avoiding hyperextension. Anteroposterior and lateral fluoroscopic images should be checked after positioning to ensure adequate visualization of the treated level. The patient's shoulders should be taped down if necessary to visualize the lower cervical levels (C6 and C7).

The surgical method utilizes the well-described Smith-Robinson exposure.[8] After the skin is cut with a transverse incision based on anatomic landmarks and/or radiologic guidance, the platysma is exposed and incised. The deep cervical fascia is then exposed and incised anterior to the anterior border of the anterior belly of the sternocleidomastoid muscle. After palpating the carotid pulse and remaining medial to it, the surgeon uses blunt dissection to palpate the cervical spine. After the anterior cervical spine is adequately visualized, this structure is divided to expose the prevertebral fascia underneath. This is also divided vertically in the midline of the cervical spine. The midline is denoted by the gap seen by the medial borders of the longus colli.

Once the midline is adequately identified radiographically and marked, the longus colli muscles are elevated bilaterally (Tips from the Masters 1-1). After the proper disk space is identified, the exposure of the disk space is completed laterally to the uncovertebral joints bilaterally.

Tips from the Masters 1-1 • Identifying the midline is essential to appropriate implant placement.

After placement of craniocaudal distractors (Caspar-type pins in the vertebral body above and below the disk space) and self-retaining lateral retractors under the longus colli, diskectomy is performed (Tips from the Masters 1-2).

Tips from the Masters 1-2 • Careful attention must be paid to creating parallel end plates for implant insertion while minimizing weakening of the subchondral bone of the vertebral end plates.

In certain instances, contracture of the posterior longitudinal ligament (PLL) may limit parallel distraction of the vertebral end plates, which is typically required for appropriate prosthesis positioning, and thus division or removal of the PLL is necessary. If removal of the PLL or central osteophytes is required to effect neural decompression, this should be performed. When a TDR is carried out, the end plates should be preserved to avoid subsidence and heterotopic bone formation. A curette may be used to remove cartilaginous tissue to ensure parallel end plates. Use of a bur should be avoided to ensure minimal disruption of the end plates. Once the end plates are adequately prepared, careful attention is paid to the affected cervical foramina, and adequate foraminal decompression is ensured with curettes and/or Kerrison rongeurs to remove any residual posterior uncovertebral spurs (Tips from the Masters 1-3). Adequate foraminal decompression is essential to relieving radiculopathy and minimizing recurrent symptoms in cervical disk replacement (Tips from the Masters 1-4).

Tips from the Masters 1-3 • Unlike after fusion, after total disk replacement motion will continue, so that symptoms will not be relieved unless complete direct foraminal decompression is achieved at surgery.

Tips from the Masters 1-4 • In most instances, the prosthesis should be placed posteriorly in the disk space to allow for more normal kinematics.

Once the decompression is complete and the end plates prepared, attention is turned toward instrumentation. Using trial spacers, the implant of proper height and width is obtained. The widest implant able to be safely implanted should be selected to reduce the risks of subsidence. "Overstuffing" of the disk space will reduce implant motion, so the shortest implant (in a cranial-caudal direction) that is stable within the disk space should be used. Most trials have specific rotational specifications that require strict centering of the implant at the midline. After the properly fitted trial implant is placed, it is useful to obtain anteroposterior (AP) and lateral fluoroscopic images to confirm adequate positioning of the implant. After thorough irrigation and trialing, the TDR implant is placed, with careful attention to rotation, angulation, and depth. Whereas rotation is largely assessed with direct visualization and is based on identification of the midline at exposure, angulation and depth are best assessed with fluoroscopic guidance.

Postoperative course: The patient left the hospital on postoperative day 1, tolerating a soft diet. Upright cervical spine radiographs were obtained before discharge (Figure 1-4). He wore his soft collar for 1 week and was seen for a clinical recheck at 2 weeks. His radiculopathy and neck pain resolved, and by 3 months after surgery he had resumed all usual activities. He required no pain medications. He was seen again at 3 months, 6 months, 12 months, 15 months, and 24 months. He was working in an unlimited capacity at 3 months; he was performing all of his recreational activities—including horseback riding and playing tennis—by 6 months. His motor strength and sensation returned to normal on the left side by his 6-month visit. Plain radiographs were taken at all visits and demonstrated a well-fixed prostheses with no evidence of lucency or migration (Figure 1-5). As part of the FDA study, a CT scan was performed at 2 years (Figure 1-6), which demonstrated osseous ingrowth and no evidence of lucency, migration, or osteolysis.

DISCUSSION OF BEST EVIDENCE

For the treatment of cervical radiculopathy, ACDF is a successful procedure for relief of neck and arm symptoms.[9,10] With greater than 90% fusion success using modern instrumentation techniques, it has become a reliable option in patients requiring surgery.[11] Clinical outcomes have been good for pain relief, return to work, and patient satisfaction.[12] With minimal morbidity in most cases, it has become one of the most common spine procedures performed. Despite the overall success of the procedure, however, there are potential disadvantages. Hilibrand and colleagues[13] reported an

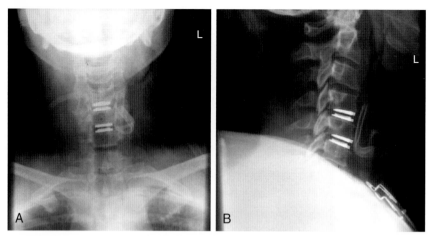

FIGURE 1-4 Radiographs taken immediately after surgery. **A,** AP view. **B,** Lateral view.

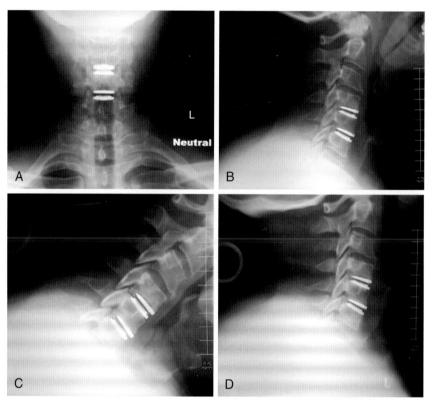

FIGURE 1-5 Radiographs obtained at 2-year follow-up. **A,** AP view. **B,** Lateral view. **C,** Flexion. **D,** Extension.

incidence of degeneration at segments adjacent to a fusion of 2.9% per year, with 25.6% of patients having symptomatic cervical disk disease within 10 years of ACDF. In a number of instances, degeneration of adjacent segments results in the need for additional surgery that carries a higher risk of complications, including dysphagia, pseudarthrosis, and dysphonia.[14,15] The potential for preserving motion and avoiding degeneration of adjacent segments has resulted in an increased interest in cervical TDR over the past decade.

Patients with congenital cervical stenosis should not be considered for disk replacement, because the retrovertebral compression will not be adequately

FIGURE 1-6 Follow-up CT scan at 2 years after surgery.

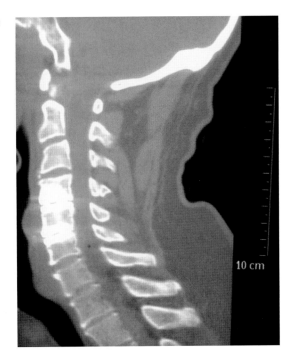

addressed with diskectomy only. Patients who have undergone prior laminectomies or have posterior column instability due to trauma or rheumatoid arthritis should not be considered for cervical disk replacement, because disk replacement in these patients may create an unstable cervical motion segment.[16] Patients with ankylosing spondylitis or diffuse idiopathic skeletal hyperostosis should not undergo cervical disk replacement because of the tendency to ankylosis. Patients with ossification of the PLL should not undergo cervical disk replacement, because motion preservation at the level of the cervical disk replacement may lead to further ossification of the PLL and thus result in cord compression. TDR is contraindicated in patients with active or chronic infections of the cervical spine.

Facet arthrosis is a contraindication to cervical TDR, because the procedure may not result in relief of symptoms due to ongoing motion at the diseased facet joint. Patients with advanced spondylosis, severe disk space collapse, and a relatively immobile segment are not considered good candidates for TDR. Osteoporosis increases the risk for implant subsidence and represents a contraindication to TDR. Finally, axial neck pain without radiculopathy or myelopathy has not been studied in sufficient detail to warrant cervical disk replacement in these patients at this time.[17] Further studies providing outcome measures and quality of life data are required to support recommendation in this patient population.[16,18]

Over the past 5 years, three cervical disk replacement devices have been approved by the FDA to treat cervical disk disease: the Prestige (Medtronic Spinal and Biologics, Memphis), Bryan (Medtronic Spinal and Biologics), and ProDisc-C (Synthes Spine, West Chester, Pa.). Several more designs are under investigation by the FDA and may be approved in the near future.[19] For the purposes of this general review, the focus is on peer-reviewed published data concerning the use of these three FDA-approved cervical disk replacement devices.

The first FDA-approved cervical disk replacement device was the Prestige, approved in 2007. The Prestige cervical disk has a ball-and-trough design that allows relatively unconstrained motion (Figure 1-7).[20] The Prestige ST is a stainless steel implant with a 2.5-mm anterior faceplate, whereas the Prestige LP is a titanium-ceramic composite that has a lower profile without the anterior

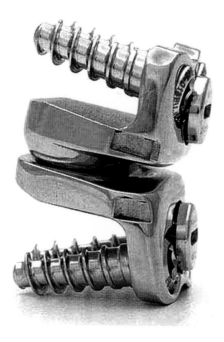

FIGURE 1-7 Prestige ST cervical disk replacement device. *(Courtesy Medtronic Spinal and Biologics, Memphis)*

faceplate and allows easier viewing on CT and MRI scans.[21,22] **Prospective, randomized trial** results at 12 months and 24 months have been reported for the Prestige ST.[23] Five hundred forty-one patients with single-level cervical disease and radiculopathy were enrolled at 32 sites and randomly assigned to undergo cervical disk replacement or ACDF. A greater improvement in the Neck Disability Index (NDI) score, a higher rate of neurologic success, and a lower rate of secondary revision surgeries were reported in the cervical disk replacement patients in the initial study. These patients also showed more improvement in their scores on the Short Form 36 (SF-36) Health Survey, experienced more improvement in their neck pain, and returned to work faster than patients undergoing ACDF. There were no cases of implant failure or migration. Although the clinical significance of the differences remains controversial, these results indicate that disk replacement using the Prestige ST device is at least comparable to ACDF at 2 years and can be considered as safe as ACDF over the short term (up to 24 months). More recently, 5-year outcomes from this trial have been reported and are similar to those seen at 2 years, with no evidence of implant migration.[24]

The Bryan disk is a one-piece, biarticulating, metal-on-polymer implant.[25] The component is made up of two titanium shells with an intervening polyurethane nucleus in a saline-contained sheath (Figure 1-8). This gives the component a hydraulic cushioning effect, which dampens axial loads. Two-year results have been recently reported for a **prospective, randomized, multicenter trial** of cervical disk replacement using the Bryan disk.[26] Four hundred sixty-three patients were randomly assigned to undergo either ACDF or cervical disk replacement with the Bryan disk. Analysis of data 12 and 24 months postoperatively showed improvement in all clinical outcome measures for both groups; however, 24 months after surgery, the patients in the investigational group receiving the artificial disk had a statistically greater improvement in NDI scores and overall success. The replacement group had a *lower* rate of implant-associated adverse events (1.7% vs. 3.2%). There was no statistical difference between the two groups with regard to the rate of secondary surgical procedures performed subsequent to the index procedure. Two-year follow-up results indicate that cervical disk replacement is a viable alternative to ACDF in patients with persistently symptomatic, single-level cervical disk disease. More recently, 4-year outcomes from this trial have been reported

FIGURE 1-8 Bryan cervical disk replacement device. *(Courtesy Medtronic Spinal and Biologics, Memphis)*

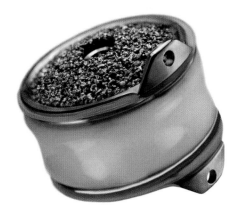

FIGURE 1-9 ProDisc-C cervical disk replacement device. *(Courtesy Synthes Spine, West Chester, Pa.)*

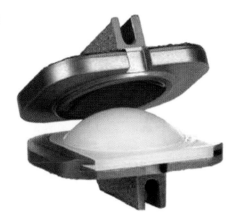

nationally and are similar to those seen at 2 years, with cervical disk replacement results statistically better than ACDF.[27,28]

The ProDisc-C is a ball-and-socket joint, with cobalt chrome alloy end plates and an ultra-high-molecular-weight polyethylene articulating insert.[29] Fixation is based on slotted keels and a titanium plasma spray coating to allow for bone ingrowth.[30,31] It is a nonconstrained implant that limits translation (Figure 1-9). Two-year follow-up results have recently been reported from the FDA Investigational Device Exemption (IDE) study involving the ProDisc-C.[32] In this **prospective, randomized, multicenter trial,** 209 patients were randomly assigned to undergo either ACDF or cervical disk replacement with the ProDisc-C device. NDI scores, SF-36 scores, and neurologic success were similar in both groups. VAS-assessed neck pain intensity and frequency as well as VAS-assessed arm pain intensity and frequency were significantly improved but were no different between treatment groups. At 24 months after surgery, 84% of patients receiving the ProDisc-C device achieved 4 degrees of motion or more at the operated level. There was a statistically significant difference in the number of secondary surgeries, with 8.5% of patients undergoing ACDF needing reoperation, revision, or supplemental fixation within the 24 months after the initial surgery, compared with only 1.8% of patients undergoing disk replacement with the ProDisc-C device. At 24 months, there was a statistically significant difference in medication usage, with 90% of patients in the ProDisc-C group not taking strong narcotics or muscle relaxants, compared with 82% of those in the ACDF group. Based on these data, it appears that disk replacement using the ProDisc-C device is safe and effective in treating single-level cervical disk disease and may have advantages when compared with ACDF. More recently, 5-year results from this study have been reported nationally and demonstrate outcomes similar to those seen at 2 years, with cervical disk replacement results statistically better than ACDF results, but functional and clinical outcomes appear to be equivalent compared with those for ACDF. The decreased rate of subsequent surgeries in the ProDisc-C group appears to be clinically significant.[33]

Although cervical disk replacements have been shown to provide near-physiologic motion in cadaver specimens and in vitro models,[20,25,34,35] it is unclear if these **cadaveric biomechanical data** are reproduced in the clinical setting. Moreover, what happens to motion at the level of the cervical replacement over time is still unclear. These questions are slowly being answered with radiographic and clinical follow-up data.

As for **patient biomechanical data,** in patients receiving the Prestige disk device, Mummaneni and colleagues[23] demonstrated an average of 7 degrees of motion at the level of the replacement as measured by angulation of the disk space on flexion-extension radiographs. Similarly, in patients implanted with the ProDisc-C device, Bertagnoli and associates[31] demonstrated an average of 4 to 12 degrees of motion at the level of the replacement at the 24-month follow-up. In a subset of patients enrolled in the trial of the Bryan disk, Sasso and Best[36] demonstrated increased motion in those undergoing single-level disk replacement compared with those undergoing single-level ACDF. Using flexion, extension, and neutral lateral radiographs obtained preoperatively, immediately postoperatively, and at regular intervals up to 24 months, range of motion, translation, and center of rotation were calculated using quantitative motion analysis software. Significantly more flexion-extension motion was retained in the disk replacement group than the fusion group at the index level. The disk replacement group retained an average of 6.7 degrees of motion at 24 months. In contrast, the average range of motion in the fusion group was 2.0 degrees at the 3-month follow-up and gradually decreased to 0.6 degrees at 24 months. Thus, as expected, the short-term results seem to indicate preservation of motion at the level of the replacement, especially when compared with ACDF. Longer-term follow-up is needed to determine if this motion is preserved over a longer period of time and if it can prevent degeneration of adjacent segments.

Although cervical disk replacement can be subject to many of the same complications as other commonly performed anterior-based cervical procedures,[37] there are a few potential complications unique to TDR. Implant migration and subsidence have been infrequently reported.[26,28,32] Another complication limiting successful motion after cervical disk replacement has been heterotopic fusion across the implant or involved motion segment.[38] Cervical kyphosis has been reported by multiple investigators across the level of the TDR,[39] potentially affecting some implant designs more than others. Furthermore, partial dislocation of the implant also has been noted, albeit rarely.[39] Finally, rare cases of hypersensitivity to metal ions and reaction to other wear debris have been reported.[40] Further long-term studies are needed to determine the true incidence of these adverse events and their effects on long-term outcomes in TDR.

Results reported for the U.S. IDE trials involved patients who underwent single-level cervical disk replacement for isolated disk disease. These studies do not address the concerns regarding two-level disk degeneration. Given the young age of the patient in the case presented earlier, performing an ACDF at one level would have left a degenerative disk susceptible to even further accelerated adjacent-segment degeneration. Fusing both levels via a two-level ACDF would address both of the patient's affected segments, but might leave the adjacent levels above and below the two-level fusion mass at an even greater risk of accelerated degeneration given the increased stresses exerted by the longer fusion construct.[41] Thus, conceptually, a two-level cervical disk replacement appears more appealing than a two-level ACDF, and cervical disk replacement may be a better option than ACDF in multilevel degenerative disk disease.

Surgeons have been increasingly performing multilevel cervical disk replacements in selected patients and/or combining cervical disk replacement at one level with ACDF at another level.[42] Recently, Phillips and colleagues[43] reported on a **prospective study** comparing results for patients who had cervical TDR adjacent to a prior fusion with results for patients who underwent total primary disk replacement.

The findings of this study demonstrated similar outcomes at short-term follow-up. Pimenta and colleagues[44] reported on a **prospective series** comparing outcomes for 71 patients who underwent single-level cervical replacement with outcomes for 69 patients who underwent multilevel cervical replacement. Of these 69 patients, 53 underwent two-level replacement, 12 underwent three-level replacement, and 4 underwent four-level replacement. The self-assessment outcomes, NDI scores, and VAS scores obtained up to 36 months of follow-up all showed significantly greater improvement for the patients undergoing multilevel procedures. The rates of reoperation and serious adverse events were similar in those undergoing single-level and multilevel replacement. Although longer-term follow-up is needed, these findings have potentially created another set of possibilities for surgeons treating patients with multilevel cervical disk disease, with perhaps another unique set of problems.[45]

Cervical disk replacement has undergone a renaissance over the past decade, with improved implant technology and better patient selection criteria. With the longer-term data now available for the three FDA-approved implants, surgeons have a better understanding of the long-term effects of ACDF as well as the potential advantages of cervical disk replacement. Although by most functional and clinical outcome measures, cervical disk replacement appears to be equivalent to ACDF, there may be significant advantages for replacement in particular patients and situations (e.g., multilevel cervical disk degeneration). Over the next few years, as nondeveloper surgeons perform more cervical disk arthroplasties, as more surgeons perform multilevel arthroplasties, and as researchers help identify the replacement design that provides the optimal kinematics, the spine surgery community will continue to refine the design and application of this new technology.

COMMENTARY

Cervical TDR has emerged as a viable surgical alternate to fusion in the treatment of degenerative cervical conditions. FDA IDE trials have confirmed that single-level TDR performed by expert cervical spinal surgeons in a carefully selected cohort of patients produces clinical results that are at least equivalent to and in some instances surpass those reported for cervical fusion. Cervical TDR, however, may produce potential complications that are distinct from those seen with fusion, and these have been highlighted in the chapter. For cervical TDR to become generally accepted, this technology must be shown to provide value over existing treatments in terms of improved function, enhanced patient productivity, or a reduction in future or current health care needs (such as adjacent-level treatments) at a cost that is commensurate with its potential advantages.

REFERENCES

1. Polston DW: Cervical radiculopathy, *Neurol Clin* 25:373–385, 2007.
2. Matz PG, Anderson PA, Holly LT, et al: The natural history of cervical spondylotic myelopathy, *J Neurosurg Spine* 11:104–111, 2009.
3. Rao R: Neck pain, cervical radiculopathy, and cervical myelopathy: pathophysiology, natural history, and clinical evaluation, *Instr Course Lect* 52:479–488, 2003.
4. Carette S, Fehlings MG: Clinical practice. Cervical radiculopathy, *N Engl J Med* 353:392–399, 2005.
5. An HS, Simpson JM, Glover JM, et al: Comparison between allograft plus demineralized bone matrix versus autograft in anterior cervical fusion. A prospective multicenter study, *Spine* 20:2211–2216, 1995.
6. Buchowski JM, Anderson PA, Sekhon L, et al: Cervical disc replacement compared with arthrodesis for the treatment of myelopathy. Surgical technique, *J Bone Joint Surg Am* 91(Suppl 2):223–232, 2009.
7. Goldberg EJ, Singh K, Van U, et al: Comparing outcomes of anterior cervical discectomy and fusion in workman's versus non–workman's compensation population, *Spine J* 2:408–414, 2002.
8. Chesnut RM, Abitbol JJ, Garfin SR: Surgical management of cervical radiculopathy. Indication, techniques, and results, *Orthop Clin North Am* 23:461–474, 1992.
9. Anderson PA, Subach BR, Riew KD: Predictors of outcome after anterior cervical discectomy and fusion: a multivariate analysis, *Spine* 34:161–166, 2009.
10. Angevine PD, Zivin JG, McCormick PC: Cost-effectiveness of single-level anterior cervical discectomy and fusion for cervical spondylosis, *Spine* 30:1989–1997, 2005.
11. Samartzis D, Shen FH, Matthews DK, et al: Comparison of allograft to autograft in multilevel anterior cervical discectomy and fusion with rigid plate fixation, *Spine J* 3:451–459, 2003.

12. Moreland DB, Asch HL, Clabeaux DE, et al: Anterior cervical discectomy and fusion with implantable titanium cage: initial impressions, patient outcomes and comparison to fusion with allograft, *Spine J* 4:184–191, discussion, 91; 2004.

13. Hilibrand AS, Carlson GD, Palumbo MA, et al: Radiculopathy and myelopathy at segments adjacent to the site of a previous anterior cervical arthrodesis, *J Bone Joint Surg Am* 81:519–528, 1999. **This classical study describes the incidence, prevalence, and radiographic progression of symptomatic adjacent-segment disease in a consecutive series of 374 patients over a minimum 10-year period. Symptomatic adjacent-segment disease occurred at a relatively constant incidence of 2.9% per year during the 10 years after the operation. Survivorship analysis predicted that 25.6% of the patients who had an anterior cervical arthrodesis would have new disease at an adjacent level within 10 years after the operation.**

14. Bartolomei JC, Theodore N, Sonntag VK: Adjacent level degeneration after anterior cervical fusion: a clinical review, *Neurosurg Clin N Am* 16:575–587, v 2005.

15. Park JB, Cho YS, Riew KD: Development of adjacent-level ossification in patients with an anterior cervical plate, *J Bone Joint Surg Am* 87:558–563, 2005. **This study is a retrospective review of lateral radiographs of the cervical spine of 118 patients who had a solid fusion following an anterior cervical arthrodesis with a plate for the treatment of a degenerative cervical condition. There was a positive association between adjacent-level ossification following anterior cervical plate procedures and the plate-to-disk distance. The authors recommend that surgeons place anterior cervical plates at least 5 mm away from the adjacent disk spaces in order to decrease the likelihood of moderate-to-severe adjacent-level ossification.**

16. Fehlings MG, Arvin B: Surgical management of cervical degenerative disease: the evidence related to indications, impact, and outcome, *J Neurosurg Spine* 11:97–100, 2009.

17. Lin EL, Wang JC: Total disk replacement, *J Am Acad Orthop Surg* 14:705–714, 2006.

18. Orr RD, Postak PD, Rosca M, et al: The current state of cervical and lumbar spinal disc replacement, *J Bone Joint Surg Am* 89(Suppl 3):70–75, 2007.

19. Baaj AA, Uribe JS, Vale FL, et al: History of cervical disc replacement, *Neurosurg Focus* 27:E10, 2009.

20. Traynelis VC: The Prestige cervical disc replacement, *Spine J* 4:310S–314S, 2004.

21. Mummaneni PV, Robinson JC, Haid RW Jr: Cervical replacement with the Prestige LP cervical disc, *Neurosurgery* 60:310–314, discussion, 4–5; 2007.

22. Sekhon LH, Duggal N, Lynch JJ, et al: Magnetic resonance imaging clarity of the Bryan, ProDisc-C, Prestige LP, and PCM cervical replacement devices, *Spine* 32:673–680, 2007.

23. Mummaneni PV, Burkus JK, Haid RW, et al: Clinical and radiographic analysis of cervical disc replacement compared with allograft fusion: a randomized controlled clinical trial, *J Neurosurg Spine* 6:198–209, 2007. **This is a prospective, randomized, multicenter study in which the results of cervical disk arthroplasty were compared with anterior cervical diskectomy and fusion (ACDF) in patients treated for symptomatic single-level cervical degenerative disk disease (DDD). The PRESTIGE ST Cervical Disc System maintained physiological segmental motion at 24 months after implantation and was associated with improved neurological success, improved clinical outcomes, and a reduced rate of secondary surgeries compared with ACDF.**

24. Burkus JK, Haid RW, Traynelis VC, Mummaneni PV: Long-term clinical and radiographic outcomes of cervical disc replacement with the Prestige disc: results from a prospective randomized controlled clinical trial, *J Neurosurg Spine* 13(3):308–318, 2011.

25. Papadopoulos S: The Bryan cervical disc system, *Neurosurg Clin N Am* 16:629–636, vi, 2005.

26. Heller JG, Sasso RC, Papadopoulos SM, et al: Comparison of Bryan cervical disc replacement with anterior cervical decompression and fusion: clinical and radiographic results of a randomized, controlled, clinical trial, *Spine* 34:101–107, 2009.

27. Sasso RC, Anderson PA, Riew KD, Heller JG: Results of cervical arthroplasty compared with anterior discectomy and fusion: four-year clinical outcomes in a prospective, randomized controlled trial, *J Bone Joint Surg Am* 93(18):1684–1692, 2011.

28. Garrido BJ, Taha TA, Sasso RC: Clinical outcomes of Bryan cervical disc replacement: a prospective, randomized, controlled, single site trial with 48-month follow-up, *J Spinal Disord Tech* 23(6):367–371, 2010. **This is a prospective, randomized, single-center study in which the results of cervical disk arthroplasty were compared with anterior cervical diskectomy and fusion (ACDF) in patients treated for symptomatic single-level cervical degenerative disk disease (DDD). In this study, 47 patients were randomized to ACDF versus disk arthroplasty. At 48 months, cervical arthroplasty with the Bryan cervical disk prosthesis continued to compare favorably with ACDF. There was no degradation of functional outcomes from 24 to 48 months for NDI, VAS of neck and arm, and SF-36. There was a lower incidence of secondary surgeries for the Bryan arthroplasty cohort.**

29. Chi JH, Ames CP, Tay B: General considerations for cervical replacement with technique for ProDisc-C, *Neurosurg Clin N Am* 16:609–619, vi, 2005.

30. Bertagnoli R, Duggal N, Pickett GE, et al: Cervical total disc replacement, part two: clinical results, *Orthop Clin North Am* 36:355–362, 2005.

31. Bertagnoli R, Yue JJ, Pfeiffer F, et al: Early results after ProDisc-C cervical disc replacement, *J Neurosurg Spine* 2:403–410, 2005.

32. Murrey D, Janssen M, Delamarter R, et al: Results of the prospective, randomized, controlled multicenter Food and Drug Administration investigational device exemption study of the ProDisc-C total disc replacement versus anterior discectomy and fusion for the treatment of 1-level symptomatic cervical disc disease, *Spine J* 9:275–286, 2009. **This is a prospective, randomized, multicenter study in which the results of cervical disk arthroplasty were compared with anterior cervical diskectomy**

and fusion (ACDF) in patients treated for symptomatic single-level cervical degenerative disk disease (DDD). The results of this clinical trial demonstrate that ProDisc-C is a safe and effective surgical treatment for patients with disabling cervical radiculopathy because of single-level disease. By all primary and secondary measures evaluated, clinical outcomes after ProDisc-C implantation were either equivalent or superior to those same clinical outcomes after fusion.

33. Murrey D, Janssen ME, Delamarter RB, et al: *Five-year results of the prospective, randomized, multicenter FDA Investigational Device Exemption (IDE) ProDisc C TDR clinical trial.* Paper presented at the Cervical Spine Research Society annual meeting, Salt Lake City, 2009.

34. Galbusera F, Bellini CM, Brayda-Bruno M, et al: Biomechanical studies on cervical total disc replacement: a literature review, *Clin Biomech (Bristol, Avon)* 23:1095–1104, 2008.

35. Puttlitz CM, DiAngelo DJ: Cervical spine replacement biomechanics, *Neurosurg Clin N Am* 16: 589–594, v, 2005.

36. Sasso RC, Best NM: Cervical kinematics after fusion and Bryan disc replacement, *J Spinal Disord Tech* 21:19–22, 2008.

37. Daniels AH, Riew KD, Yoo JU, et al: Adverse events associated with anterior cervical spine surgery, *J Am Acad Orthop Surg* 16:729–738, 2008.

38. Mehren C, Suchomel P, Grochulla F, et al: Heterotopic ossification in total cervical artificial disc replacement, *Spine* 31:2802–2806, 2006.

39. Pickett GE, Sekhon LH, Sears WR, et al: Complications with cervical replacement, *J Neurosurg Spine* 4:98–105, 2006.

40. Cavanaugh DA, Nunley PD, Kerr EJ 3rd, et al: Delayed hyper-reactivity to metal ions after cervical disc replacement: a case report and literature review, *Spine* 34:E262–E265, 2009.

41. Mummaneni PV, Kaiser MG, Matz PG, et al: Cervical surgical techniques for the treatment of cervical spondylotic myelopathy, *J Neurosurg Spine* 11:130–141, 2009.

42. Barbagallo GM, Assietti R, Corbino L, et al: Early results and review of the literature of a novel hybrid surgical technique combining cervical arthrodesis and disc replacement for treating multilevel degenerative disc disease: opposite or complementary techniques? *Eur Spine J* 18(Suppl 1):29–39, 2009.

43. Phillips FM, Allen TR, Regan JJ, et al: Cervical disc replacement in patients with and without previous adjacent level fusion surgery: a prospective study, *Spine* 34:556–565, 2009. This multicenter trial reports outcomes from patients with and without previous ACDF receiving the porous coated motion (PCM) artificial cervical disk. In this trial, 126 patients who underwent disk replacement were compared with 26 patients who had disk replacement adjacent to a prior cervical fusion. The early clinical results of disk replacement adjacent to a prior fusion are good and comparable to the outcomes after primary disk replacement surgery. However, in view of the small study population and short-term follow-up, continued study is mandatory.

44. Pimenta L, McAfee PC, Cappuccino A, et al: Superiority of multilevel cervical replacement outcomes versus single-level outcomes: 229 consecutive PCM prostheses, *Spine* 32:1337–1344, 2007.

45. Datta JC, Janssen ME, Beckham R, et al: Sagittal split fractures in multilevel cervical replacement using a keeled prosthesis, *J Spinal Disord Tech* 20:89–92, 2007.

Chapter 2   Multilevel Anterior Cervical Diskectomy and Fusion: Bone-Grafting Options

Sheeraz A. Qureshi, Andrew C. Hecht, Scott D. Boden

Degenerative cervical spondylosis is a common cause of multilevel cervical stenosis that can result in symptomatic radiculopathy or myelopathy depending on the location of compression. The indications for surgical management include persistent or worsening symptoms despite a trial of appropriate nonoperative treatment options. The primary goal of surgical treatment is physical decompression of the neurologic elements. This can be accomplished posteriorly using laminectomy or laminoplasty techniques, or anteriorly through corpectomy or diskectomy approaches.

The decision to decompress anteriorly or posteriorly depends not only on surgeon preference, but also on several key factors, including location of the stenosis, alignment of the cervical spine, and number of levels involved. One of the primary settings in which a surgeon will choose an anterior approach is a case in which anterior compressive structures are present in a patient with a kyphotic cervical spine. In this scenario an anterior approach allows for direct decompression as well as restoration of spinal alignment.

Once the decision has been made to proceed with anterior decompression for multilevel cervical stenosis, the surgeon must choose between multilevel diskectomies and vertebral corpectomy. Although no consensus exists with regard to which option is appropriate in which circumstance, it is the feeling of many that in most cases the same degree of decompression can be achieved through multilevel diskectomy as through vertebral corpectomy.[1] In addition, one of the advantages of multilevel cervical diskectomy is that it provides multiple distraction points, which can permit more effective restoration of lordosis than a long, straight corpectomy graft such as a fibula.

Although decompression of the neurologic elements is the primary goal in the treatment of radiculopathy and myelopathy, successful fusion and maintenance of normal cervical spinal alignment are critical to the long-term success of most operative treatment options for multilevel cervical stenosis. The reported rates of fusion for single-level anterior cervical diskectomy and fusion (ACDF) procedures are extremely high, reaching 97% in some studies.[2] Unfortunately, as the number of operative levels increases, the fusion rates for ACDF decrease.[3] Studies that have compared multilevel cervical diskectomy and fusion to cervical corpectomy and fusion have found that although there are higher fusion rates in patients undergoing corpectomy, there are also higher rates of graft extrusion resulting in loss of spinal alignment.[4] The addition of an anterior cervical plate not only can improve stability, but also has been shown to enhance fusion rates in multilevel ACDF operations.[5]

The ultimate goal of multilevel ACDF surgery is decompression of the neurologic elements, restoration of spinal alignment, and achievement of fusion. Often, the ability to achieve fusion is the most difficult part, with rates of pseudoarthrosis ranging from 2.5% to 44%.[6,7] Although there are several factors that can contribute to pseudoarthrosis (nicotine usage, inadequate end-plate preparation, excessive distraction, improper graft positioning, etc.), the type of graft used is an important variable. This chapter presents the different bone-grafting options available when performing multilevel ACDF and reviews the indications for inclusion of posterior fusion.

CASE PRESENTATION

A 39-year-old right-hand-dominant woman came for treatment after 4 months of severe neck pain radiating into both upper extremities. Her condition had failed to improve after several months of physical therapy and management with multiple medications. At the time of presentation she reported severe paresthesias throughout her left upper extremity and worsening left arm weakness. The patient reported no problems with balance or fine motor control and did not suggest any changes in bowel or bladder habits.

- PMH: Unremarkable
- PSH: Unremarkable
- Exam: On physical examination, the patient was quite tender to palpation along the posterior cervical spine. She had limited range of motion of the cervical spine due to pain. She had 4/5 weakness in the left upper extremity in the deltoid, biceps, triceps, and hand intrinsics. Her reflexes were diminished in the biceps, brachioradialis, and triceps in the left upper extremity. No abnormal reflexes were present. Her gait pattern was normal.
- Imaging: Preoperative imaging evaluation revealed a neutral to slightly kyphotic alignment of the cervical spine. Magnetic resonance imaging (MRI) of the cervical spine showed multilevel cervical spinal cord compression secondary to ventral compression at C3-4, C4-5, C5-6, and C6-7 (Figures 2-1 and 2-2). Computed tomographic (CT) scanning was ordered, and the findings confirmed that the compressive elements were soft herniations.

SURGICAL OPTIONS

Interbody grafts in multilevel ACDF serve several purposes. Perhaps the two most important goals for the graft are to provide structural support and to allow solid fusion to be achieved. The most commonly used interbody options are autogenous bone grafts, allogeneic bone grafts, and anterior cervical cages. When the surgeon is deciding on what type of graft to use, important considerations include the number of levels being fused, the quality of the host bone, medical comorbidities, and the smoking status of the patient.

After discussion of management options, a decision was made to proceed with multilevel ACDF given the lack of cervical lordosis and the ventral nature of compression, which was all at the level of the disk spaces.

The patient underwent successful multilevel ACDF from C3 to C7 using freeze-dried machined allograft with recombinant human bone morphogenetic protein-2 and an anterior cervical plate.

Postoperatively the patient experienced complete resolution of her neck and arm symptoms and her strength normalized. Successful fusion was achieved both clinically and radiographically (Figure 2-3).

FUNDAMENTAL TECHNIQUE

When a multilevel ACDF operation is performed the patient is positioned supine on a radiolucent operating table with a roll placed between the shoulder blades to allow for neck extension (Tips from the Masters 2-1 and 2-2). Gardner-Wells tongs can be applied to allow controlled distraction. The amount of distraction can be increased at the discretion of the surgeon. Distal traction through the shoulders is applied using wide tape to help with fluoroscopic visualization.

Tips from the Masters 2-1 • Make sure the majority of neurologic compression is occurring ventral to the thecal sac and is at the level of the disk space.

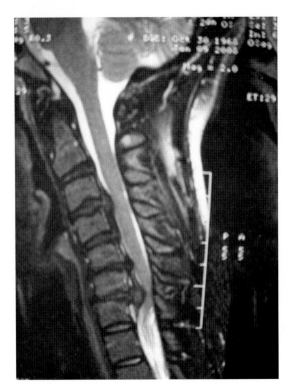

FIGURE 2-1 Preoperative sagittal T2-weighted MRI scan showing multilevel disk herniations causing spinal cord compression.

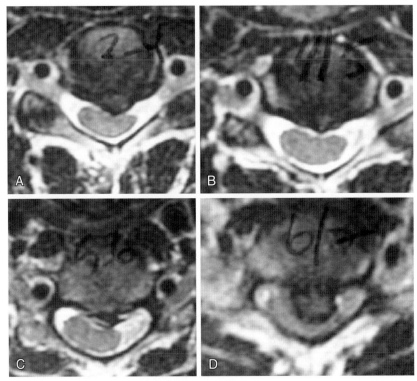

FIGURE 2-2 Preoperative axial T2-weighted MRI scan showing central and left posterolateral herniations with multilevel cervical stenosis at C3-4 (**A**), C4-5 (**B**), C5-6 (**C**), and C6-7 (**D**).

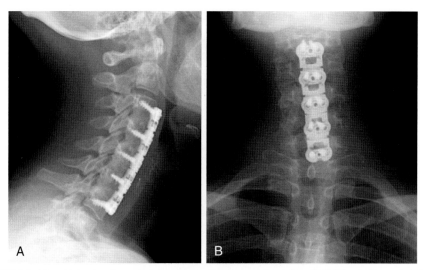

FIGURE 2-3 AP and lateral radiographs taken 1 year after surgery consisting of C3-C7 anterior cervical diskectomies with fusion using allograft, recombinant human bone morphogenetic protein-2, and an anterior cervical plate.

FIGURE 2-4 Distraction pins placed at the disk level that is going to be addressed.

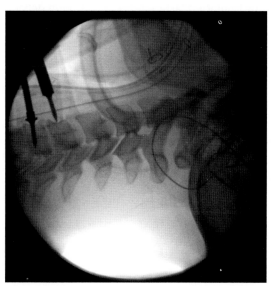

Tips from the Masters 2-2 • Always make sure the patient is positioned so that cervical lordosis is restored and all disk spaces can be visualized fluoroscopically.

The preference is to use a left-sided approach to the anterior cervical spine. However, a right-sided approach can also be used if the surgeon is more comfortable with this. Placement of a longitudinal incision along the medial border of the sternocleidomastoid can allow for easier visualization proximally and distally. However, a horizontal incision centered over the center vertebra or disk space is more cosmetically pleasing.

After confirming the appropriate disk levels, many surgeons tend to work from distal to proximal in performing the diskectomies. Distraction pins are used sequentially at each disk level to help in opening the disk space and performing a complete diskectomy (Figure 2-4). It is common practice to resect the posterior longitudinal ligament in all cases (Tips from the Masters 2-3).

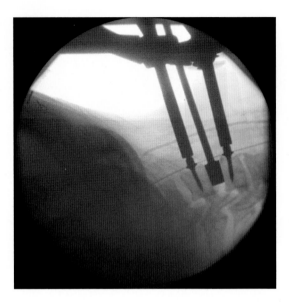

FIGURE 2-5 Sizing of disk space while distraction is applied to obtain an appropriate height.

Tips from the Masters 2-3 • A thorough decompression is critical to the relief of neurologic symptoms.

Tips from the Masters 2-4 • Prepare the end plates to reveal points of bleeding cancellous bone, which can be created with a small angled currette punched through the end plates at multiple points.

After each diskectomy is completed the end plates are prepared using a high-speed bur to reach bleeding cancellous bone (Tips from the Masters 2-5). The disk space is then sized and packed with a hemostatic agent such as surgical foam (Figure 2-5). Attention is then turned to the next proximal disk space and the steps are repeated until all diskectomies are performed, end plates prepared, and disk spaces sized (Tips from the Masters 2-6).

Tips from the Masters 2-5 • A graft that is at least 2 mm larger, but not more than 4 mm larger, than the resting disk height should be placed to allow for restoration of foraminal height without risking nonunion or overdistraction of the facet joints.

Tips from the Masters 2-6 • Interbody grafts should be slightly recessed and all anterior vertebral osteophytes removed for appropriate plate placement.

At this point allograft bone (or whichever interbody graft material is chosen) is placed sequentially into each disk space. It is important to apply controlled distraction to each disk space as the graft is being placed so that foraminal height can be restored without overdistracting the facet joints posteriorly. Each disk space should be resized before placement of the interbody fusion device so that the most appropriate size can be chosen (Figure 2-6).

Once all interbody grafts are in place and slightly recessed, all distraction is removed to obtain a press fit. Each graft should be checked at this point to ensure that it is solidly locked into place (Tips from the Masters 2-7).

Tips from the Masters 2-7 • Remove all distraction before placing an anterior cervical plate.

FIGURE 2-6 Appropriately sized allograft bone placed in each disk space and slightly recessed.

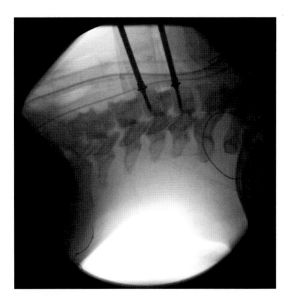

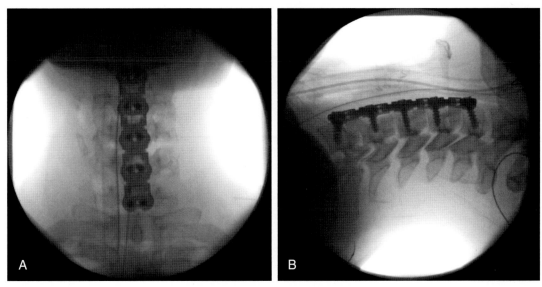

FIGURE 2-7 Anterior cervical plate applied from C3 to C7 with unicortical screws placed bilaterally at each vertebral level.

An anterior cervical plate is then applied. For multilevel ACDF operations, use of a translational plate is preferred to allow for controlled compression across the graft sites. However, the surgeon should choose whatever plate he or she is most comfortable using (Figure 2-7).

During the placement of a long anterior cervical plate, a common pitfall is using a plate that is too long. The shortest plate that allows purchase of the subchondral bone in a trajectory that allows the screw threads to purchase cancellous bone is optimal and provides the best pullout strength. If the plate is too long, screws may enter the adjacent disk space or canal (Figure 2-8). Before the plate is secured onto the anterior cervical spine surface, it is imperative to adequately prepare the bony surfaces by removing anterior osteophytes. Failure to do so will cause the plate to be raised in areas adjacent to osteophytes and will place stress on the screws that are not flush with bone (Figure 2-9).

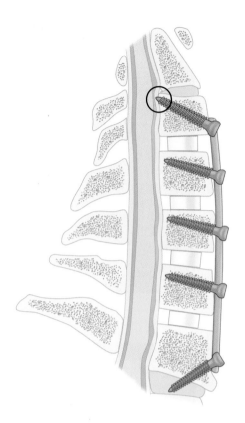

FIGURE 2-8 A common pitfall in multilevel plating is using a plate that is too long, so that either the superior or inferior screws enter the adjacent disk space. This can be avoided by choosing the shortest plate possible. It is acceptable, and perhaps desirable, for the initial screw entry point to be in the subchondral bone of the vertebral body, provided the screw trajectory is appropriate and the remaining threads of the screw will capture cancellous bone. Moreover, the purchase of subchondral bone is significantly stronger than that of cancellous bone, and screw pullout strength is increased. (*Adapted from McLaughlin M, Haid R, Rodts G:* Atlas of cervical spine surgery, *Philadelphia, 2005, Saunders, p 80.*)

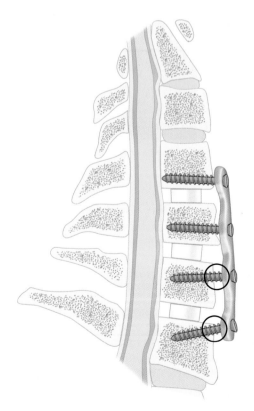

FIGURE 2-9 Another common pitfall is suboptimal trimming of the anterior osteophytes before performing the diskectomy. If an osteophyte is still present, the plate will not sit flush on the face of the vertebral bodies. This can create stress risers and can decrease screw purchase at adjacent levels. (*Adapted from McLaughlin M, Haid R, Rodts G:* Atlas of cervical spine surgery, *Philadelphia, 2005, Saunders, p 80.*)

DISCUSSION OF BEST EVIDENCE

Autogenous Bone Grafts

Autogenous bone graft can be harvested from the iliac crest, fibula, or rib. In multilevel ACDF procedures in which autogenous bone graft is to be used, the anterior iliac crest is the most common site from which bone graft is harvested. Autogenous tricorticocancellous graft from the iliac crest remains the gold standard against which all other fusion devices must be compared. Autogenous iliac crest bone graft is osteoinductive, osteoconductive, and osteogenic; carries no risk of disease transmission or graft rejection; and has excellent compressive strength to support physiologic loads.

The use of iliac crest autograft in single-level ACDF is associated with fusion rates near 100%.[2] Unfortunately, as the number of graft-bone surfaces that must heal increases, the rate of fusion decreases, even when autograft bone is used. The rate of fusion for two-level ACDF using iliac crest autograft without plate fixation has been reported to be 87%.[8] In a **retrospective study,** the rate of successful fusion for two-level ACDF using iliac crest autograft with an anterior cervical plate has been reported to be as high as 100%.[6] For three-level ACDF using iliac crest autograft without plate fixation the reported rate of fusion falls to 57.6%.[8] Whether adding an anterior cervical plate promotes fusion is controversial, with some studies showing no benefit[9] and others showing rates of fusion of over 95%.[6]

Autogenous bone grafts are the gold standard with regard to promoting fusion but do have disadvantages. Schnee and colleagues[10] reported on the complications of anterior iliac bone graft harvest for use in anterior cervical surgery. There was one permanent injury to the lateral femoral cutaneous nerve. Other complications included wound complications in 5.6%, reoperation in 4%, poor cosmesis in 3.5%, and chronic donor site pain in 2.8%.

Allogeneic Bone Grafts

The use of allograft bone in anterior cervical spine surgery has become commonplace. Allograft bone is osteoconductive and only weakly osteoinductive. Allograft bone used in anterior cervical spine surgery is harvested from a human cadaver and preserved to remove some of its antigenicity. Structural allograft bone is treated by freezing or freeze-drying. Fresh frozen allograft bone is collected with sterile techniques and then stored at −60 degrees F to prevent enzymatic breakdown. Fresh frozen allograft retains good structural integrity but has a significantly higher antigen load than freeze-dried bone, which is dehydrated and stored at room temperature. Although the freeze-drying process decreases the antigen load, it also decreases graft strength. Gamma irradiation and ethylene oxide are generally not used in the sterilization process for allograft bone to be used in the anterior cervical spine because they significantly weaken the bone.

Rates of fusion in single-level ACDF procedures using allograft and an anterior cervical plate have been reported to be between 90% and 100%.[11] For two-level ACDF using allograft without a plate the fusion rates drop to 37% to 72%.[12,13] The addition of an anterior cervical plate when performing a two-level ACDF using allograft increases the rate of fusion to nearly 100%.[6,14] In a **retrospective review,** Wang and associates[5] reported a pseudoarthrosis rate of 37% in patients undergoing unplated three-level ACDF procedures using allograft bone, which declined to 18% with application of an anterior cervical plate. Corticocancellous machined allografts and ring allografts that are filled in the middle with a substance such as DBM are both excellent options. There has been no evidence to assess differences between the two, and the rates of usage are likely equal.

Risk of disease transmission from allograft is extremely low. Donor bone is screened by evaluating the donor's complete medical history, and serologic testing is performed to assess for human immunodeficiency virus (HIV) infection, hepatitis B, and hepatitis C.[15] Use of structural allograft for multilevel ACDF has been associated with reduced length of hospitalization and earlier return to work compared with use of autograft.[16]

Synthetic Interbody Spacers

Synthetic interbody spacers can potentially be made in any shape or size. They are most commonly metallic or made of polyetheretherketone (PEEK). There has been interest in the use of synthetic interbody devices in anterior cervical fusion procedures because of continued concerns about donor site morbidity with autograft harvesting and the theoretical risks of allograft disease transmission and potentially limited supply of allografts.

Rigid metallic cages showed early promise; however, longer-term follow-up demonstrated high subsidence rates.[17] There is also an inherent difficulty in assessing fusion radiographically given the radiopaque properties of metallic cages. Perhaps of greatest concern is the increased stress shielding, and thus decreased contact surface, that can occur with the use of metallic cages and can lead to a higher rate of pseudoarthrosis as shown in a **prospective, randomized study.**[18]

Cancellous autograft, cancellous allograft, or a demineralized bone matrix plug can be placed inside the cages, whether they are made of titanium or PEEK. PEEK is a nonresorbable, semicrystalline, aromatic polymer that can be used to create a structural bone graft with a modulus of elasticity resembling that of bone.[19] The purported advantages of PEEK cages include the fact that they are nonresorbable, radiolucent, and MRI compatible, and elicit minimal to no inflammatory response. Early literature reports favorable results with regard to maintenance of foraminal height and achievement of high fusion rates. Although it appears that PEEK cages will be an acceptable alternative to autograft and allograft, there are no studies to date specifically addressing the rate of successful fusion using PEEK cages in multilevel ACDF procedures.

Recombinant Human Bone Morphogenetic Protein-2

Since the reported success of recombinant human bone morphogenetic protein-2 (rhBMP-2) in achieving anterior lumbar fusions, there has been significant interest in its use in other areas, including the anterior cervical spine (Tips from the Masters 2-8). A **prospective, randomized study** has reported 100% fusion rates in one- or two-level fusions when rhBMP-2 is used in combination with allograft bone and an anterior cervical plate.[20] Recently, Riew's group reported on the pseudoarthrosis rates in multilevel ACDF (at least three levels) with rhBMP-2 and allograft. For this series of 127 patients with a minimum 2-year follow-up, the investigators reported a pseudoarthrosis rate of 10.2%. Subset analysis showed that the rate was 4% for three-level fusion, 17.4% for four-level fusion, and 22.2% for five-level fusion.[21]

Despite the high rate of successful fusion with the use of rhBMP-2 in anterior cervical spine surgery, there is significant concern regarding the possibility of serious complications such as airway swelling. Shields and colleagues[22] and Smucker and associates[23] have reported complication rates of 23.2% and 27.5%, respectively. This led to a U.S. Food and Drug Administration (FDA) warning on the usage of rhBMP-2 in anterior cervical spine surgery in 2008. The FDA noted having received at least 38 reports of complications over 4 years with the use of rhBMP in cervical spine fusion. According to the report, the complications were associated with swelling of neck and throat tissue resulting in compression of the airway and/or neurologic structures in the neck, which in some cases led to difficulty in swallowing, breathing, or speaking. Severe dysphagia after cervical spine fusion using rhBMP products has also been reported in the literature.

Many believe that administration of perioperative steroids combined with placement of rhBMP-2 within a contained vessel (i.e., allograft or PEEK cage) substantially reduces the risk of anterior neck swelling postoperatively. Surgeons using rhBMP-2 in anterior cervical spine surgery should discuss the potential risks and benefits with the patient and should be extremely cautious with its use.

Tips from the Masters 2-8 • When considering the use of a fusion enhancer such as rhBMP-2, have a detailed discussion with the patient regarding the risks and benefits and consider having the patient sign a separate consent form for its use.

Need for Posterior Fusion

Adding a posterior cervical fusion can increase the rate of successful anterior cervical fusion when a multilevel anterior cervical procedure is performed. The potential advantages of additional posterior fusion include greater construct stability and larger surface area for fusion.

For patients with symptomatic pseudoarthrosis following an anterior cervical fusion, posterior fusion leads to a high rate of success while avoiding the previous surgical site.[24] In a **retrospective study,** a concomitant posterior approach has also been shown to increase fusion rates in multilevel cervical fusion procedures; however, it is technically demanding and leads to longer operating times and increased blood loss.[25]

Despite the increased rate of fusion success, the addition of posterior cervical fusion is not advocated for most patients undergoing multilevel ACDF. It is recommended that posterior cervical fusion be used in patients with traumatic conditions that have resulted in disruption of the posterior ligamentous complex and in patients who have significant dorsal compression requiring additional posterior decompression. The preferred practice is also to treat all symptomatic pseudoarthroses of previous anterior cervical fusions with posterior cervical fusion.

When posterior fusion is added, the use of lateral mass instrumentation with posterior iliac crest autograft or allograft bone is recommended. Spinous process wiring can be added at the discretion of the surgeon.

COMMENTARY

There are many bone grafting options for multilevel anterior cervical arthrodesis. In making choices the surgeon should keep in mind a balance among known efficacy, risks, and cost. The choice of bone graft substitutes should be individualized and also based on patient factors (e.g., smoking, steroid or chemotherapy exposure, diabetes) that can impede bone healing. For multilevel fusions in patients with potential impaired healing due to host factors, one must consider the addition of a posterior fusion or use of one of the more potent osteoinductive bone graft substitutes.

REFERENCES

1. Hillard VH, Apfelbaum RI: Surgical management of cervical myelopathy: indications and techniques for multilevel cervical discectomy, *Spine J* 6:242S–251S, 2006.
2. Bishop RC, Moore KA, Hadley MN: Anterior cervical interbody fusion using autogeneic and allogeneic bone graft substrate: a prospective comparative analysis, *J Neurosurg* 85:206–210, 1996.
3. Bohlman H, Emery S, Goodfellow D, et al: Robinson anterior cervical discectomy and arthrodesis for cervical radiculopathy, *J Bone Joint Surg Am* 75:1298–1307, 1993. This retrospective study evaluated the results of using the Robinson method of ACDF with placement of autogenous iliac crest bone grafts at one to four levels in 122 patients who had cervical radiculopathy. A one-level procedure was performed in 62 of the 122 patients; a two-level procedure in 48; a three-level procedure in 11; and a four-level procedure in 1. The average duration of clinical and radiographic follow-up was 6 years (range, 2 to 15 years). The average age was 50 years (range, 25 to 78 years). Lateral radiographs of the cervical spine, made in flexion and extension, showed a pseudoarthrosis at 24 of 195 operatively treated segments. The risk of pseudoarthrosis was significantly greater after a multilevel arthrodesis than after a single-level arthrodesis ($P < .01$). The results of this study suggest that the Robinson ACDF with an autogenous iliac crest bone graft for cervical radiculopathy is a safe procedure that can relieve pain and lead to resolution of neurologic deficits in a high percentage of patients. However, as the number of fusion levels increases, so does the risk of pseudoarthrosis.
4. Hilibrand AS, Fye MA, Emery SE, et al: Increased rate of arthrodesis with strut grafting after multilevel anterior cervical decompression, *Spine* 27:146–151, 2002.
5. Wang JC, McDonough PW, Kanim LE, et al: Increased fusion rates with cervical plating for three-level anterior cervical discectomy and fusion, *Spine* 26:643–647, 2001. This retrospective review looked at patients surgically treated by a single surgeon with a three-level ACDF with and without anterior plate fixation. The primary purpose of this study was to compare the clinical and radiographic success of anterior three-level diskectomy and fusion performed with and without anterior cervical plate fixation. After previous studies of multilevel cervical diskectomies and fusions had shown that

fusion rates decrease as the number of surgical levels increases, this study assessed whether the addition of anterior cervical plate stabilization can provide more stability and potentially increase fusion rates for multilevel fusions. Fifty-nine patients were treated surgically with a three-level ACDF by the senior author over 7 years. Cervical plates were used in 40 patients, whereas 19 underwent fusions with no plates. The fusion rates were improved with the use of a cervical plate. Patients treated with cervical plating had overall better results compared with those treated without cervical plates. According to the authors, although the use of cervical plates decreased the pseudoarthrosis rate, a three-level procedure was still associated with a high rate of nonunion, and other strategies to increase fusion rates should be explored.

6. Samartzis D, Shen F, Matthews D, et al: Comparison of allograft to autograft in multilevel anterior cervical discectomy and fusion with rigid plate fixation, *Spine J* 3:451–459, 2003. The purpose of this retrospective radiographic and clinical review was to determine the efficacy of allograft versus autograft with regard to fusion rate and clinical outcome in patients undergoing two- and three-level ACDF with rigid anterior plate fixation. Fusion rate and postoperative clinical outcome were assessed in 80 patients. Seventy-eight patients (97.5%) achieved solid arthrodesis. Pseudoarthrosis occurred in two patients who received allografts for two-level and three-level fusions. Nonsegmental screws were used in the two-level nonunion case. The authors reported that a high fusion rate of 97.5% was obtained for multilevel ACDF with rigid plating with either autograft or allograft.

7. Emery SE, Fisher JR, Bohlman HH: Three-level anterior cervical discectomy and fusion: radiographic and clinical results, *Spine* 22:2622–2624, 1997. This study is a retrospective review of 16 patients who underwent the modified Robinson ACDF at three operative levels. The purpose of this study was to provide long-term follow-up data on the surgical success and patient outcome of three-level anterior cervical diskectomies and fusions using autograft bone. The critical finding of this study is that the success of arthrodesis for anterior cervical fusion depends on several factors, including the number of surgical levels. This was also the first study to provide long-term follow-up on arthrodesis rate and outcomes for patients who specifically underwent three-level diskectomy and fusion procedures In this study, only 9 (56%) of the 16 patients went on to achieve solid arthrodesis at all three levels. Of the seven patients with pseudoarthrosis, two had severe pain and required revision; two had moderate pain; and three no pain. The conclusion of this study was that a three-level modified Robinson cervical diskectomy and fusion results in an unacceptably high rate of pseudoarthrosis. Although not all pseudoarthroses are painful, the data suggested that those with a successful fusion have a better outcome. The authors recommended that these patients undergo additional or alternative measures to achieve arthrodesis consistently.

8. Nirala AP, Husain M, Vatsal DK: A retrospective study of multiple interbody grafting and long segment strut grafting following multilevel anterior cervical decompression, *Br J Neurosurg* 18:227–232, 2004.

9. Bolesta MJ, Rechtine GR, Chrin AM: Three- and four-level anterior cervical discectomy and fusion with plate fixation: a prospective study, *Spine* 25:2040–2044, 2000.

10. Schnee CL, Freese A, Weil RJ, et al: Analysis of harvest morbidity and radiographic outcome using autograft for anterior cervical fusion, *Spine* 22:2222–2227, 1997.

11. Wang JC, McDonough PW, Endow KK, et al: The effect of cervical plating on single-level anterior discectomy and fusion, *J Spinal Disord* 12:467–471, 1999.

12. Zdeblik TA, Ducker TB: The use of freeze-dried allograft bone for anterior cervical fusion, *Spine* 6:726–729, 1991.

13. DiAngelo DJ, Foley KT, Vossel KA, et al: Anterior cervical plate reverses load transfer through multilevel strut-grafts, *Spine* 25:783–795, 2000.

14. Wang JC, McDonough PW, Endow KK, et al: Increased fusion rates with cervical plating for two-level anterior cervical discectomy and fusion, *Spine* 25:41–45, 2000.

15. Anderson DG, Albert TJ: Bone grafting, implants, and plating options for anterior cervical fusions, *Orthop Clin N Am* 33:317–328, 2002.

16. Shapiro S: Banked fibula and the locking anterior cervical plate in anterior cervical fusions following cervical discectomy, *J Neurosurg* 84:161–165, 1996.

17. Wilke HJ, Kettler A, Goetz C, et al: Subsidence resulting from simulated postoperative neck movements: an in vitro investigation with a new cervical fusion cage, *Spine* 25:2762–2770, 2000.

18. Vavruch L, Hedlund R, Javid D: A prospective randomized comparison between the Cloward procedure and a carbon fiber cage in the cervical spine: a clinical and radiologic study, *Spine* 27:1694–1701, 2002.

19. Hee HT, Kudnani V: Rationale for use of polyetheretherketone polymer interbody cage device in cervical spine surgery, *Spine J* 10:66–69, 2010.

20. Baskin DS, Ryan P, Sonntag V, et al: A prospective, randomized, controlled cervical fusion study using recombinant human bone morphogenetic protein-2 with the CORNERSTONE-SR allograft ring and ATLANTIS anterior cervical plate, *Spine* 28:1219–1225, 2003.

21. Shen H, Buchowski J, Yeom J, et al: Pseudoarthrosis in multilevel anterior cervical fusion with rhBMP-2 and allograft: analysis of one hundred twenty-seven cases with minimum two-year follow-up, *Spine* 35:747–753, 2010. This consecutive case series analyzed the pseudoarthrosis rate after rhBMP-2–augmented multilevel (three or more levels) anterior cervical fusion. Data for a large number of patients with cervical spondylosis and/or disk herniation who underwent anterior cervical fusion with rhBMP-2, structural allograft, and plate fixation and had a minimum of 2 years of follow-up were examined by experienced, independent spine surgeons. A total of 127 patients, 54 men and 73 women with a mean age of 54 ± 10 years (range, 32 to 79 years), were included. Seventy-five patients (59.1%) underwent a three-level fusion, 34 (26.7%) underwent a four-level fusion, and 18 (14.2%)

underwent a five-level fusion. Of the 451 fusion segments, 14 segments (3.1%) in 13 of 127 patients (10.2%) had evidence of pseudoarthrosis 6 months after surgery. The only statistically significant risk factor for developing a pseudoarthrosis was the number of fusion levels. In this large series of rhBMP-2–augmented multilevel fusions, the pseudoarthrosis rate was 10.2% at 6 months after surgery. The authors concluded that since the risk of pseudoarthrosis increases with the number of fusion levels, a long fusion lever arm may biomechanically overwhelm the biologic advantage of rhBMP-2 treatment. Although rhBMP-2 is known to enhance fusion rates, it does not guarantee fusion in all situations.

22. Shields LB, Raque GH, Glassman SD, et al: Adverse effects associated with high-dose recombinant human bone morphogenetic protein-2 use in anterior cervical spine fusion, *Spine* 31:542–547, 2006.

23. Smucker JD, Rhee JM, Singh K, et al: Increased swelling complications associated with off-label usage of rhBMP-2 in the anterior cervical spine, *Spine* 31:2813–2819, 2006.

24. Brodsky AE, Khalil MA, Sassard WR, et al: Repair of symptomatic pseudoarthrosis of anterior cervical fusion: posterior versus anterior repair, *Spine* 17:1137–1143, 1992.

25. Sembrano J, Mehbod A, Garvey T, et al: A concomitant posterior approach improves fusion rates but not overall reoperation rates in multilevel cervical fusion for spondylosis, *J Spin Disord* 22:162–169, 2009. This retrospective comparative study of two approaches to multilevel fusion for cervical spondylosis in patients treated at a single institution was carried out to provide justification for a concomitant posterior approach in multilevel cervical fusion for spondylosis by demonstrating decreased pseudoarthrosis and reoperation rates. Seventy-eight consecutively treated patients who underwent multilevel cervical fusion at a single institution and for whom a minimum of 2 years of follow-up data were available were divided into an anterior-only group (n = 55) and an anteroposterior (AP) group (n = 23). Results showed a significant difference between the two groups in pseudoarthrosis rates (anterior, 38% vs. AP, 0%; $P < .001$) and rates of reoperation for pseudoarthrosis (anterior, 22% vs. AP, 0%; $P = .01$). There were no differences in overall reoperation rates (anterior, 36% vs. AP, 30%; $P = .62$) and in early reoperation rates (anterior, 15% vs. AP, 26%; $P = .13$), but the rate of late reoperations was increased in the anterior-only group (anterior, 24% vs. AP, 4%; $P = .043$). A concomitant posterior fusion significantly reduced the incidence of pseudoarthrosis (0% vs. 38%) and pseudoarthrosis-related reoperations (0% vs. 22%) compared with traditional anterior-only fusion. However, this did not translate into a difference in overall reoperation rates.

Chapter 3   Ossification of the Posterior Longitudinal Ligament: Anterior Versus Posterior Approach

Garrick W. Cason, Edward R. Anderson III, Harry N. Herkowitz

Ossification of the posterior longitudinal ligament (OPLL) in the cervical spine as a diagnosis leading to myelopathy and serious impairment has been studied extensively. Inconsistencies in the findings of different investigators and disparities in prevalence in the community, especially in Japan, has led to the formation of the Investigation Committee on Ossification of the Spinal Ligaments and the Investigation Committee on OPLL organized by the Japanese Ministry of Public Health and Welfare. Recent investigations of long-term outcomes associated with various treatment methods have yielded insight into the natural history, prognostic factors, and optimal preoperative evaluations, and provide best evidence–based information for surgical decision making. This chapter presents the case of a myelopathic patient with OPLL and discusses techniques of the primary treatment methods. Recent literature provides the best evidence regarding treatment and prognosis for counseling patients with OPLL.

CASE PRESENTATION

A 58-year-old man had a chief complaint of mild neck pain and bilateral hand paresthesias. His upper extremity paresthesias had become worse over the previous 6 months and no longer responded to nonsteroidal antiinflammatory drugs. The paresthesias were constant and did not change with alteration of arm or head position. He reported no gait abnormalities or bowel or bladder dysfunction. When questioned, he commented that he frequently drops objects and said that he wears pullover shirts due to difficulty with buttons.

- PMH: Hypertension and diabetes mellitus

- PSH: Unremarkable

- Exam: The patient showed good range of motion of the cervical spine without exacerbation of his neck pain or upper extremity symptoms. His upper extremity examination reveals 5/5 strength with diminished sensation to light touch from C6 to C8 dermatomes bilaterally. His biceps and brachioradialis reflexes were 4/5 bilaterally, and when the brachioradialis reflex was tested his thumb, index, and long fingers flexed (inverted radial reflex). His attempts to rapidly open and close his fists revealed significant spasticity (dysdiadochokinesia). The Hoffman sign was positive bilaterally. Lower extremity examination revealed normal gait stride and cadence with 5/5 strength and sensation intact to light touch from L2 to S1 myotomes and dermatomes, respectively. Patellar and Achilles reflexes were 4/5 bilaterally. There was no spasticity with range of motion of the knees, but six beats of clonus bilaterally. His toes were down turning on testing of the plantar reflex.

- Imaging: Sagittal computed tomographic (CT) scans (Figure 3-1) demonstrated mixed-type OPLL from C3 to C7 with increased ossification posterior to C5-6, and lordotic alignment. Axial CT images (Figure 3-2) demonstrated OPLL and

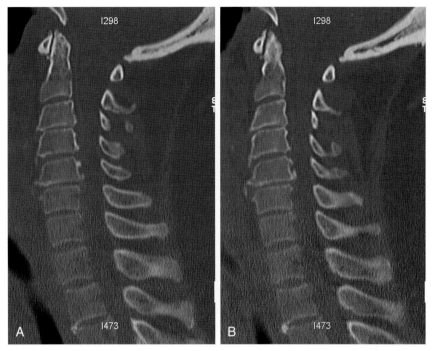

FIGURE 3-1 Preoperative sagittal CT scans demonstrating mixed-type OPLL from C3 to C7 with an increase posterior to C5-6.

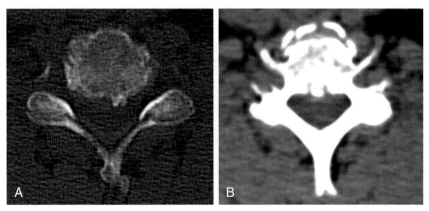

FIGURE 3-2 Axial CT scans demonstrating OPLL intrusion into the spinal canal.

diminished canal dimension. Sagittal and axial magnetic resonance (MRI) images (Figure 3-3) show spinal cord compression by the ossified lesions.

SURGICAL OPTIONS

Surgical options for the treatment of OPLL depend on the site of compression, the number of levels involved, nuchal sagittal balance, the potential for the cord to drift posteriorly, the presence or absence of congenital stenosis, and the morphologic type of the OPLL. Anterior surgical options include multilevel anterior cervical diskectomy and fusion (ACDF) or multilevel anterior cervical corpectomy and fusion (ACCF). Posterior options include laminectomy with or without fusion or laminoplasty. In certain cases circumferential treatment is necessary that combines anterior decompression and fusion with supplemental posterior instrumented fusion.

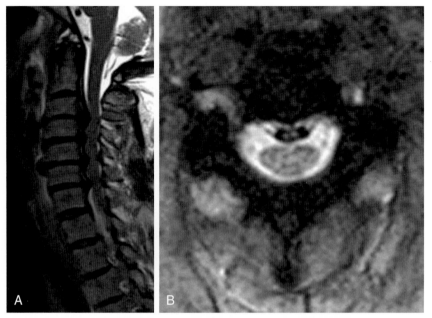

FIGURE 3-3 Sagittal and axial MRI images of OPLL effacing cerebrospinal fluid signal and compressing the spinal cord.

The 58-year-old patient with mixed-type OPLL from C3 to C7 and a lordotic cervical spine was determined to be a good candidate for a C3-C7 laminectomy and fusion. Postoperative anteroposterior (AP) and lateral radiographs (Figure 3-9) demonstrated slight loss of lordosis with maintenance of decompression. Clinically the patient's myelopathic symptoms improved along with his radicular hand symptoms.

Postoperative course: The patient was admitted to the hospital after surgery for pain control and physical and occupational therapy. Findings of the immediately postoperative physical examination were stable relative to those of the preoperative examination, and after a 3-day uneventful hospital course he was discharged home. Maintenance of strength and resolution of upper extremity sensory deficits as well as clonus was demonstrated at 6- and 12-month follow-up. The patient has had no progression of OPLL. He maintains an independent lifestyle and performs activities of daily living himself. He is a community ambulator.

FUNDAMENTAL TECHNIQUE

Multilevel Cervical Diskectomies and/or Corpectomies

The Smith-Robinson approach is the principal surgical approach for the performance of anterior cervical fusions. A left-sided exposure is used primarily because the course of the recurrent laryngeal nerve is more predictable and protected in the left tracheoesophageal groove. The presence of a kyphotic deformity necessitates consideration of preoperative and/or intraoperative cervical traction. Preoperatively, cervical range of motion must be assessed by the anesthesia and surgical teams. Hyperextension of the cervical spine should be avoided during intubation and patient positioning. In patients with myelopathy, awake fiberoptic intubation and neurophysiologic monitoring of transcranial motor evoked potentials (tcMEPs) and somatosensory evoked potentials (SSEPs) should be considered. OPLL beyond the margins of the disk space causing retrovertebral compression warrants either a partial or complete corpectomy.

The level of the skin incision can be assessed using the palpable subcutaneous landmarks corresponding to the adjacent vertebral bodies (Figure 3-4). The hyoid

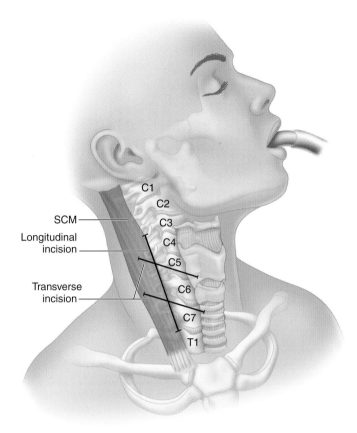

FIGURE 3-4 Palpable landmarks to identify the appropriate level of surgical incision for the anterior approach to the cervical spine. The hyoid bone is at C3, the thyroid cartilage corresponds to C4-5, and the Chassaignac tubercle and cricoid cartilage correspond to C6.

corresponds to C3, the thyroid cartilage to C4-C5, and the cricoid to C6. In addition, the carotid tubercle of C6 can often be palpated. An oblique incision paralleling the anterior margin of the sternocleidomastoid is often utilized for multilevel procedures because it grants access to more levels than does the more cosmetically appealing transverse incision that corresponds to Langer lines. Sharp dissection is performed down to the platysma, and it is divided transversely. Flaps are raised proximally and distally deep to the platysma. The sternocleidomastoid is identified. Dissection is performed bluntly, anterior and medial to the anterior edge of the sternocleido-mastoid, through the deep cervical fascia where the omohyoid is encountered. Care must be taken to keep the carotid sheath and its contents lateral to the plane of dissection (Tips from the Masters 3-1). The middle layer of the deep cervical fascia between the omohyoid and the sternocleidomastoid is bluntly dissected. The omo-hyoid may be divided if necessary to extend the exposure over multiple levels. The deep layer of the deep cervical fascia is incised vertically over the midline of the ver-tebral bodies and disks. Radiographic documentation of the appropriate diskectomy or corpectomy level is obtained by placing a spinal needle or marker within either a disk or vertebral body. The longus colli is elevated for 3 to 4 mm off the adjacent disk spaces and vertebral bodies.

Tips from the Masters 3-1 • The carotid sheath and its contents should be kept lateral to the plane of dissection, which is toward the anterior cervical spine.

The disk material is extricated and the uncinate processes are identified to delin-eate the lateral limits of the decompression or corpectomy. The decompression

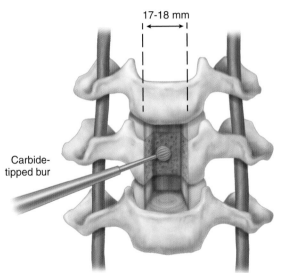

17-18 mm

Carbide-tipped bur

FIGURE 3-5 A depiction of a corpectomy trough that has been widened posteriorly to provide adequate decompression of the spinal cord. (Truumees E HH: Anterior cervical corpectomy. In Haher T, Merola A, editors: *Surgical techniques for the spine,* New York, 2003, Thieme, pp 29–35.)

includes removal of the posterior disk-osteophyte complexes, identification and removal, or "floating," of the ossified PLL, and foraminal decompression via removal of uncovertebral osteophytes.

If the surgical plan involves a corpectomy, the disks cephalad and caudad to the planned vertebrectomy level, along with any intervening disk in the case of a multi-level procedure, are completely excised before the vertebrectomy is performed. The decompression should be extended so as to completely alleviate elements leading to spinal cord deformation and compression.

When OPLL is the source of compression, caution must be exercised in removal of the ossification, and corpectomies are often necessary (Tips from the Masters 3-2). The presence of the double layer sign (a rim of ossification surrounding the hypodense ligament) on radiographic workup of OPLL is suggestive of dural penetration.[1] The two layers represent ossification of the ventral PLL and ossification that invests the dura with an intervening space of less dense PLL. This increases the risk of neurologic injury and iatrogenic durotomy if complete débridement of the OPLL is performed. An alternative to complete resection of the OPLL is the anterior floating method, which involves a transverse decompression of 20 to 25 mm to the joints of Luschka and release of the OPLL around the region that invests or replaces the dura to allow sufficient 4 to 5 mm of anterior migration of the ossification.[2] In the event of a dural defect, a primary repair should be attempted, and adjuncts such as dural grafts and fibrin glue sealant can be applied to prevent cerebrospinal fluid (CSF) leaks. The patient can be kept in an upright position to diminish the buildup of CSF pressure across the anterior cervical spinal cord. Persistent leaks have been successfully treated with lumboperitoneal shunts and lumbar drains to prevent CSF fistulas.[3]

Tips from the Masters 3-2 • Electrocautery exposure of anterior osteophytes facilitates complete removal, which improves visualization of the posterior vertebral body and allows for anatomic placement of anterior plates.

Orientation to the midline must be maintained during the decompression. As demonstrated by An and colleagues[4], the risk of vertebral artery injury increases as one moves rostrally in the subaxial cervical spine. At C3 a 15-mm-wide central decompression, and at C6 a 19-mm-wide decompression, yields a 5-mm margin of safety for the transverse foramen and vertebral artery[5] (Figure 3-5). Goto and associates[6] reported in 1993 that the central decompression should be at least 16 mm. This can be achieved by maintaining C3 15-mm and C6 19-mm-wide central decompressions at the level of the vertebral artery and expanding the decompression dorsally as the canal is approached. After the decompression is completed, the focus shifts to reconstruction and grafting of the corpectomy defect. Fibular strut allografts and cages filled with local autograft are principally used to reconstruct the corpectomy defects. Before anterior cervical instrumentation became standard, postoperative graft dislodgment was a significant risk. Several authors have recommended that the treatment of OPLL involving one- or two-level corpectomies consist of allograft strut grafting and anterior plating.[7-9] Multilevel OPLL involving three or more levels should be addressed with multilevel corpectomies, allograft strut grafting, anterior plating, and supplemental posterior fixation and fusion. This approach has been associated with few, if any, graft-related complications.[7-9]

Laminectomy with or without Fusion

Posterior surgical approaches to treat myelopathy due to OPLL include laminectomy with or without fusion and laminoplasty (Tips from the Masters 3-3). The patient can be placed prone in a Mayfield pin headrest or in a halo ring vest to maintain alignment and avoid pressure on the central retinal artery. Reverse Trendelenburg positioning helps reduce bleeding and improve visualization for the surgeon. Neurophysiologic monitoring (measurement of SSEPs and tcMEPs, electromyography) is generally recommended.

Tips from the Masters 3-3 • Preoperative administration of steroids can help mitigate neurologic injury.

Landmarks for the posterior midline dissection include the palpable spinous processes of C2 and C7. Bilateral subperiosteal dissection of the posterior elements is carried out to the facets of the levels involved. Complete exposure and packing of the most cephalad levels initially, followed by sequential exposure and packing of the caudal levels in addition, improves visualization and reduces bleeding. Careful dissection should avoid removal of the C2 attachments of the erector spinae and suboccipital triangle muscles, because they contribute to stability and resist kyphosis at this level.

After adequate exposure of the involved levels is obtained, a high-speed bur is used to create a trough at the facet-lamina junction bilaterally (Figure 3-6, *A*). A Kerrison rongeur is used to release the ligamentum flavum and complete the troughs. The lamina is then removed en bloc (Figure 3-6, *B*). After completion of the laminectomy (Figure 3-6, *C*), foraminotomies can be performed as indicated. Decompression of the exiting nerve roots is assessed with a small nerve hook or probe.

Laminectomy is often carried out from C3 to C7 to ensure that decompression is sufficient to prevent dorsal kinking of the spinal cord and resultant neurologic deficit (Tips from the Masters 3-4). In addition, removal of the T1 lamina can destabilize the cervicothoracic junction and result in postoperative deformity.

Tips from the Masters 3-4 • Avoid complete facetectomy to prevent iatrogenic destabilization and assess foraminal decompression with a right-angled nerve probe.

Instrumented fusion, using lateral mass screws in the subaxial cervical spine, generally accompanies laminectomy. Starting points for the screws should be 1 mm medial to the coronal and sagittal midpoints (Figure 3-7, *A*). A 2-mm bur is used to initiate the starting points, which should be in line with each other. A 2.5-mm drill with a 12- to 14-mm stop is used to drill the holes to orient the screws 30 degrees laterally and 15 to 30 degrees cephalad (Figure 3-7, *B* and *C*). Following drilling, the holes should be probed, measured, tapped, and probed again (Tips from the Masters 3-5). After the lateral mass screws are placed, a longitudinal rod is measured, cut, contoured, and definitively fixed to the rod-screw construct. The lateral masses are then decorticated, graft material is placed laterally to the rod-screw construct, and the incision is closed in layers over a drain.

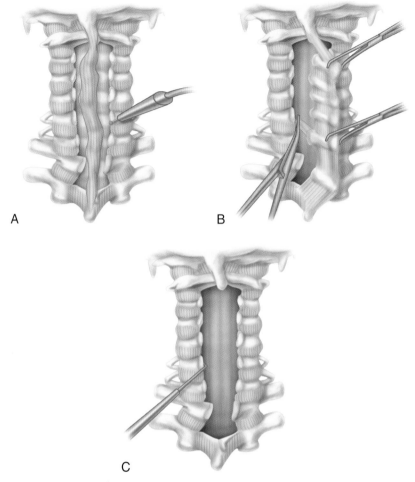

A

B

C

FIGURE 3-6 Posterior view of a cervical spine laminectomy. **A,** Use of high-speed bur to create a laminec-tomy trough. **B,** Incision of the ligamentum flavum and en bloc resection of the lamina from C3 to C7. **C,** Completed laminectomy with spinal cord decompressed.

Tips from the Masters 3-5 • If a unilateral violation of the vertebral artery occurs during drilling or tapping of lateral mass screw holes, pack the hole with bone wax and place the screw for hemostasis, and do not instrument the contralateral side.

Laminoplasty

Laminoplasty is an alternative to laminectomy. After a dissection and exposure simi-lar to that for laminectomy are performed, a bur is used to make a full-thickness trough on the opening side at the lamina-facet junction. Then a partial-thickness gutter is made on the hinge side to prevent the hinge from becoming unstable or disjointed (Figure 3-8, *A* and *B*). A small or micro Kerrison rongeur is used to complete the trough on the opening side. The opening side should be the more symptomatic side demonstrating radicular symptoms so that foraminotomies may be performed. The ligamentum flavum at the rostral and caudal ends of the laminar door is removed transversely. While the gutter on the hinge side is deepened, the surgeon should gradually apply an opening force to the spinous processes (Tips from the Masters 3-6). When the laminoplasty door is ready to be opened, stay sutures from the intact facet capsules around the bases of the spinous processes (Figure 3-8, *C* and *D*), allograft bone, or specially designed plates can be used to keep the door open as the free edge is elevated.

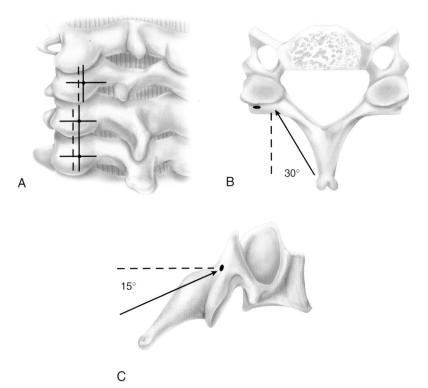

FIGURE 3-7 Placement of cervical lateral mass screws. **A,** Entry points for lateral mass screws 1 mm medial to the midpoint of the lateral mass. **B,** Coronal plane trajectory of 30° from midsagittal of the facet joint. **C,** Sagittal plane trajectory of 15° cephalad.

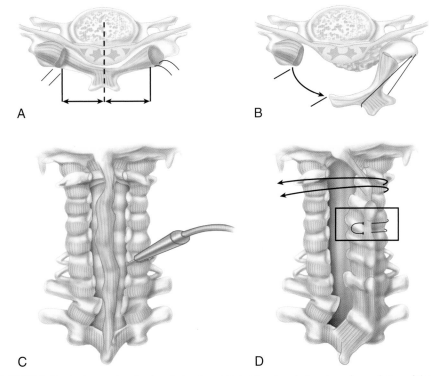

FIGURE 3-8 Cervical open-door laminoplasty. **A** and **C,** Axial and posterior view of completion of the laminoplasty trough on the opening side and deepening of the gutter on the hinge side. **B** and **D,** Axial and posterior view of opening of the laminoplasty door and closure of the hinge side held in place with sutures from the intact facets around the base of the spinous processes.

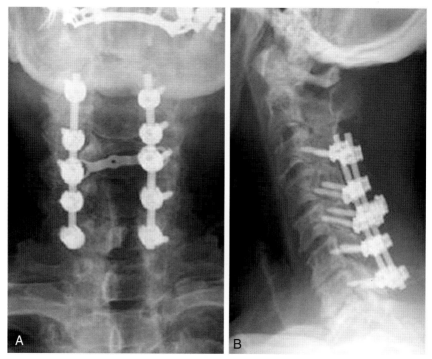

FIGURE 3-9 AP and lateral radiographs of a laminectomy and instrumented spinal fusion.

Tips from the Masters 3-6 • If hinge fracture occurs, a complete laminectomy should be performed.

DISCUSSION OF BEST EVIDENCE

The discussion of current best evidence in the evolving field of treating OPLL should begin with some basic science and natural history of the disease. OPLL is heterotopic lamellar bone formed from enchondral and intramembranous ossification. It may have woven bone at its margins.[10] The prevalence of OPLL is highest in the Japanese population (1.9% to 4.3% in patients older than 30 years). The prevalence in Taiwan, China, and Korea ranges from 0.6% to 2.8%. The United States and Germany have much lower rates ranging from 0.1% to 0.7%. There is an association of OPLL with ankylosing spondylitis and diffuse idiopathic skeletal hyperostosis.[11] Diabetes mellitus is an independent risk factor for OPLL, and the degree of abnormal insulin secretory response is positively associated with the extent of OPLL.[12] OPLL more often occurs in the cervical spine of men older than age 40 and frequency increases in the 50s. It can occur in the upper and middle thoracic spine and may be associated with ossification of the ligamentum flavum. OPLL can penetrate the dura, which eliminates the epidural space. En bloc excision of this area of OPLL can result in a dural defect, CSF leakage, and possible neurologic injury.[1] Variations in the pattern of OPLL have been classified as *continuous, segmental, mixed,* and *other* types. Static compression of the spinal cord is thought to be the main cause of myelopathy in OPLL, yet dynamic factors can play a role in further deterioration.

Regarding the natural history of OPLL, Matsunaga and colleagues[13-15] reported a 71% myelopathy-free rate after 30 years. They noted that 100% of patients with greater than 60% stenosis or less than 6 mm of space available for the cord developed myelopathy. Those patients who had an available cord space of between 6 mm and 14 mm and had an increased C2-C7 range of motion were also more likely to develop myelopathy. In addition to increased cervical range of motion, the presence of the segmental type of OPLL, age older than 50 years, and high signal intensity in the spinal cord on T2-weighted MRI are risk factors for the development of myelopathy.[16]

TABLE 3-1   Nurick Grade for Cervical Myelopathy

Grade	Description
0	Signs or symptoms of root involvement but without evidence of spinal cord disease
1	Signs of spinal cord disease, but no difficulty in walking
2	Slight difficulty in walking that does not prevent full-time employment
3	Difficulty in walking that prevents full-time employment or the ability to do all housework, but that is not so severe as to require someone else's help to walk
4	Able to walk only with someone else's help or with the aid of a walking frame
5	Chair bound or bedridden

Adapted from Nurick S: The pathogenesis of the spinal cord disorder associated with cervical spondylosis, *Brain* 95(1):87–100, 1972.

In a patient with OPLL, the presentation may range from neck pain, to an insidious onset of myelopathy or myeloradiculopathy, to an acute onset from minor trauma. Physical examination may demonstrate radiculopathy and sensory disturbances of the upper extremities, spasticity and hyperreflexia of upper or lower extremities, gait abnormalities, and other long-tract signs. The examination should be thorough and should attempt to rule out other sources of pathology such as tumor, spondylosis, or trauma. Special physical examination tests, which are beyond the scope of this chapter, may be necessary to appreciate very mild myelopathic changes. Both Nurick grade and Japanese Orthopaedic Association (JOA) score (Tables 3-1 and 3-2) should be determined, because results of previous outcome studies have been inconsistent with regard to which assessment tool has been used to evaluate the severity of myelopathy upon presentation and to evaluate the improvement or deterioration after surgical interventions. Most current long-term outcome studies limit postoperative evaluations to the upper extremity and trunk, since lumbar pathology often coexists or develops over the course of follow-up and can obscure comparative results.

Radiographic evaluation of patients with OPLL should begin with plain radiographs, including flexion and extension lateral projections of the cervical spine to assess alignment and instability, classify the type of OPLL, quantify the C2-C7 range of motion, and calculate the occupying ratio of OPLL. CT myelography should be performed to better elucidate the characteristics of OPLL for punctate calcifications, "pearls" of bone, and signs of dural penetration such as the double layer sign, which is pathognomonic for dural penetration. Thin-slice bone window CT scanning with sagittal and axial reformations is the best modality to diagnose and characterize the morphology of OPLL and identify the presence of dural penetration. It has been demonstrated that 50% of nonsegmental types of OPLL are associated with dural penetration and 52% to 88% of cases in which scans demonstrate the double layer sign have been shown to have dural penetration.[17-19] This preoperative information aids in directing treatment and helps minimize the risk of neurologic injury due to manipulation of ossified dura and CSF leaks. CT may also be used to calculate the space-occupying ratio of OPLL, which is the ratio of maximum AP thickness of OPLL to the AP diameter of the spinal canal at that level. CT myelography should be considered if the plan is for surgical intervention via anterior resection or use of the floating method. MRI should be performed to evaluate for nerve root impingement, spinal cord flattening, intrinsic signal changes indicating edema, myelomalacia, and demyelination.[17-21]

Current best evidence in the treatment of OPLL via the anterior approach suggests that an anterior approach is often indicated in the segmental type of OPLL rather than in the continuous or mixed type.[22] A kyphotic cervical spine is also best treated via the anterior approach unless the kyphosis is corrected, because the spinal cord is less likely to drift posteriorly. Correction of kyphosis and maintenance of lordosis are better when addressed anteriorly. Yamaura and colleagues[2] followed 107 patients treated using the anterior floating method for at least 3 years. They found 84% to have better than 50% recovery rate and 100% fusion with external immobilization. The anterior migration occurred over 4 to 8 weeks with no proliferation of ossification. Tateiwa and colleagues[23] reported on 27 patients with OPLL treated with multilevel subtotal

TABLE 3-2   Japanese Orthopaedic Association (JOA) Score for Cervical
Myelopathy

JOA Assessment for Cervical Myelopathy	Chiles Modification of the JOA Assessment Scale
Motor Dysfunction Scores of the Upper Extremity	
0 Inability to feed oneself	
1 Inability to handle chopsticks; ability to eat with a spoon	Inability to use knife and fork, or eat with a spoon
2 Ability to handle chopsticks, but with much difficulty	Ability to use knife and fork, but with much difficulty
3 Ability to handle chopsticks, but with slight difficulty	Ability to use knife and fork with slight difficulty
4 None	
Motor Dysfunction Scores of the Lower Extremity	
0 Inability to walk	
1 Ability to walk on flat floor with walking aid	
2 Ability to walk up and/or down stairs with hand rail	
3 Lack of stability and smooth reciprocation	
4 None	
Sensory Deficit Scores of the Upper Extremity	
0 Severe sensory loss or pain	
1 Mild sensory loss	
2 None	
Sensory Deficit Scores of the Lower Extremity	
0 Severe sensory loss or pain	
1 Mild sensory loss	
2 None	
Sensory Deficit Scores of the Trunk	
0 Severe sensory loss or pain	
1 Mild sensory loss	
2 None	
Sphincter Dysfunction Scores	
0 Inability to void	
1 Marked difficulty in micturition	
2 Difficulty in micturition	
3 None	
Total individual item scores for assessment of severity	

Adapted from Ogino H, Tada K, Okada K, et al: Canal diameter, anteroposterior compression ratio, and spondylotic myelopathy of the cervical spine, *Spine* 8(1):1–15, 1983; and Chiles BW 3rd, Leonard MA, Choudhri HF, et al: Cervical spondylotic myelopathy: patterns of neurological deficit and recovery after anterior cervical decompression, *Neurosurgery* 44(4):762–769, 1999; discussion, 769–770.

corpectomy, fibular strut graft, and halo immobilization, demonstrating a 62% recovery rate at an average 8-year follow-up. These patients maintained their lordosis without progression of OPLL, which resulted in a 100% fusion rate and only two transient C5 root palsies. A **retrospective review** of data for patients with OPLL treated with anterior corpectomies, fibular strut grafting, and halo immobilization has shown 56% to 80% good or excellent results with few complications and reoperations at 6- to 10-year follow-up. These results proved better than those for laminoplasty for hill-type OPLL lesions when the occupying ratio was more than 60%.[24,25] Severe OPLL can narrow the AP diameter of the spinal canal by more than 50%, which makes decompression more technically demanding. Chen and colleagues[26] performed ACCF with titanium mesh cages filled with local autograft and an anterior plate for severe multilevel OPLL, reporting 84% good or excellent results, significant improvement of cervical lordosis, increased canal diameter, and a myelopathy improvement rate of 62%. A multiple logistic regression analysis of prognostic factors affecting outcomes for 47 patients with OPLL treated with ACCF, fibular strut allograft, and anterior plating found that patients with diabetes mellitus had worse outcomes.[27] Rajshekar and colleagues[28] reported, in their study of a **prospective series** of 72 patients managed with corpectomy and uninstrumented iliac crest autograft fusions, that those whose symptoms had been present for 12 months or less had better rates of functional improvement and cure. Of note, patients with cervical spondylotic myelopathy had better functional improvement than those with OPLL.

Indications for treating myelopathy due to OPLL via a posterior approach include OPLL extending for more than three levels, an occupying ratio greater than 50% to 60%, OPLL above C2 or below C7, and continuous or mixed-type OPLL over several levels in a straight or lordotic spine.[22,29] The prerequisite for a nonkyphotic spine is that the sagittal alignment be able to be corrected and better maintained via an anterior approach.[26] Postlaminectomy kyphosis is more frequent and severe when preoperative cervical alignment is not lordotic.[29] Assessment of cervical alignment, relative to the OPLL, using the K-line can provide the prognosis for neurologic improvement. Fujiyoshi defined the K-line by marking the midpoint of the spinal canal at C2 and C7, and then drawing a line connecting the points (Figure 3-10). If the connecting line intersects the OPLL, then alignment is termed *K-line (−)* and there is insufficient cord shift and poorer neurologic recovery, whereas if the line is posterior to the OPLL, then alignment is K-line (+) and neurologic recovery is significantly better after posterior decompression.[30] Kato and associates[31] presented findings after long-term follow-up of 14 years in patients undergoing laminectomy for the treatment of myelopathy due to OPLL, reporting a recovery rate of 43% at 1 year and 32% at 10 years, with 23% of patients experiencing late neurologic deterioration related to trauma or ossification of the ligamentum flavum. Seventy percent of patients in this series had OPLL progression and 47% showed progressive kyphosis, neither of which contributed to neurologic changes. Postoperative neurologic improvement was greater in those with higher JOA scores and younger age at surgery. In a **retrospective review** of surgical techniques to treat cervical spondylotic myelopathy, Mummaneni and co-workers[32] discussed the Level III evidence that laminectomy alone can be associated with late deterioration and that

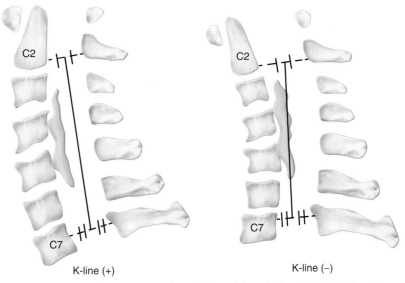

FIGURE 3-10 The K-line is a line connecting the midpoint of the spinal canal behind C2 and the midpoint of the canal behind C7. K-line (+) is when the line does not intersect the OPLL and thus indicates lordotic alignment. K-line (−) is when the line intersects the OPLL and thus represents more kyphotic alignment.

instrumented fusion should be added, especially in younger patients. Chen and associates[29] reported a **prospective study** with long-term follow-up of 83 patients who underwent laminectomy and instrumented fusion for the treatment of OPLL with an average improvement in JOA score of 5 points and maintenance of lordotic alignment, which correlated with clinical prognosis. Complication rates for laminectomy with or without fusion range from 5% to 12%, and complications most commonly involve transient cervical root palsies.[29,31,32]

Expansive open-door laminoplasty has been studied extensively as a treatment for OPLL, demonstrating improved results in those with lordotic spines before surgery. Postoperative loss of lordosis does not appear to affect outcome.[33] Recovery rates are 60% to 63% at 5 to 10 years and diminish to 40% to 50% at 10 to 13 years.[33,34] Postoperative progression of OPLL is 40% for the segmental type and 64% to 70% for continuous and mixed types, but does not affect clinical outcomes.[33-36] Ogawa and associates found in a **retrospective review** that 15% of patients have late-onset deterioration at 10 years as evidenced by a JOA score decrease of 2 points or more, and that segmental-type OPLL can result in deterioration of more than 1 point in the JOA score in 70% of patients. Furthermore, this correlates with increased C2-C7 range of motion and poorer outcomes compared with continuous or mixed types of OPLL.[33,35] Range of motion after laminoplasty has been shown to progressively decrease and plateau by 18 months, and autofusion occurs in 85% to 97% of patients by 5 to 10 years.[33,36,37] Iwasaki and colleagues found that older age at surgery and lower preoperative JOA scores were predictive of lower postoperative JOA scores.[34] Iwasaki and associates found in a **retrospective review** that the most significant predictor of poor outcome after laminoplasty was hill-shaped OPLL.[38] Complication rates for laminoplasty range from 5% to 9%, and complications most commonly include transient C5 or C6 nerve root palsies.[33,34,36,38]

COMMENTARY

The approach to treating OPLL should be determined by cervical alignment, type and location of the OPLL, evidence of dural penetration, and surgeon experience. Factors such as age, duration of symptoms, and severity of preoperative myelopathy should be weighed with the knowledge that studies have yielded conflicting results as to their effect on surgical and clinical outcome. The anterior approach to the cervical spine is familiar to most spine surgeons. Performing a technically sound anterior decompression and fusion operation for OPLL may sacrifice motion, but would likely give better results than a poorly performed posterior operation undertaken in an effort to retain motion. Attempts to preserve motion with laminectomy alone or laminoplasty must be tempered by the knowledge that postlaminectomy kyphosis can lead to deterioration and the possible need for further surgery, and that many patients lose motion or even experience autofusion after laminoplasty. This summary of recent best evidence can provide surgeons with a sound foundation for gauging prognosis and making surgical decisions to determine the optimal approach to treatment of patients with OPLL. The surgical techniques and tips from the masters presented in this chapter should enhance surgeons' skills in performing these operations to yield a better surgical and clinical outcome for their patients.

REFERENCES

1. Min JH, Jang JS, Lee SH: Significance of the double-layer and single-layer signs in the ossification of the posterior longitudinal ligament of the cervical spine, *J Neurosurg Spine* 6(4):309–312, 2007. **A retrospective review in Korea of medical records for 197 patients with OPLL and preoperative CT scans. The authors found that 52% with a double layer sign had dural penetration and 50% of those with nonsegmental-type OPLL had dural penetration.**
2. Yamaura I, Kurosa Y, Matuoka T, et al: Anterior floating method for cervical myelopathy caused by ossification of the posterior longitudinal ligament, *Clin Orthop Relat Res* 359:27–34, 1999.
3. Epstein N: Identification of ossification of the posterior longitudinal ligament extending through the dura on preoperative computed tomographic examinations of the cervical spine, *Spine* 26(2):182–186, 2001.
4. An HS, Vaccaro A, Cotler JM, et al: Spinal disorders at the cervicothoracic junction, *Spine* 19(22): 2557–2564, 1994.

5. Vaccaro AR, Ring D, Scuderi G, et al: Vertebral artery location in relation to the vertebral body as determined by two-dimensional computed tomography evaluation, *Spine* 19(23):2637–2641, 1994.
6. Goto S, Mochizuki M, Watanabe T, et al: Long-term follow-up study of anterior surgery for cervical spondylotic myelopathy with special reference to the magnetic resonance imaging findings in 52 cases, *Clin Orthop Relat Res* 291:142–153, 1993.
7. Epstein N: Anterior approaches to cervical spondylosis and ossification of the posterior longitudinal ligament: review of operative technique and assessment of 65 multilevel circumferential procedures, *Surg Neurol* 55:313–324, 2001.
8. Chen Y, Chen D, Wang X, et al: Anterior corpectomy and fusion for severe ossification of posterior longitudinal ligament in the cervical spine, *Int Orthop* 33:477–482, 2009.
9. Choi S, Lee S, Lee J, et al: Factors affecting prognosis of patients who underwent corpectomy and fusion for treatment of cervical ossification of the posterior longitudinal ligament, *J Spinal Disord Tech* 18(4):309–314, 2005.
10. Ono K, Yonenobu K, Tada K, et al: Pathology of ossification of the posterior longitudinal ligament and ligamentum flavum, *Clinical Orthop* 359:18–26, 1999.
11. Kim T, Bae K, Uhm W, et al: Prevalence of ossification of the posterior longitudinal ligament of the cervical spine, *Joint Bone Spine* 75:471–474, 2008.
12. Li H, Jiang L, Dai L: A review of prognostic factors for surgical outcome of ossification of the posterior longitudinal ligament of cervical spine, *Eur Spine J* 17:1277–1288, 2008.
13. Matsunaga S, Sakou T, Taketomi E, et al: Clinical course of patients with ossification of the posterior longitudinal ligament: a minimum 10 year cohort study, *J Neurosurg Spine* 100:245–248, 2004. **A retrospective study in Japan of 450 patients with OPLL. Risk factors for progression to myelopathy included greater than 60% stenosis and increased range of motion between C1 and C7. The authors also found a myelopathy-free rate of 71% at 30 years.**
14. Matsunaga S, Kukita M, Hayashi K, et al: Pathogenesis of myelopathy in patients with ossification of the posterior longitudinal ligament, *J Neurosurg Spine* 96:168–172, 2002.
15. Matsunaga S, Nakamura K, Seichi A, et al: Radiographic predictors for the development of myelopathy in patients with ossification of the posterior longitudinal ligament: a multicenter cohort study, *Spine* 33:2648–2650, 2008.
16. Mochizuki M, Aiba A, Hashimoto M, et al: Cervical myelopathy in patients with ossification of the posterior longitudinal ligament, *J Neurosurg Spine* 10:122–128, 2009. **A Japanese study of 21 patients with OPLL and mild or no myelopathy. The 6 without myelopathy remained in neurologically stable condition. Among the 15 with mild myelopathy, 8 experienced improvement, the condition of 6 remained unchanged, and the myelopathy of 1 worsened during the 4-year follow-up period.**
17. Chen Y, Guo Y, Chen D, et al: Diagnosis and surgery of ossification of posterior longitudinal ligament associated with dural ossification in the cervical spine, *Eur Spine J* 18:1541–1547, 2009.
18. Epstein N: Posterior approaches in the management of cervical spondylosis and ossification of the posterior longitudinal ligament, *Surg Neurol* 58:194–208, 2002.
19. Min J, Jang J, Lee S: Significance of the double-layer and single-layer signs in the ossification of the posterior longitudinal ligament of the cervical spine, *J Neurosurg Spine* 6:309–312, 2007.
20. Epstein N: Anterior approaches to cervical spondylosis and ossification of the posterior longitudinal ligament: review of operative technique and assessment of 65 multilevel circumferential procedures, *Surg Neurol* 55:313–324, 2001.
21. Mizuno J, Nakagawa H, Matuso N, et al: Dural ossification associated with cervical ossification of the posterior longitudinal ligament: frequency of dural ossification and comparison of neuroimaging modalities in ability to identify disease, *J Neurosurg Spine* 2:425–430, 2005.
22. Mizuno J, Nakagawa H: Ossified posterior longitudinal ligament: management strategies and outcomes, *Spine J* 6:282s–288s, 2006.
23. Tateiwa Y, Kamimura M, Itoh H, et al: Multilevel subtotal corpectomy and interbody fusion using a fibular bone graft for cervical myelopathy due to ossification of the posterior longitudinal ligament, *J Clin Neurosci* 10(2):199–207, 2003.
24. Onari K, Akiyama N, Kondo S, et al: Long-term follow-up results of anterior interbody fusion applied for cervical myelopathy due to ossification of the posterior longitudinal ligament, *Spine* 26(5):488–493, 2001.
25. Iwasaki M, Okuda S, Miyauchi A, et al: Surgical strategy for cervical myelopathy due to ossification of the posterior longitudinal ligament. Part 2: Advantages of anterior decompression and fusion over laminoplasty, *Spine* 32(6):654–660, 2007. **A Japanese retrospective review comparing outcomes for 27 patients treated with anterior decompression and fusion (ADF) with those for 66 patients treated with laminoplasty for OPLL. Patients with occupying ratios of more than 60% had better neurologic outcomes with ADF than with laminoplasty. This more technically demanding approach was associated with a higher incidence of surgery-related complications.**
26. Chen Y, Chen D, Wang X, et al: Anterior corpectomy and fusion for severe ossification of the posterior longitudinal ligament in the cervical spine, *Int Orthop* 33:477–482, 2009.
27. Choi S, Lee S, Lee J, et al: Factors affecting prognosis of patients who underwent corpectomy and fusion for treatment of cervical ossification of the posterior longitudinal ligament: analysis of 47 patients, *J Spinal Disord Tech* 18(4):309–314, 2005.
28. Rajshekar V, Kumar G: Functional outcome after central corpectomy in poor grade patients with cervical spondylotic myelopathy or ossified posterior longitudinal ligament, *Neurosurgery* 56(6):1279–1285, 2005. **A prospective study in India including 12 patients with OPLL treated with central corpectomy. The authors reported 100% fusion with greater improvement in Nurick scores for patients with cervical spondylotic myelopathy than for those with OPLL.**

29. Chen Y, Guo D, Wang X, et al: Long-term outcome of laminectomy and instrumented fusion for cervical ossification of the posterior longitudinal ligament, *Int Orthop* 33:1075–1080, 2009. **A Japanese prospective 4.8-year evaluation of 83 patients with OPLL extending more than three levels and occupying more than 50% of the canal between C2 and C7 who were treated with laminectomy and instrumented fusion. Seventy-one percent of patients had a good prognosis, and the authors found that lordotic alignment allows a better decompressive effect.**

30. Fujiyoshi T, Yamazaki M, Kawabe J, et al: A new concept for making decisions regarding the surgical approach for cervical ossification of the posterior longitudinal ligament: the K-line, *Spine* 33: E990–E993, 2008. **Japanese study evaluating the kyphotic alignment of the cervical spine (K-line) as a line connecting the midpoints of the canal behind C2 and C7. If the line intersects the OPLL, then the alignment is termed *K-line (−)* and there will be insufficient posterior drift of the spinal cord for neurologic improvement. In K-line (+) alignment the line is posterior to OPLL and recovery rates were 66% versus 13.9% in the K-line (−) group.**

31. Kato Y, Iwasaki M, Fuji T, et al: Long-term follow-up results of laminectomy for cervical myelopathy caused by ossification of the posterior longitudinal ligament, *J Neurosurg* 89:217–223, 1998.

32. Mummaneni P, Kaiser M, Matz P, et al: Cervical surgical techniques for the treatment of cervical spondylotic myelopathy, *J Neurosurg Spine* 11:130–141, 2009.

33. Ogawa Y, Toyama Y, Chiba K, et al: Long-term results of expansive open-door laminoplasty for ossification of the posterior longitudinal ligament of the cervical spine, *J Neurosurg Spine* 1(2): 168–174, 2004. **A Japanese retrospective review of 72 patients with OPLL treated with open-door laminoplasty. The authors reported a 63% recovery rate at 5 to 10 years. Sixty-four percent of patients experienced OPLL progression and 21% lost lordosis, neither of which affected outcome; 97% experienced autofusion of more than one segment.**

34. Iwasaki M, Kawaguchi Y, Kimura T, et al: Long-term results of expansive laminoplasty for ossification of the posterior longitudinal ligament of the cervical spine: more than 10 years follow up, *J Neurosurg* 96(2 Suppl):180–189, 2002.

35. Ogawa Y, Chiba K, Matsumoto M, et al: Long-term results after expansive open door laminoplasty for segmental type of ossification of the posterior longitudinal ligament of the cervical spine: a comparison of nonsegmental type lesions, *J Neurosurg Spine* 3:198–204, 2005. **A Japanese study of 57 patients with OPLL treated with laminoplasty who were followed for a minimum of 7 years. Clinical results (JOA scores) were found to be better for those with nonsegmental-type (mixed and continuous) OPLL than for those with segmental-type OPLL. C2-C7 hypermobility was associated with late deterioration.**

36. Chiba K, Ogawa Y, Ishii K, et al: Long-term results of expansive open door laminoplasty for cervical myelopathy—average 14 year follow-up study, *Spine* 31(26):2998–3005, 2006.

37. Hyun S, Rhim S, Roh S, et al: The time course of range of motion loss after cervical laminoplasty: a prospective study with minimum two-year follow up, *Spine* 34(11):1134–1139, 2009.

38. Iwasaki M, Okuda S, Miyauchi A, et al: Surgical strategy for cervical myelopathy due to ossification of the posterior longitudinal ligament. Part 1: Clinical results and limitations of laminoplasty, *Spine* 32(6):647–653, 2007.

Chapter 4   Minimally Invasive Approaches to Thoracic Disk Herniations

Alfred T. Ogden, Michael G. Kaiser, Richard G. Fessler

Thoracic disk herniations are uncommon surgical lesions that exist along a continuum of surgical complexity from the relatively straightforward to the extremely challenging depending on their anatomic relationship to the spinal cord and their intrinsic tissue characteristics. Several different approaches are available to spine surgeons, some of which are not incorporated into common clinical practice. Historically, poor results following laminectomy, particularly with central, calcified herniations, led to the use of posterolateral and transthoracic approaches that allow more direct access to the herniation but are associated with significant approach-related morbidity. Minimally invasive techniques offer the advantages of these approaches while mitigating the exposure-related morbidity.

CASE PRESENTATION

A 63-year-old woman came for treatment after experiencing several months of leg weakness, gait instability, pain, and paresthesias in her anterolateral right thigh, and urinary urgency with intermittent incontinence. Her symptoms progressed over several months despite physical therapy.

- PMH: Unremarkable
- PSH: Unremarkable
- Exam: Neurologic examination revealed mild bilateral leg weakness to confrontation, disproportionately increased reflexes in the legs, and a mildly spastic gait. On her initial office visit/neurologic examination, the patient had noticeable progression of leg extensor weakness, had a progressive foot drop, and had developed a sensory deficit at the midthoracic level.
- Imaging: magnetic resonance imaging (MRI) and computed tomography (CT) imaging showed a ventral T7-8 thoracic disk herniation with partial calcification and cord compression (Figure 4-1, *A* and *B*).

Tips from the Masters 4-1 • Thoracic disk herniations are heterogeneous with respect to internal consistency and relationship to the thecal sac and spinal cord. Before any particular approach is elected, careful assessment of these characteristics with MRI and CT is required.

Given the patient's pathologic features and neurologic progression, she was offered surgical decompression.

MINIMALLY INVASIVE SURGICAL OPTIONS

Transfacet Approach

Several variations of the transfacet approach to a thoracic disk herniation have been described.[1-4] These vary in terms of muscle dissection, retractor type (self-retaining or tubular), method of operative visualization (microscope vs. endoscope),

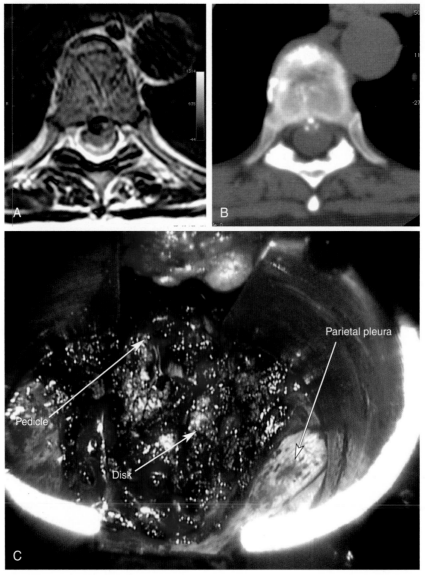

FIGURE 4-1 A, Preoperative magnetic resonance imaging scan demonstrating a T7-8 left paracentral disk herniation. **B,** Computed tomography scan of the area showing partial calcification. **C,** Exposure afforded through the minimally invasive retropleural approach.

and extent of facet resection (lateral, partial, or "window"). This approach is similar to the more familiar approach for resection of a lumbar disk herniation. The advantages of this approach are a direct exposure over the lateral disk that affords a small incision and minimal muscle disruption, complete or relative sparing of the pedicle of the inferior vertebral segment, and disk removal without risk of entering the thoracic cavity.

The main disadvantage of this approach is its dorsal angle of attack, which can be problematic with central and/or calcified disks. Soft lateral, contiguous disk herniations that extend beyond the edge of the thecal sac are the ideal indication for this approach. Such fragments can be delivered into the foramen with minimal retraction on the thecal sac. For the patient described in the Case Presentation, the calcified nature and the central location of the disk herniation were felt to be contraindications to this approach.

Tips from the Masters 4-2 • Transfacet approaches are most suitable for lateral and preferably soft disk herniations that can be removed with minimal manipulation of the thecal sac.

Thoracoscopic Approach

The thoracoscopic approach[5] takes advantage of a more anterior approach that provides an advantageous angle of attack for midline lesions. The evolution of specialized instrumentation developed for thoracic surgery has mitigated the morbidity of an open thoracotomy. The placement of three working ports through several small incisions between the intercostal muscles provides access into the thoracic cavity after the ipsilateral lung has been deflated. A camera is placed through one port, while instruments for the resection of the disk are inserted through the remaining two ports. The approach is then similar to that with an open thoracotomy, with dissection of the parietal pleura and removal of the rib head overlying the disk space. The superior edge of the inferior pedicle may be drilled away for orientation and improved exposure.

The major advantages of this approach are the direct line of sight and angle of resection that allow for the safe resection of a calcified midline disk, particularly when the spinal cord is draped over the disk. The disadvantages include the potential approach-related pulmonary complications, two-dimensional viewing screen, possible surgeon inexperience with thoracoscopic instruments, and the requirement for an approach surgeon.

Minimally Invasive Retropleural Approach

Because of the ventral position of the disk herniation and its partial calcification in the patient described in the Case Presentation, an approach that offered a lateral angle of attack was felt to be more suitable. The retropleural approach described by Otani and colleagues[6] and McCormick and colleagues[7] affords a lateral approach without pleural violation or the need for single lung ventilation, but still requires a relatively large exposure with extensive soft tissue manipulation. Utilizing the benefits of minimally invasive tubular retractor systems, a modification is presented that minimizes the morbidity of the traditional retropleural approach.

Tips from the Masters 4-3 • Midline and calcified disk herniations are relative indications for lateral or anterolateral approaches such as the minimally invasive retropleural approach and thoracoscopic approaches.

FUNDAMENTAL TECHNIQUE

Tips from the Masters 4-4 • Depending on the spine level of the disk and the patient's individual anatomy, the initial thoracotomy in the minimally invasive retropleural approach may be at the level, or a level above, the disk space of the patient's lesion. The more distal the segment, the more caudally angulated the rib, and the more likely that the initial thoracotomy will need to be performed at the level above.

Tips from the Masters 4-5 • If greater exposure is needed, the minimally invasive retropleural approach is easily converted into an open retropleural thoracotomy.

The patient was placed in the standard lateral position for an open retropleural approach, with the ipsilateral arm positioned above the head to elevate the scapula. As is true in most patients, a lateral fluoroscopic image demonstrated that the T7 rib covered the site of the pathology, that is, the T7-8 disk space that articulates with the T8 rib head. This is a result of caudal angulation of the rib from its costovertebral articulation. A 4-cm incision was made over the T7 rib. The exposed rib was dissected free of its muscle insertions, with care taken to preserve the T7 neurovascular bundle. A2 to 3 cm section of the rib was resected without violation of the parietal pleura. Using blunt dissection, the parietal pleura was elevated off the ventral surface of the proximal rib. With account taken of the caudal rib angulation, a direct lateral approach to the anterolateral surface of the spine allowed exposure of the T7-8 disk space. Once the anterolateral spine was identified, the dissection cavity was extended to allow visualization of the proximal T8 rib and rib head. The parietal pleura over the T8 rib head, the T7-8 disk space, and the lateral aspect of the T8 vertebral body was mobilized and reflected ventrally. A thin malleable retractor was placed over the reflected parietal pleura to protect and retract the lung, which continued to be ventilated. An expandable tubular retractor was placed through the mini-thoracotomy, docked over the rib head and disk space, and locked into position (see Figure 4-1, *C*). The procedure was performed through the tubular retractors using the intraoperative microscope for visualization. The rib head was removed with a drill and rongeurs providing exposure of the disk space. The canal was defined using the T8 pedicle as the principal landmark. The diskectomy was performed with standard techniques using curettes, rongeurs, and drill with modifications for minimally invasive spine surgery.

Tips from the Masters 4-6 • A narrow, malleable retractor is a useful adjunct to a tubular retractor to protect the lung and keep it out of the operative field, which obviates the need for lung deflation during surgery.

Tips from the Masters 4-7 • Drilling of the rib head and the posterolateral end plates of the vertebral bodies is useful to provide additional exposure and space in which to deliver the disk herniation.

Postoperative course: The patient did not require a chest tube and had an uneventful postoperative recovery. Because of her gait disorder, she was discharged to an acute inpatient rehabilitation facility on postoperative day 3. She was discharged home after 2 weeks and was seen 1 month after surgery. At this time she had had modest improvement in her neurologic symptoms and was taking a small amount of narcotic pain medication. At last follow-up, 3 months after surgery, she had stopped taking all narcotics and had experienced a significant improvement in leg strength and gait as well as resolution of her urinary dysfunction.

DISCUSSION OF BEST EVIDENCE

The history of surgery for thoracic disk herniations reflects disaffection with the dismal neurologic outcomes from a purely dorsal approach (i.e., laminectomy) and the subsequent adoption of lateral or posterolateral approaches (transpedicular, lateral extracavitary, retropleural) that resulted in excellent neurologic outcomes but were more invasive.[6-9] The subsequent development of less invasive approaches stemmed from a desire to mitigate postoperative pain and recovery time while maintaining excellent outcomes. To date, the best evidence regarding minimally invasive approaches to thoracic diskectomy is confined to small **retrospective** surgical series and descriptions of operative techniques.[3,5] These reports illustrate the feasibility and initial efficacy of less invasive approaches for this pathologic condition in selected patients. The evidence cannot begin to elucidate the superiority of one approach over another. Indeed, given the relative rarity of this lesion, and the case-to-case heterogeneity, such comparisons will be difficult and perhaps inappropriate. The decision of whether to use a less invasive approach over a more invasive one and which approach to select is likely to remain primarily influenced by the constraints of the pathologic features present and the training and expertise of the individual surgeon.

COMMENTARY

Thoracic disk herniations are extremely heterogeneous with respect to presenting symptoms, anatomic relationship to the spinal cord, and intrinsic physical properties. This explains to a large degree why there is such an array of approaches for what is a relatively rare surgical disease. The extremes illustrate this point. What is required of a surgical approach for the safe, effective removal of a soft lateral disk herniation causing a radiculopathy bears little resemblance to what is required for a calcified midline disk or osteophyte causing myelopathy. The foremost consideration is the ability to safely remove the lesion regardless of the invasiveness of the exposure. Having said this, there are clearly some thoracic disk herniations that do not require extensive exposures. As is often the case in spine surgery, judicious selection of the approach based on the nature of the lesion and the surgeon's own expertise is paramount, as is a back-up plan should the initial surgical approach prove unfeasible.

REFERENCES

1. Isaacs RE, Podichetty VK, Sandhu FA, et al: Thoracic microendoscopic discectomy: a human cadaver study, *Spine* 30:1226–1231, 2005.
2. Jho HD: Endoscopic transpedicular thoracic discectomy, *J Neurosurg* 91:151–156, 1999.
3. Perez-Cruet MJ, Kim BS, Sandhu F, et al: Thoracic microendoscopic discectomy, *J Neurosurg Spine* 1:58–63, 2004. **A retrospective review of data for seven patients with soft disk herniations who underwent diskectomy via the transfacet approach using a muscle-splitting tubular retractor and endoscopic visualization. Outcomes were excellent, and no complications were reported.**
4. Stillerman CB, Chen TC, Day JD, et al: The transfacet pedicle-sparing approach for thoracic disc removal: cadaveric morphometric analysis and preliminary clinical experience, *J Neurosurg* 83:971–976, 1995. **This study describes the transfacet approach to thoracic diskectomy with a unilateral muscle dissection and the authors' experience with the approach in cadavers and six patients. The authors reported excellent outcomes and decreased perioperative morbidity compared with other approaches.**
5. Rosenthal D, Dickman CA: Thoracoscopic microsurgical excision of herniated thoracic discs, *J Neurosurg* 89:224–235, 1998. **A retrospective review comparing outcomes for 55 patients who underwent thoracoscopy for thoracic disk herniations with outcomes for 18 patients who underwent thoracotomy and 15 patients who underwent costotraversectomy. Neurological outcomes were similar. However, patients in the thoracoscopy group had fewer pulmonary complications, less pain, and shorter length of hospital stay than those in the thoracotomy group.**
6. Otani K, Yoshida M, Fujii E, et al: Thoracic disc herniation. Surgical treatment in 23 patients, *Spine* 13:1262–1267, 1988.
7. McCormick PC: Retropleural approach to the thoracic and thoracolumbar spine, *Neurosurgery* 37:908–914, 1995. **This study describes in detail the retropleural approach to the thoracic spine and the author's initial experience in treating a range of pathologic conditions, including thoracic disks.**
8. Benzel EC: The lateral extracavitary approach to the spine using the three-quarter prone position, *J Neurosurg* 71:837–841, 1989.
9. Patterson RH Jr, Arbit E: A surgical approach through the pedicle to protruded thoracic discs, *J Neurosurg* 48:768–772, 1978.

Chapter 5

Lumbar Disk Herniation with Mild Neurologic Deficit: Microdiskectomy Versus Conservative Treatment

Kelli L. Crabtree, Paul M. Arnold

Sciatica is one of the most common reasons patients seek medical attention in the United States and around the world. Sciatica, a radiculopathy arising when one or more lumbosacral nerve roots become compressed, can lead to radiating leg pain, as well as sensory and motor deficits in some cases.[1,2] Sciatica is most commonly caused by disk herniation. L4-5 is the most frequently involved level, followed closely by L5-S1, then L3-4. Disk protrusion at other levels or at more than one level at any given time is rare. Other potential causes of sciatica include spondylosis, infection, neoplasm, and vascular disease. Although their clinical presentations may be similar, the management and prognosis of each of these conditions differs from that of a herniated disk and is not within the scope of this chapter.

To properly evaluate a patient presenting with a lumbosacral radiculopathy, it is important to understand the anatomy of the lumbar spine, with particular attention to the relationships of the lumbar intervertebral spaces and foramina, nerve roots, and pedicles. Each lumbosacral nerve root exits the spinal canal via the neural foramen at the disk space below its respective vertebral body and is typically compressed by a herniation of the disk immediately above this vertebral body. For example, the L5 nerve root exits through the neural foramen at the level of the L5-S1 disk space; L5 nerve root compression is generally caused by an L4-5 posterolateral disk herniation, although a large medial disk herniation at the level of L3-4 (Figure 5-1) or a far-lateral L5-S1 herniated nucleus pulposus can also be responsible.

Although sciatica was initially described around 2000 BC, the relationship between lumbar disk disease and sciatica was not fully understood until the early part of the twentieth century.[3-5] Once an effective surgical treatment of sciatica was described in 1934,[4] surgery began to be offered routinely to a small subset of patients whose symptoms persisted after a period of nonsurgical management, since this treatment alone would lead to the resolution of symptoms in most patients.[6,7] The ideal length of time that nonoperative treatment should be tried before surgery is considered is still under debate. Finding the optimal balance between conservative care and surgical treatment is critical, because sciatica can be completely debilitating to individuals and can negatively affect the economy through a combination of hospital costs, work absenteeism, and disability.[6-8]

CASE PRESENTATION

A 29-year-old man had a 12-week history of progressively worsening lower back pain radiating down the lateral portion of his right leg into his foot. Complaints included an intermittent tingling sensation on the dorsal surface of his right foot. He reported no weakness, numbness, or change in bowel or bladder habits. The patient noted that the pain interfered with his job as a warehouse stocker, although he recalled no specific inciting event and had no history of trauma. He had tried both ibuprofen and tramadol for pain relief without success. He took no other medications. A complete review of symptoms yielded negative findings except for lower back pain rated 4 on a scale of 10 and right radicular leg pain rated 7 out of 10. The patient underwent a trial of physical therapy, which did not alleviate his pain.

- PMH: Hypertension and diabetes mellitus
- PSH: Unremarkable
- Exam: On neurologic examination, cranial nerves II through XII and cerebellar function were found to be intact. Results of the motor examination were 5/5 in bilateral upper and lower extremities, with very mild weakness of dorsiflexion on the right. His reflexes were normal. The patient had slightly decreased sensation to pinprick on the dorsum of his right foot; otherwise his sensation was intact. He was slightly tender to palpation of the lower lumbar spine and had a positive result on the straight leg raise test on the right. Gait was normal. No other abnormalities or deformities were noted.
- Imaging: Magnetic resonance imaging (MRI) of the lumbar spine showed a large lateral disk herniation at the level of L4-5 (Figures 5-2 and 5-3). After discussion of all the therapeutic options, the patient selected surgery.

The patient underwent a standard L4 hemilaminectomy with L4-5 microdiskectomy. The patient did well postoperatively and was discharged on postoperative day 1. The patient was seen in the clinic for follow-up 2 weeks later and was doing well, with significant improvement in his lower back pain and right radicular leg pain. He has had moderate improvement of his right foot paresthesia.

TREATMENT OPTIONS

Any effective treatment plan should focus on alleviating pain, ameliorating symptoms, and improving the quality of the patient's life. Since the natural history of sciatica secondary to disk herniation is favorable and typically self-limited, symptomatic therapy is usually used early on, with the goal of providing adequate pain relief while the underlying disease process resolves over time. The time it takes for symptoms to improve can vary, although most patients experience an improvement of leg pain within the first 7 to 10 days and a complete resolution of all symptoms within 8 weeks.[9-11] Some patients will continue to have severe or intolerable, progressive symptoms (pain, weakness, or numbness) after several weeks or months. Once a course of conservative care has failed, surgery becomes a good option to adequately address the abnormality and improve both pain and/or neurologic symptoms in most patients requiring surgery. Although multiple studies have shown that the long-term outcomes of nonsurgical treatment and surgical management are comparable, surgery consistently provides the most effective, immediate relief for many patients.[12-15]

FIGURE 5-1 Mechanism of radiculopathy secondary to disk herniation. The herniated disk is compressing the exiting nerve root.

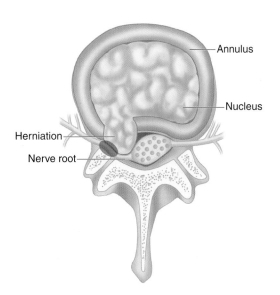

Annulus

Nucleus

Herniation

Nerve root

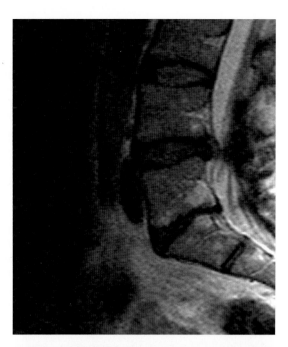

FIGURE 5-2 T2-weighted sagittal MRI scan showing L4-5 herniated disk.

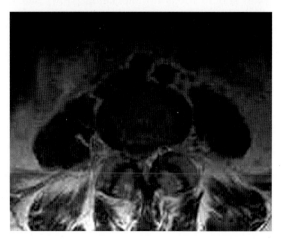

FIGURE 5-3 T2-weighted axial MRI scan showing right-sided herniated disk with nerve root compression.

Tips from the Masters 5-1 • Multiple randomized trials have shown that patients with lumbar disk herniation and persistent radiculopathy who choose surgery experience a substantial improvement in their symptoms sooner than do patients undergoing nonsurgical treatment.

Conservative Treatment

The mainstay of conservative care includes a short-term (4-week) trial of nonnarcotic analgesics, such as nonsteroidal antiinflammatory drugs (NSAIDs) or acetaminophen, in addition to activity modification. Although NSAIDs are the analgesic of choice for most patients, acetaminophen can be used in patients who cannot tolerate NSAIDs. Although these medications are universally used as the initial nonsurgical management of sciatica, evidence supporting their effectiveness in sciatica is lacking.[16-19]

Activity modification is a critical part of nonsurgical management, because it aims to minimize nerve root compression and avoid any activities that generate significant pain. Modification of activity does not equate to continual bed rest. As soon as acute symptoms lessen, which generally occurs within the first week, patients should resume modest physical activity, since multiple studies have shown that prolonged bed rest is of no benefit.[20] Many patients with persistent symptoms also try physical therapy even though there is insufficient evidence evaluating this treatment.[10] Additional studies are needed to assess the optimal timing and duration of visits, as well as the effectiveness of therapy in cases of lumbosacral radiculopathy. Given the favorable natural history of sciatica, it is currently recommended that physical therapy be delayed until symptoms have persisted for 3 weeks, since many patients will experience improvement on their own during this time.

Opioids and muscle relaxants are commonly used to treat patients with an acute radiculopathy when their pain is severe and insufficiently controlled by nonopioid analgesics. The use of opiates or muscle relaxants for acute radiculopathy is a matter of clinical judgment, due to the paucity of data regarding the efficacy of these medications. If prescribed, opioids should be used on a fixed schedule for a limited time and should not be combined with muscle relaxants due to the additive sedating effects. Systemic and epidural glucocorticoids are also treatment options for patients with persistent severe radicular pain refractory to NSAIDs, acetaminophen, and activity modification. The most recent American Pain Society[21] practice guidelines concluded that systemic glucocorticoids are an ineffective treatment for low back pain with sciatica, whereas epidural steroid injections are moderately effective as a short-term treatment for persistent lumbosacral radiculopathy secondary to lumbar disk herniation, but are not indicated for use during the acute phase.

Although further randomized studies will be required to effectively evaluate all of the nonsurgical treatment options discussed here, the benign natural history of sciatica will continue to make accurate data collection and interpretation extremely difficult in future trials. Unfortunately, other confounders, such as the placebo effect and patient social issues, also interfere with study designs and subsequent result analysis, further hindering the selection of the most effective treatments for sciatica. Thus, it is critical to determine the optimal length of time that conservative management should be offered before surgery is considered.

Surgical Treatment

The main goal of surgery for symptomatic lumbar disk herniation is to alleviate unremitting radicular pain and/or persistent neurologic deficit caused by compression of lumbosacral nerve roots. This is done by removing either a portion of, or the entire, herniated disk. Although severe, progressive neurologic decline is an indication for urgent evaluation and potentially emergent surgical intervention, this is not commonly caused by a herniated lumbar disk. The most common indication for diskectomy is persistent or worsening radicular leg pain, but it is critical that the distribution of the radicular pain correspond to the nerve root compression seen on preoperative imaging for the operation to have the best outcome. Neurologic signs (slight weakness and/or pain on straight leg raise) are often more confirmatory of the level than the reason, per se, for surgery. Although lumbar microdiskectomy is a very successful procedure that relieves radicular leg pain in 85% to 90% of appropriately selected patients,[22-25] the adequacy of relief of back pain after surgery is unpredictable.[26,27] The importance of proper patient selection cannot be overemphasized, because complications and poor outcomes can arise when patients are not chosen carefully.[28]

Early referral for surgery does not improve outcomes in patients with lumbar disk herniation and radiculopathy who do not have severe or progressive motor weakness, or symptoms of cauda equina syndrome. Referral for surgery should be an elective option for patients with persistent disabling symptoms after at least 4 to 6 weeks of standard nonsurgical management. Multiple studies have shown that these patients have a more favorable outcome after microdiskectomy than nonsurgically treated patients at short-term follow-up, but outcomes are equivalent at 1 to 2 years.[12-15] The American Pain Society[21] treatment guidelines currently recommend that physicians consider surgery in patients who have both persistent, disabling radiculopathy and a corresponding herniated lumbar disk on imaging. These patients generally experience a moderate improvement almost immediately after surgery, even though their total overall improvement at 1 to 2 years may be equivalent to that of patients managed conservatively.

Tips from the Masters 5-2 • Surgery provides effective short-term relief in these patients, but this benefit lessens over time because both surgical and nonsurgical groups eventually report similar overall improvements.

There is no clear correlation between the size of the herniated disk or nerve compression and the amount of pain or nerve root injury. In fact, small compressive lesions can produce extensive, irreversible nerve damage if they affect the nerve's arterial blood supply. Unfortunately, these ischemic nerve roots are not likely to improve after the compressive lesion is removed during surgery. Overall, microdiskectomy continues to be a reasonable option for patients with incessant disabling radicular symptoms lasting 4 to 6 weeks who are good surgical candidates and desire surgery.

Lumbar Diskectomy

A variety of diskectomy techniques are currently used by orthopedic and neurologic surgeons. The procedure chosen is typically based on the surgeon's preference and experience. The conventional open diskectomy involves use of a standard surgical incision to obtain adequate visualization and illumination, then frequently performance of a hemilaminotomy to relieve pressure on the nerve roots and visualize the protruded disk, followed by a diskectomy to remove the herniated nuclear disk material. Microdiskectomy, the most common diskectomy procedure, is a modification of the open diskectomy technique that can be performed on an outpatient basis. A smaller incision is made in the back, visualization through loupes or an operating microscope is required, and a hemilaminectomy is performed with removal of the disk fragment compressing the affected nerve roots (Figures 5-4 through 5-6).

Tips from the Masters 5-3 • Results appear to be equivalent for minimally invasive surgery and open microdiskectomy. The results of laser diskectomy are not compelling.

Minimally invasive techniques use very small incisions, so indirect visualization techniques are required to help perform the diskectomy. Multiple minimally invasive options exist and include tubular diskectomy, laser diskectomy, percutaneous manual nucleotomy, automated percutaneous lumbar diskectomy, endoscopic diskectomy, and coblation nucleoplasty[29] (see Figure 5-6). It is thought that use of these techniques could potentially lead to quicker recovery after surgery than with open or microdiskectomy techniques, but this potential advantage has not been supported in randomized controlled trials. Overall, major postoperative complications are rare after any of the diskectomy procedures,[13,15] and outcomes are the same for patients undergoing microdiskectomy and minimally invasive diskectomy.

FUNDAMENTAL TECHNIQUE

Anatomic landmarks and/or preincision needle localization films can be used to determine the correct site of exposure. Once local anesthetic is injected, make the skin incision with a No. 10 blade. Subcutaneous dissection is achieved with bovie electrocautery down to the thoracolumbar fascia. Then make a midline or paramedial facial incision. Subperiosteal dissection can be performed quickly using electrocautery or a large periosteal elevator, although the latter tends to create more bleeding and thus is not commonly used. A localizing film should be done at this point to assess the correct level. Once verified, begin the hemilaminectomy by finding the soft interspace between the laminaes of interest. Thin out the lamina cortical bone down to cancellous bone. Complete the laminectomy with Kerrison rongeurs and an up-going curette. To identify the thecal sac, insert a sharp right-angled instrument into the ligamentus flavum and use it to pull up dorsally from the thecal sac while cutting along the instrument with a No. 15 blade. Carefully continue the dissection until the thecal sac is seen. Then remove the ligamentum flavum with a rongeur to create the largest working area possible.

Once an adequate working window is obtained, explore the epidural space and identify the nerve root. The nerve root may be displaced medially or laterally depending on the size and location of the disk herniation, but it is imperative that

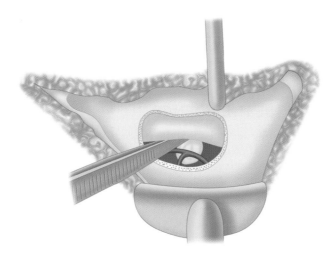

FIGURE 5-4 Extruded fragment is visible beneath the epidural vein at the level of the interspace.

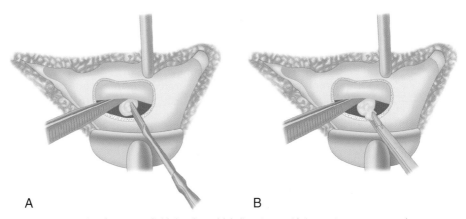

A   B

FIGURE 5-5 Dissection from a medial (**A**) to lateral (**B**) direction avoids increasing pressure on the nerve root.

FIGURE 5-6 Endoscopic view of the nerve root.

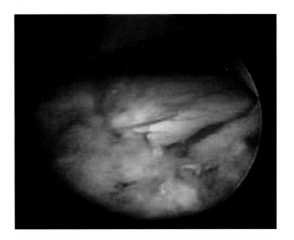

it is identified prior to removing any portion of the disk. Epidural veins should be individually coagulated with bipolar cautery on a low setting. Avoid excessive use of cautery in the epidural space. Using a nerve root retractor, gently retract the nerve root medially. This will expose the underlying disk herniation. Remove any free fragments of disk material if present. Then incise the posterior longitudinal ligament and annulus with a No. 11 blade. Disk material will often extrude spontaneously. Use a pituitary rongeur to remove this disk material. Push any paracentral disk material down into the now decompressed disk space with a curette. Copiously irrigate and control any sources of bleeding prior to closure. Ensure a watertight, dry closure using a layer of 0-size interrupted sutures. Superficial fascial closure can be done with 2-0 inverted, interrupted sutures. Skin closures vary and are based on the surgeon's preference.

DISCUSSION OF BEST EVIDENCE

It is universally accepted that the majority of patients with sciatica will improve within 8 weeks of symptom onset with conservative management alone.[9-11] The issue currently under debate is what to do for the small percentage of patients who have unremitting symptoms after this time. Multiple, **prospective, randomized trials** have shown that patients with lumbar disk herniation and persistent radiculopathy who choose surgery experience a substantial improvement in their symptoms in a shorter amount of time compared with patients undergoing nonsurgical treatment.[12-15,30] It should be noted that similar improvements are seen in surgical patients regardless of whether a standard open diskectomy or a microdiskectomy is performed.[31-34]

Surgery provides effective short-term relief in these patients, but this benefit lessens over time because both surgical and nonsurgical groups eventually report similar overall improvements. The time it takes the conservative treatment group to catch up with the surgically treated group with regard to overall symptom relief and outcome varies slightly across studies.[12-15,30] The Spine Patient Outcomes Research Trial (SPORT) assessing therapeutic options for lumbar disk prolapse with radiculopathy found that surgical treatment does not provide any additional pain relief or improvement in function compared with nonsurgical treatment after 3 months.[15] These findings are supported by the results of two other **randomized prospective studies** that compare the outcomes of early microdiskectomy, specifically, with nonoperative treatment in patients with lumbar disk herniation and radiculopathy.[12-14] A cost-utility analysis performed in conjunction with the larger of these two trials found that early microdiskectomy is cost effective from a societal viewpoint, since the actual costs of this surgery are less than those of nonoperative management once savings gained by early patient productivity have been factored into the equation.[14,35] This study also found that patients undergoing early microdiskectomy have increased quality-adjusted life years compared with those in the nonoperative group.[35]

Important limitations must be considered when analyzing the data from these randomized trials. One key factor is that these studies are not blinded, since sham procedures are not performed on the nonsurgical group. Therefore, patients know which treatment group they belong to and thus could develop personal expectations of outcomes that could alter the results of a study. Another potential confounder is the significant crossover that occurs between treatment conditions, with up to half of the patients assigned to nonsurgical management eventually undergoing surgery, and vice versa.[12-15,30] This makes the long-term outcomes of these two therapeutic interventions difficult to evaluate and could result in an underestimation of the benefits that surgical treatment may provide.

Although outcomes data are available for open diskectomy and microdiskectomy, evidence supporting the effectiveness of surgery using minimally invasive techniques in cases of lumbar disk herniation with persistent radiculopathy is lacking. Of the randomized controlled studies that do currently exist, most have focused on comparing percutaneous tubular diskectomy with standard microdiskectomy.[36-38] Only one of these percutaneous tubular diskectomy trials had a double-blind design; it is also the largest and most recently published of all of the studies.[36] In contrast to the findings of previous studies, the results of this **randomized prospective trial** did not show that patients undergoing tubular diskectomy recovered faster than those undergoing conventional microdiskectomy. It did find that improvement in both leg and back pain was slightly better in the microdiskectomy group than in the tubular diskectomy group, as were 1-year disability scores.[36] There are a few small studies evaluating other minimally invasive techniques, such as automated percutaneous diskectomy,[39] percutaneous manual nucleotomy,[40] and endoscopic diskectomy,[41] but these studies are insufficient. Currently no research trial has been conducted to evaluate laser diskectomy, coblation nucleoplasty, or other minimally invasive techniques compared with open diskectomy, microdiskectomy, or nonsurgical therapy. Until more data are available to suggest a significant benefit to using any of these minimally invasive techniques, it is recommended that either microdiskectomy or open diskectomy be performed on patients with sciatica secondary to lumbar disk prolapse who are appropriate surgical candidates.

COMMENTARY

Lumbar radiculopathy remains one of the most common and most challenging causes of disability in the Western world. It often presents a management dilemma to the treating spine physician as well. It is clear that most cases of lumbar radiculopathy due to herniated disk will resolve spontaneously or with nonsurgical treatment, but some cases will require surgical intervention. Although the science has become straightforward, the art of managing this clinical problem remains elusive.

When surgical intervention is required, with the patient experiencing either neurologic deficit or intractable pain, surgical results are often predictable, whether the procedure is done in an open operation or through a minimally invasive approach. At this point it appears that the results are equivalent for minimally invasive surgery and open microdiskectomy. The results of laser diskectomy are not compelling.

There is currently no evidence in the literature that one surgical procedure is better than another for resection of a herniated lumbar disk. It is not clear that a randomized trial will be able to sort out this issue, because both procedures have good outcomes and are associated with minimal complications. The good news for patients affected by this problem is that there is often a solution, either surgical or nonsurgical.

ACKNOWLEDGMENT

The authors are grateful to Karen K. Anderson, BS, for her assistance with manuscript preparation.

REFERENCES

1. Cherkin DC, Deyo RA, Loeser JD, et al: An international comparison of back surgery rates, *Spine* 19(11):1201–1206, 1994.
2. Tarlov E, D'Costa D: *Back attack*, ed 1, Boston, 1985, Little, Brown.
3. Ehni G: Effects of certain degenerative diseases of the spine, especially spondylosis and disk protrusion, on the neural contents, particularly in the lumbar region. Historical account, *Mayo Clin Proc* 50(6):327–338, 1975.
4. Mixter WJ, Barr JS: Rupture of intervertebral disc with involvement of the spinal canal, *N Engl J Med* 211:210–215, 1934.
5. Dandy WE: Loose cartilage from intervertebral disc simulating tumor of the spinal cord, *Arch Surg* 19:660–672, 1929.
6. Luijsterburg PA, Verhagen AP, Braak S, et al: Do neurosurgeons subscribe to the guideline lumbosacral radicular syndrome? *Clin Neurol Neurosurg* 106(4):313–317, 2004.
7. Vader JP, Porchet F, Larequi-Lauber T, et al: Appropriateness of surgery for sciatica: reliability of guidelines from expert panels, *Spine* 25(14):1831–1836, 2000.
8. van Tulder MW, Koes BW, Bouter LM: A cost-of-illness study of back pain in the Netherlands, *Pain* 62(2):233–240, 1995.
9. Vroomen PC, de Krom MC, Wilmink JT, et al: Lack of effectiveness of bed rest for sciatica, *N Engl J Med* 340(6):418–423, 1999.
10. Hofstee DJ, Gijtenbeek JM, Hoogland PH, et al: Westeinde sciatica trial: randomized controlled study of bed rest and physiotherapy for acute sciatica, *J Neurosurg* 96(Suppl 1):45–49, 2002.
11. Awad JN, Moskovich R: Lumbar disc herniations: surgical versus nonsurgical treatment, *Clin Orthop Relat Res* 443:183–197, 2006.
12. Osterman H, Seitsalo S, Karppinen J, et al: Effectiveness of microdiscectomy for lumbar disc herniation: a randomized controlled trial with 2 years of follow-up, *Spine* 31(21):2409–2414, 2006.
13. Peul WC, van Houwelingen HC, van den Hout WB, et al: Leiden-The Hague Spine Intervention Prognostic Study Group: Surgery versus prolonged conservative treatment for sciatica, *N Engl J Med* 356(22):2245–2256, 2007. **The results of this high-quality study comparing early microdiskectomy with nonoperative management showed that patients undergoing early surgery had quicker relief of pain and faster rates of perceived recovery, even though overall 1-year outcomes were comparable in the two treatment groups.**

14. Peul WC, van den Hout WB, Brand R, et al: Leiden-The Hague Spine Intervention Prognostic Study Group: Prolonged conservative care versus early surgery in patients with sciatica caused by lumbar disc herniation: two year results of a randomised controlled trial, *BMJ* 336(7657):1355–1358, 2008.

15. Weinstein JN, Tosteson TD, Lurie JD, et al: Surgical vs nonoperative treatment for lumbar disk herniation: the Spine Patient Outcomes Research Trial (SPORT): a randomized trial, *JAMA* 296(20): 2441–2450, 2006. **This multicenter randomized controlled trial found no difference between surgery, either open diskectomy or microdiskectomy, and nonsurgical treatment with regard to pain relief and functional improvement after 3 months. Study findings are complicated by high rates of patient crossover between treatment groups, which may potentially underestimate the long-term benefits of surgery.**

16. Weber H, Holme I, Amlie E: The natural course of acute sciatica with nerve root symptoms in a double-blind placebo-controlled trial evaluating the effect of piroxicam, *Spine* 18(11):1433–1438, 1993.

17. Dreiser RL, Le Parc JM, Vélicitat P, et al: Oral meloxicam is effective in acute sciatica: two randomised, double-blind trials versus placebo or diclofenac, *Inflamm Res* 50(Suppl 1):S17–S23, 2001.

18. Goldie I: A clinical trial with indomethacin (Indomee®) in low back pain and sciatica, *Acta Orthop Scand* 39(1):117–128, 1968.

19. Roelofs PD, Deyo RA, Koes BW, et al: Non-steroidal anti-inflammatory drugs for low back pain, *Cochrane Database Syst Rev* (1), 2008:CD000396.

20. Hagen KB, Hilde G, Jamtvedt G, et al: Bed rest for acute low-back pain and sciatica, *Cochrane Database Syst Rev* (4), 2004:CD001254.

21. Chou R, Loeser JD, Owens DK, et al: American Pain Society Low Back Pain Guideline Panel: Interventional therapies, surgery, and interdisciplinary rehabilitation for low back pain: an evidence-based clinical practice guideline from the American Pain Society, *Spine* 34(10):1066–1077, 2009.

22. Ehni BL, Benzel EC, Biscup RS: Lumbar discectomy. In Benzel EC, editor: *Spine surgery*, ed 2, Philadelphia, 2005, Churchill Livingstone, pp 601–618.

23. Daneyemez M, Sali A, Kahraman S, et al: Outcome analyses in 1072 surgically treated lumbar disc herniations, *Minim Invasive Neurosurg* 42(2):63–68, 1999.

24. Davis RA: A long-term outcome analysis of 984 surgically treated herniated lumbar discs, *J Neurosurg* 80(3):415–421, 1994.

25. McCulloch JA: Focus issue on lumbar disc herniation: macro- and microdiscectomy, *Spine* 21(Suppl 24):45S–56S, 1996.

26. Weber H: The natural history of disc herniation and the influence of intervention, *Spine* 19(19): 2234–2238, 1994.

27. Yorimitsu E, Chiba K, Toyama Y, et al: Long-term outcomes of standard discectomy for lumbar disc herniation: a follow-up study of more than 10 years, *Spine* 26(6):652–657, 2001.

28. Tarlov EC, Magge SN: Microsurgery of ruptured lumbar intervertebral disc. In Schmidek HH, Roberts DW, editors: *Schmidek and Sweet operative neurosurgical techniques: indications, methods, and results*, ed 5, Philadelphia, 2006, Saunders, pp 2055–2071.

29. Maroon JC: Current concepts in minimally invasive discectomy, *Neurosurgery* 51(Suppl 5):S137–S145, 2002.

30. Weber H: Lumbar disc herniation. A controlled, prospective study with ten years of observation, *Spine* 8(2):131–140, 1983. **This early study comparing standard open diskectomy with nonsurgical therapy concluded that patient outcomes were better 1 year out in the surgical treatment group, but this difference in outcome was no longer present after 4 years.**

31. Henriksen L, Schmidt K, Eskesen V, et al: A controlled study of microsurgical versus standard lumbar discectomy, *Br J Neurosurg* 10(3):289–293, 1996.

32. Lagarrigue J, Chaynes P: Comparative study of disk surgery with or without microscopy. A prospective study of 80 cases, *Neurochirurgie* 40(2):116–120, 1994.

33. Katayama Y, Matsuyama Y, Yoshihara H, et al: Comparison of surgical outcomes between macro discectomy and micro discectomy for lumbar disc herniation: a prospective randomized study with surgery performed by the same spine surgeon, *J Spinal Disord Tech* 19(5):344–347, 2006.

34. Tullberg T, Isacson J, Weidenhielm L: Does microscopic removal of lumbar disc herniation lead to better results than the standard procedure? Results of a one-year randomized study, *Spine* 18(1): 24–27, 1993.

35. van den Hout WB, Peul WC, Koes BW, et al: Leiden-The Hague Spine Intervention Prognostic Study Group: Prolonged conservative care versus early surgery in patients with sciatica from lumbar disc herniation: cost utility analysis alongside a randomised controlled trial, *BMJ* 336(7657):1351–1354, 2008.

36. Arts MP, Brand R, van den Akker ME, et al: Leiden-The Hague Spine Intervention Prognostic Study Group (SIPS): Tubular diskectomy vs conventional microdiskectomy for sciatica: a randomized controlled trial, *JAMA* 302(2):149–158, 2009.

37. Righesso O, Falavigna A, Avanzi O: Comparison of open discectomy with microendoscopic discectomy in lumbar disc herniations: results of a randomized controlled trial, *Neurosurgery* 61(3):545–549, 2007.

38. Ryang YM, Oertel MF, Mayfrank L, et al: Standard open microdiscectomy versus minimal access trocar microdiscectomy: results of a prospective randomized study, *Neurosurgery* 62(1):174–181, 2008.

39. Chatterjee S, Foy PM, Findlay GF: Report of a controlled clinical trial comparing automated percutaneous lumbar discectomy and microdiscectomy in the treatment of contained lumbar disc herniation, *Spine* 20(6):734–738, 1995.

40. Mayer HM, Brock M: Percutaneous endoscopic discectomy: surgical technique and preliminary results compared to microsurgical discectomy, *J Neurosurg* 78(2):216–225, 1993.

41. Ruetten S, Komp M, Merk H, et al: Full-endoscopic interlaminar and transforaminal lumbar discectomy versus conventional microsurgical technique: a prospective, randomized, controlled study, *Spine* 33(9):931–939, 2008.

Chapter 6

Cervical Spondylosis–Spinal Stenosis: Laminoplasty Versus Laminectomy and Fusion

Yu-Po Lee, Niraj Patel, Steven R. Garfin

Cervical spondylosis is a common cause of hospital admission and is the most frequent cause of spinal cord dysfunction in patients older than 55 years. Chronic degenerative changes of the cervical spine result in stenosis of the spinal canal and foramina, leading to cervical spondylotic myelopathy (CSM) and radiculopathy. Conservative treatments for this condition include neck immobilization, mechanical traction, and physical therapy. Surgical management is recommended for patients with neurologic (radicular) symptoms and/or signs or documented compression of the cervical nerve root or spinal cord.

Various surgical options are available through an anterior or posterior approach to the cervical spine. The optimal surgical method can vary depending on the patient's lesion, curvature of the cervical spine, and comorbid conditions, and on surgeon preference. This chapter reviews two commonly used surgical options for the treatment of cervical spondylosis that use a posterior approach: laminoplasty and laminectomy. Although various studies have compared these two methods, their findings have not led to a definitive conclusion regarding the superiority of one technique over the other. This chapter presents a classic case of cervical myelopathy, describes the surgical technique that was used, and reviews the key literature comparing the advantages and disadvantages of these two techniques.

CASE PRESENTATION

A 71-year-old woman had complaints of neck and bilateral arm pain. The patient reported that she had started experiencing numbness and tingling in both of her hands approximately 1 month earlier.

- PMH: Unremarkable
- PSH: Unremarkable
- Exam: Motor examination of the upper extremities yielded a score of 5/5 except that right wrist flexion, interosseus muscle strength, and hand grasp were diminished. Deep tendon reflexes (brachial, brachioradialis, and triceps) were 2+ and symmetric. The Hoffmann sign was positive bilaterally. Clonus and Babinski reflexes were absent and knee reflexes were 3+ and symmetric. Ankle reflexes were 2+ and symmetric.
- Imaging: Cervical spine radiographs revealed multilevel cervical disk degeneration. No instability or spondylolisthesis was noted on flexion and extension views (Figure 6-1). Review of magnetic resonance imaging (MRI) scans revealed multilevel cervical stenosis from C3 to C7. The patient had cord signal changes in the midcervical spine (myelomalacia) (Figure 6-2). In this patient, an open door laminoplasty with fibula was elected. Postoperative radiographs after C3-C7 laminoplasty showed maintenance of cervical lordosis (Figure 6-3).

SURGICAL OPTIONS

A variety of surgical options are available for the treatment of CSM and radiculopathy associated with cervical spondylosis. Ultimately, the goal of any surgical method is to alleviate pain, decompress the spinal cord and nerve roots, maintain the alignment of the cervical spine as much as possible, and stabilize if necessary.

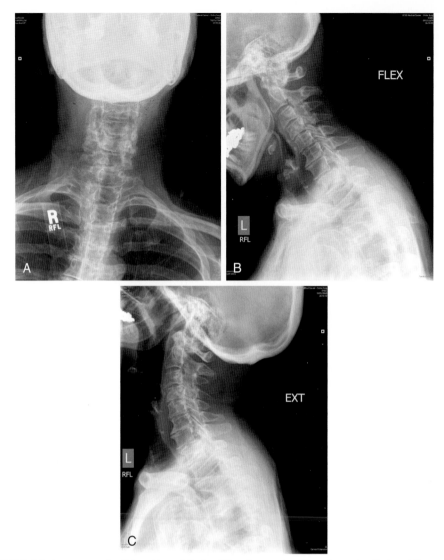

FIGURE 6-1 Anteroposterior (**A**) and lateral flexion (**B**) and extension (**C**) radiographs. No instability or spondylolisthesis is noted.

Anterior approaches to the cervical spine are generally preferred in patients who have cervical myelopathy from either a soft disk herniation or spondylotic degeneration that is limited to the disk level, or who have a kyphotic deformity of the cervical spine.[1,2] Methods include anterior cervical diskectomy and fusion, and corpectomy plus strut-cage fusion, typically with the use of anterior instrumentation. Anterior decompression and fusion have been shown to be highly successful in alleviating radicular pain and improving neurologic function in these cases.[1,2]

Patients who have contraindications to anterior cervical approaches (such as some patients with ossification of the posterior longitudinal ligament [OPLL] with dural penetration) and those with a spinal cord lesion that is diffuse or more dorsal due to buckling of the ligamentum flavum are often treated using posterior procedures.[2] Patients with preserved cervical lordosis are appropriate candidates for a posterior approach. Posterior decompression, however, can result in inadequate decompression or increased postoperative deformity in patients with cervical kyphosis.[3,4] Children are at particularly high risk for developing postlaminectomy kyphosis.[5]

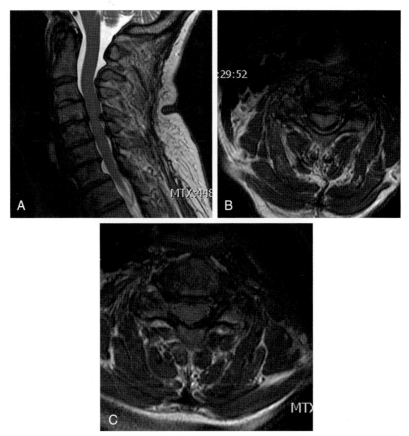

FIGURE 6-2 Magnetic resonance imaging scans of the cervical spine showing severe stenosis with myelomalacia.

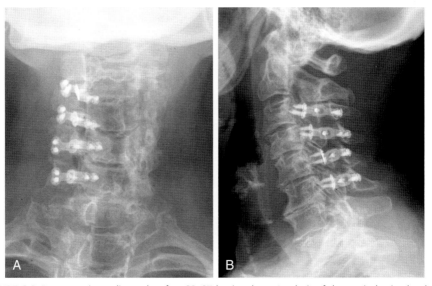

FIGURE 6-3 Postoperative radiographs after C3-C7 laminoplasty. Lordosis of the cervical spine has been maintained.

Laminectomy

Laminectomy was the first procedure developed to treat CSM.[6] Laminectomy is effective in the treatment of multilevel cervical spondylosis, OPLL, and other pathologic conditions causing cervical stenosis.[7,8] A partial facetectomy is performed with this procedure and can contribute to postoperative cervical instability and deformity.

Posterior fixation is often combined with laminectomy because it has been shown to prevent or treat instability associated with multilevel laminectomy.[9,10] In cadaver models laminectomy has been shown to significantly increase spinal cord flexibility and lead to instability.[11] This instability can have various long-term consequences, including spinal cord microtrauma. This can result in neurologic sequelae and a tendency to develop kyphosis. To maintain alignment and restore the stability that is disrupted by decompression with laminectomy and partial facetectomy, posterior instrumented fusion is often added. Although fusion slightly increases the morbidity associated with the laminectomy procedure, stabilization of the spine can arrest the progression of spondylosis and potential deformity at the affected levels.

Perez-Lopez and associates[12] compared results for 19 patients treated with laminectomy with results for 17 patients treated with laminectomy and fusion for cervical myelopathy. Similar clinical outcomes were noted in both groups as judged by Nurick scores. There was a greater increase in postoperative kyphosis in those treated with laminectomy (24%) than in those undergoing laminectomy with fusion (7%), which suggests that fusion prevents postoperative instability. The potential advantages of fusion are not certain. Hamanishi and Tanaka[13] compared outcomes for 35 patients who were treated with laminectomy and 34 patients who underwent laminectomy and fusion and noted few differences between the two groups. Clinical outcomes as judged from improvement in Japanese Orthopaedic Association (JOA) scale scores were similar in both groups (scores improved by 51% in both groups) after a mean follow-up of over 3 years. Kyphotic malalignment occurred in 17% of patients in the nonfusion group and 12% of those in the fusion group. Radiographic instability occurred in two patients who did not undergo fusion and in two patients who did.[13] However, any conclusions regarding the differences between fusion and nonfusion groups in this study are limited, because fusion was performed only in patients who were determined to have instability before surgery. Thus, the study had an inherent selection bias that steered patients whose condition was more stable toward nonfusion and those with greater instability toward fusion.

Various methods of posterior instrumented fusion have been used successfully to stabilize and fuse the spine. In the past when the posterior elements were absent, such as after a laminectomy, facet wiring with bone grafting was used as an effective method to stabilize the cervical spine.[14] Facet wiring requires removing cartilage from the facet joint, drilling a hole through the inferior facet joint through which to pass a braided titanium cable, and adding an autologous bone graft. Currently lateral mass screws are routinely used and, compared with traditional wiring techniques, provide more immediate, rigid stability and thereby promote fusion.[15,16] Cervical pedicle screws have been shown to provide better fixation and stability than lateral mass screws.[17,18] Preoperative computed tomography (CT) is recommended to help view the three-dimensional anatomy necessary for accurate pedicle screw placement. However, the use of instrumentation to stabilize the cervical spine after laminectomy increases the frequency of neurologic and vascular injury.[14-18] Thus, the benefits of improved stability with posterior instrumented fusion must be weighed against the higher risk of neurologic and/or vascular injury.

Laminoplasty

Because of the potential complications of laminectomy and posterior instrumented fusion, laminoplasty was developed in Japan in the 1970s. Various techniques for laminoplasty have been devised, but they all involve preservation of the lamina and decompression of the spinal cord by partially or completely freeing the lamina and positioning it more posteriorly. It was thought that laminoplasty would reduce the number of complications associated with postoperative spinal instability and deformity because it preserves the posterior elements of the cervical spine.

A Z-plasty laminoplasty technique was first described by Oyama.[19] In this procedure the spinous process is removed and the laminae are thinned out to the facet joint. A "Z" shaped incision is made into the thin laminae, along with lateral troughs on both sides. Thinning the laminae allows them to be manipulated and separated to expand the spinal canal. The manipulated segments of lamina are held in place with sutures or wire material (Figure 6-4).

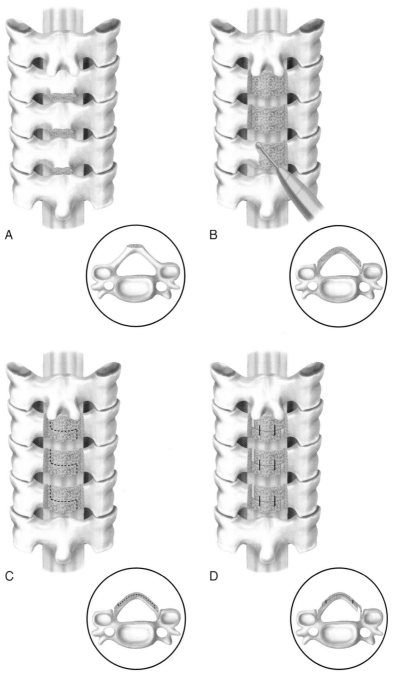

FIGURE 6-4 Original Z-plasty laminoplasty technique. The spinous processes are removed (**A**) and the laminae are then thinned (**B**). Troughs are drilled laterally (**C**). Finally, a Z-shaped cut is made between the adjacent thinned laminae (**D**). Here, the laminae are secured in an open position using sutures.

The expansive open-door laminoplasty was described by Hirayabashi and colleagues.[20] A high-speed drill is used to drill down to the ligamentum flavum on one side of the lamina that has been exposed. The facet capsules should be left intact. A trough is created on the contralateral side at the same location. Unlike on the open side, the ligamentum flavum is not reached and a thin section of the lamina anterior cortex is left intact on this side. The lamina on the open side is carefully pulled away from the spinal cord. Distraction of the lamina posteriorly expands the spinal canal. The lamina can be maintained in a more posterior position with the assistance of sutures, titanium miniplates, or small bone graft struts (Figure 6-5).[21] Herkowitz[22] combined this procedure with a unilateral foraminotomy on the open side of the laminoplasty and noted improvements in 90% of patients with cervical radiculopathy. Several variations of the open-door laminoplasty rely on instrumentation for internal fixation of the mobilized laminae (Figure 6-6). Shaffrey and associates[23] described the use of bone graft with titanium miniplates to hold the lamina in place. Gillett and colleagues[24] described a device called a *CG clip* that serves as a spacer and an attachment unit to provide stabilization of the open laminae without the need for bone grafting.

The French door laminoplasty or double-door laminoplasty was described by Kurokawa and co-workers.[25] Troughs are created bilaterally just medial to the facet joints, and the spinous process is split at the midline using a thread wire saw (T-saw) or high-speed drill. The spinous process is thus split in half and the laminae are spread apart through the midline. The laminae are held in a more posterior position with sutures attaching them to the facet capsules and wiring or ceramic spacers placed between the split spinous process (Figure 6-7).[26] In a modification of this procedure, bone graft can be harvested from the spinous process and placed as a spacer. No clear advantage over the open-door technique has been shown with this procedure, but it has been proposed that splitting at the midline allows for a more symmetric decompression of the spine.

Laminoplasty has become an increasingly popular technique for treating cervical spondylosis. As with laminectomy, several concerns and complications have been noted with this technique. Persistent axial neck pain, C5 paresis, and reduced range of motion have been reported.[27-34] Hosono and colleagues[28] observed a 60% prevalence of postoperative axial symptoms in a group of 72 patients treated for CSM. Takemitsu and associates[29] reported a 14% rate of C5 palsy in 73 patients treated with laminoplasty for CSM. The rate was much higher in the 10 patients in whom laminoplasty was combined with posterior instrumentation to treat instability and kyphosis (50% rate of C5 palsy). Tanaka and colleagues[30] noted transient C5 nerve palsy in 3 of 62 patients treated with laminoplasty despite intraoperative spinal cord monitoring with transcranial motor evoked potentials. Several studies have confirmed that laminoplasty is associated with reduced postoperative cervical range of motion. Chiba and co-workers[33] followed 80 patients who underwent open-door laminoplasty for CSM or OPLL for an average of 14 years and noted a 36% reduction in cervical range of motion. Kawaguchi and colleagues[34] followed 126 patients for longer than 10 years after laminoplasty for CSM. Range of motion decreased to 25% of preoperative range of motion. Although dural lacerations are more commonly associated with laminectomy, they have also been documented with double-door laminoplasty. Dickerman and associates[35] noted delayed dural lacerations due to dislodgment of hydroxyapatite spacers in 4 of 130 patients treated with this procedure for CSM.

Skip Laminectomy

Axial neck and shoulder pain, restriction of cervical range of motion, and the reduction of cervical lordosis have been the significant postoperative problems noted with laminoplasties of the cervical spine. To minimize the damage to the posterior musculature, skip laminectomy was developed. In this procedure, a standard laminectomy at the affected levels is combined with a partial laminectomy of the cephalad half of the laminae at other levels, at which the muscular attachments to the spinous processes are left undisturbed. This technique was first described by Shiraishi[36] in 2002.

The initial results of skip laminectomy have been very encouraging. In 2003, Shiraishi and associates[37] published a retrospective review comparing skip laminectomy with open-door laminoplasty. The authors noted increased axial neck pain in 66% of the patients undergoing laminoplasty, whereas only one patient (2%) in the skip laminectomy group developed axial neck pain. The patients in

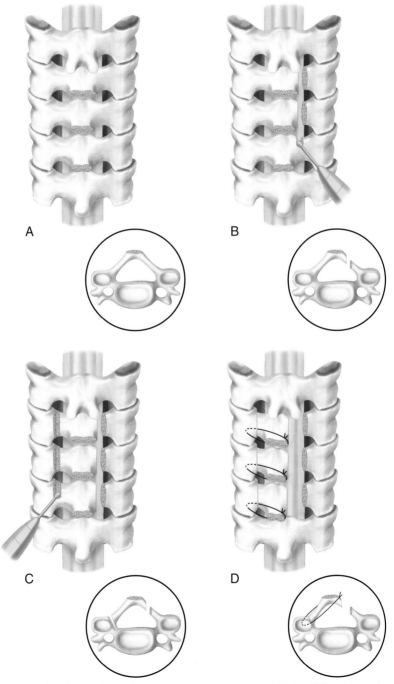

FIGURE 6-5 Open-door laminoplasty. The spinous processes are removed (**A**) and bilateral troughs created at the facet-lamina junctions (**B**). A thin rim of bone is left on one side (**C**). The laminae are elevated and, in this modification, secured to the facet using sutures (**D**).

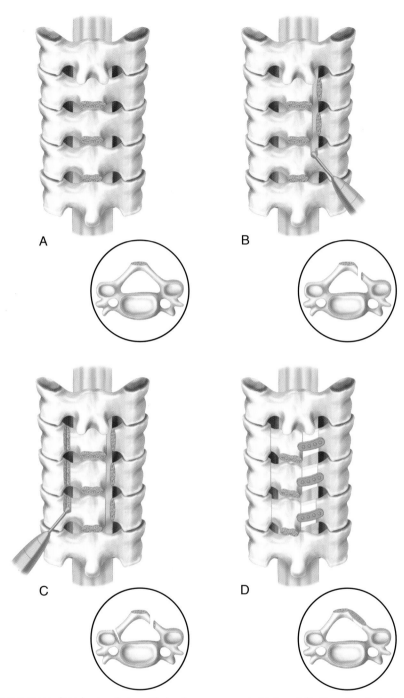

FIGURE 6-6 Open-door laminoplasty with hardware-augmented internal fixation. The techniques are similar to those in the Hirabayashi-type laminoplasty. The spinous processes are removed (**A**) and bilateral troughs created at the facet-lamina junctions (**B**). A thin rim of bone is left on one side (**C**). In the final step, as described by Shaffrey and colleagues,[23] titanium miniplates are placed to secure the elevated laminae and hold the bone graft in place (**D**).

the skip laminectomy group maintained 98% of their range of motion, whereas the patients in the laminoplasty group maintained only 61% of their range of motion.

In another study by Yukawa and associates[38], the authors conducted a prospective, randomized trial comparing laminoplasty and skip laminectomy. Forty-one patients with CSM were randomly assigned to undergo either a laminoplasty (n = 21) or skip laminectomy (n = 20) and were followed for longer than 1 year

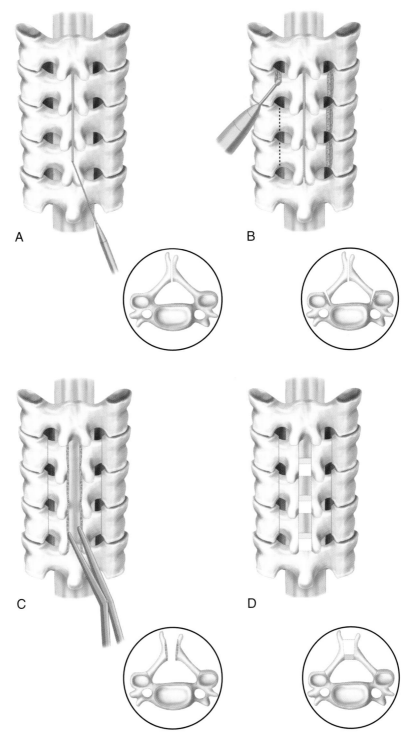

FIGURE 6-7 French door (double-door) laminoplasty. **A,** The spinous processes are split using a high-speed drill or T-saw. **B,** Troughs are drilled into the lateral aspects of the laminae and medial facets. **C,** The spinous processes are split in the midline. **D,** Wiring, bone graft, or ceramic material is used as a spacer.

(average, 28.1 months). No significant differences were seen between groups in operative invasiveness, axial neck pain, cervical alignment, or range of motion.

Hence, skip laminectomy has shown some promise, but more studies with longer follow-up are necessary before its efficacy relative to conventional laminectomy or laminoplasty can be determined.

FUNDAMENTAL TECHNIQUE

Multilevel cervical myelopathy may be effectively treated with laminoplasty in patients who have maintained a neutral or lordotic alignment in their cervical spine. Typically, laminoplasty is performed from C3 to C7. One full level above and below the area of compression is included in the laminoplasty to ensure a full decompression of the cervical spine. If necessary, a dome laminectomy or undercutting of the C2 lamina may be performed if the C2-3 level is affected. T1 may also be included in the laminoplasty caudally if the C7-T1 level is stenotic. The levels to include in the laminoplasty are determined by the patient's symptoms, radiographs, and magnetic resonance imaging (MRI) scans. Radiographs are important because the alignment of the cervical spine should be neutral or lordotic (Tips from the Masters 6-1). Also, any segmental instability should be noted because this might indicate the need to fuse one or more segments. MRI scans are valuable because they provide guidance on which levels need to be decompressed. As mentioned previously, one full level cephalad and caudal to the areas of compression are included in the laminoplasty to ensure adequate decompression. If MRI is not possible, a CT myelogram may be used to identify the areas of stenosis.

Tips from the Masters 6-1 • If the patient has a kyphotic alignment at the time of the laminoplasty, postsurgical kyphosis could result and could necessitate further surgery.

In patients with severe cervical myelopathy, an awake fiberoptic intubation should be considered. Trauma-dose steroids may also be helpful. The patient is then placed prone and secured in a Mayfield holder or on a sponge head rest. It is preferable to position the patient in a slightly flexed position because this reduces the posterior skinfolds and facilitates the exposure. Also, overlapping of the laminae is less pronounced in flexion, which makes it easier to prepare the troughs.

A standard midline exposure is performed with care taken to stay in line with the ligamentum nuchae to reduce blood loss. Placing the bed in reverse Trendelenburg position also helps reduce paravertebral and epidural venous pressure and bleeding. Care should be taken to preserve the muscular attachments to C2 (Tips from the Masters 6-2).

Tips from the Masters 6-2 • Care should be taken to preserve the muscular attachments to C2.

Subperiosteal exposure of the posterior elements is obtained out to the middle of the lateral mass on the side that will be opened and out to the lateral edge of the lamina on the side that will be booked open. An attempt should be made to preserve the facet capsules on the side that will be booked open to maximize stability (Tips from the Masters 6-3). It is recommended that the exposure continue only up to the junction of the lamina and facet on the closed side.

Tips from the Masters 6-3 • Try to preserve the facet capsules on the side that will be booked open to maximize stability and minimize facet.

The locations of the gutters along the medial border of the facets are identified (see Tips from the Masters 6-3). The side that will be opened is typically addressed first, which is usually the side where the radicular pain is worst. This also allows a foraminotomy to be performed before the lamina is hinged open. A matchstick bur is typically used to create the troughs. A marking pen can be used to identify the correct location for the trough. An initial pass is made with the bur to decorticate the dorsal lamina. Then, the cancellous portion of the lamina is encountered. It is typically easier to bur through the cancellous bone and then complete the trough by gently sweeping the bur back and forth through the ventral lamina until a give is felt. Then, attention proceeds to the next lamina and each is worked on sequentially until all the troughs are made. Alternatively, the trough can be completed through the anterior cortex using a 1-mm Kerrison punch and/or a small curette. Next the hinge side is addressed. Once again, the location for the trough is identified and a marking pen is used if needed. The bur is used to decorticate the dorsal lamina and bur through the cancellous bone until the ventral lamina is reached. The ventral lamina should not be cut through on this side. A greenstick fracture should be gently created on the hinge side by lifting up on the laminae on the open side. A curette may be used to assist the opening of the laminae by hooking it under the open side and pulling up while an assistant pulls on the spinous processes. A Kerrison punch may be used to transect the ligamentum flavum at the cephalad and caudal ends of the laminoplasty. As much of the caudal and cephalad attachments should be left as is possible, because they help lock (spring) the laminae anteriorly to hold the small lamina-facet grafts in place (Tips from the Masters 6-4). Common practice is to open the hinge 1.0 to 1.5 cm.

Tips from the Masters 6-4 • Leave as much of the caudal and cephalad attachments as possible, because they help lock the laminae anteriorly and help hold the grafts in place.

Once the laminoplasty has been hinged open, hemostasis is obtained by coagulating the epidural bleeders with bipolar cauterization. Now, attention is turned toward keeping the laminoplasty open. Many techniques have been described to accomplish this. Sutures, allograft spacers, autograft, and plates have all been used successfully. The tips of the spinous processes may be removed and used as graft material, or they may be left in place depending on the surgeon's preference. Some surgeons like to use specially contoured plates that can be fixed to the lateral mass and lamina. Small allograft struts with a central hole that allows a screw to go through the strut and the plate may also be added. After a plate of appropriate size has been selected, the plate is first hooked or held to the lamina and secured to the lateral mass. Once the plate has been fixed to the lateral mass with screws, additional screws may be used to fix the plate to the lamina. If a small graft is wedged in place, the spinous process at each fixation level can be pushed to help lock the graft in place before the screws are inserted. A drain may be used, and the wound is closed in layers.

DISCUSSION OF BEST EVIDENCE

Several studies have directly compared complications as well as clinical, radiographic, and biomechanical outcomes of laminoplasty and laminectomy in an effort to determine the potential advantages of each procedure. Results of these studies have not led to a definitive conclusion regarding the benefit of one technique over the other, but a discussion of the findings of these studies is worthwhile for surgeons treating cervical spondylosis.

Two nonclinical studies have used cadaver and animal models to compare laminoplasty and laminectomy. Baisden and colleagues[39] compared **animal biomechanical data** and radiographic outcomes in a goat model. Ten live goats were treated with either C3-C5 laminectomy or open-door laminoplasty. Cervical curvature index was noted to decrease by 59% at 16 weeks and by 70% at 24 weeks in the laminectomy group, and the decrease in the laminoplasty group was not significantly different. In biomechanical testing, sagittal plane slack motion was notably increased in specimens from the laminectomy group (55 degrees) compared with that in specimens from nonoperated animals (39 degrees). No significant increase was noted in specimens from the laminoplasty group. Subramaniam and co-workers[40] compared the biomechanical effects of laminectomy and laminoplasty in **human cadavers** and modeled multilevel canal stenosis with insertion of hemispheric beads into the spinal canal. Spinal canal cross-sectional area increased 70% with laminoplasty and 101% with laminectomy. In addition, cervical range of motion was 13% greater after laminectomy than after laminoplasty.

Most direct comparisons of these techniques involve retrospective clinical studies. Two early retrospective studies did not identify an advantage of laminoplasty over laminectomy. Hukuda and colleagues[41] performed a **retrospective review** of outcomes for 18 patients treated with French window laminoplasty and 10 treated with laminectomy without posterior fixation for cervical myelopathy. No significant differences in functional outcomes or postoperative development of kyphosis, instability, or canal stenosis were noted. Among laminectomy patients, 30% developed kyphosis, 30% developed instability, and 20% developed recurrent canal stenosis. Laminoplasty did not significantly reduce these postoperative complications because 28% of laminoplasty patients developed kyphosis, 20% developed instability, and 16% developed recurrent canal stenosis. Nakano and associates[42] also found no difference between open-door laminoplasty and laminectomy for treatment of cervical myeloradiculopathy and OPLL. A **retrospective review** of data for 75 laminoplasty patients and 14 laminectomy patients revealed no difference in functional improvement between the two groups and no development of instability in either group.

Another early **retrospective** comparison by Herkowitz and co-workers[43] showed improved outcomes with laminoplasty. Forty-five patients with multilevel cervical spondylotic radiculopathy underwent either laminectomy with partial facetectomy (12 patients), open-door laminoplasty (18 patients), or anterior fusion (15 patients). Success rate was determined by functional improvement and resolution of pain. The results for laminectomy were inferior to those for laminoplasty and anterior fusion. Success rates of 92% and 86% were noted for anterior fusion and open-door laminoplasty, respectively, whereas laminectomy had a success rate of 66% in resolving symptoms of multilevel disease.

Heller and colleagues[44] noted similar results as well as reduced complications with laminoplasty in a **retrospective matched cohort analysis** of patients treated either with laminectomy with partial facetectomy and fusion or with T-saw open-door laminoplasty for multilevel cervical myelopathy. Results for 13 patients in each group were compared. Average functional improvement according to the Nurick scale and subjective improvements in strength, dexterity, numbness, pain, and gait were greater in the laminoplasty group.[45] Complications in the group undergoing laminectomy with fusion included progression of myelopathy in two patients, pseudoarthrosis in five patients, broken instrumentation in two patients, adjacent-segment degeneration in one patient, and the development of kyphosis in one patient. No complications were noted in the laminoplasty group. Although the sample size was small, the lack of complications and improved clinical outcomes demonstrate a potential advantage for the use of laminoplasty in treatment of multilevel cervical myelopathy.

Kaminsky and associates[46] also performed a **retrospective matched cohort study** involving two groups of 22 matched patients treated with laminectomy or open-door laminoplasty for multilevel spondylotic myelopathy or radiculopathy. Like Heller and associates, Kaminsky and colleagues noted greater improvement of outcomes (according to the Nurick scale) and fewer complications with laminoplasty than with laminectomy.[45] Five patients treated with laminectomy experienced postoperative development of kyphosis (two of these patients had C4-C5 subluxation). In the laminoplasty group, two patients experienced transient C5 paresis that eventually resolved. In addition, neck range of motion decreased significantly in the laminoplasty group. Hardman and co-workers[47] performed a **retrospective review** of outcomes for 72 patients who underwent laminoplasty and 49 patients who underwent laminectomy for CSM or radiculopathy and noted improved clinical outcomes in the laminoplasty group according to various clinical outcome measures, including the Rankin disability score, Glasgow Outcome Scale (GOS) score, and Karnofsky score. Shorter hospital stay was also noted with laminoplasty (6.6 days vs. 8.4 days with laminectomy).

Matsunaga and associates[48] noted another potential advantage of laminoplasty, reporting on postoperative kyphosis rates in 37 patients who underwent laminectomy and 64 patients who underwent laminoplasty. Kyphosis was reported in

34% of laminectomy patients and 7% of laminoplasty patients, with mean follow-up periods of 79 and 66 months, respectively. No functional outcomes were reported. However, the authors' findings were consistent with the concern that loss of posterior structures in laminectomy can lead to kyphotic deformity.

A new procedure called *skip laminectomy* was described in an earlier section. This procedure may be advantageous because it results in less disruption of posterior elements than with a standard laminectomy. Recently, several studies have compared this technique to laminoplasty. Otani and colleagues[49] retrospectively compared results for 26 patients undergoing skip laminectomy (also known as *segmental partial laminectomy*) with those for 13 patients undergoing open-door laminoplasty for CSM. Greater maintenance of sagittal alignment and range of motion were noted in the skip laminectomy group. In addition, 54% of laminoplasty patients reported shoulder and/or neck complaints versus 19% in the skip laminectomy group at 5-year follow-up.

A similar comparison was done by Shiraishi and associates[37], who examined outcomes after treatment of cervical myelopathy with skip laminectomy in 43 patients and after open-door laminoplasty in 51 patients. Clinical outcomes as measured by the JOA score were similar in both groups. However, several postoperative problems were noted in the laminoplasty group: 66% of laminoplasty patients experienced postoperative development or worsening of axial pain versus 2% of those undergoing skip laminectomy, and only 61% of neck range of motion was maintained in the laminoplasty group versus 98% in the skip laminectomy group.

In a **prospective randomized clinical trial,** Yukawa and colleagues[38] compared outcomes for 41 patients with CSM who underwent either a modified double-door laminoplasty (n = 21) or a skip laminectomy (n = 20). After at least 1 year of follow-up, no significant difference was noted between groups undergoing these two procedures in terms of clinical outcomes, cervical alignment, and cervical range of motion. No serious complications were noted in either group.

COMMENTARY

Laminoplasty is an excellent option to consider when treating patients with CSM. The main benefits are that the procedure is motion preserving and it avoids the additional risks of performing an instrumented fusion. However, as with most procedures in spine surgery, the success of this procedure depends on its being used for the right indications. Laminoplasty should not be used in patients who complain of significant neck pain or in patients who have a kyphotic alignment. In these patients a laminoplasty may fail and result in poor outcomes. Despite these concerns, laminoplasty is a worthwhile procedure with which all spine surgeons should be familiar because of the complexity of the diseases they treat. Only by having a wide and varied skill set can surgeons ensure that they perform (often) the proper procedure on the proper patient, thus optimizing their results.

REFERENCES

1. Dillin WHSF: Laminectomy. In Herkowitz HN, Garfin SR, Balderston RA, editors: *The spine*, Philadelphia, 1999, Saunders, pp 529–531.
2. Geck MJ, Eismont FJ: Surgical options for the treatment of cervical spondylotic myelopathy, *Orthop Clin North Am* 33(2):329–348, 2002.
3. Albert TJ, Vaccaro A: Postlaminectomy kyphosis, *Spine* 23:2738–2745, 1998.
4. Kato Y, Iwasaki M, Fuji T, et al: Long-term follow-up results of laminectomy for cervical myelopathy caused by ossification of the posterior longitudinal ligament, *J Neurosurg* 89:217–223, 1998. **This retrospective study was performed to assess the long-term results of cervical laminectomy in treating ossification of the posterior longitudinal ligament (OPLL) of the cervical spine. The authors recommend early surgical decompression for OPLL because the outcome is better for younger patients and for those with a higher score as measured by the Japanese Orthopedic Association's system.**
5. Yasuoka S, Peterson HA, MacCarty CS: Incidence of spinal column deformity after multilevel laminectomy in children and adults, *J Neurosurg* 57:441–445, 1982.
6. Wilkinson M: Historical introduction. In Brain WR, Wilkinson M, editors: *Cervical spondylosis and other disorders of the cervical spine*, Philadelphia, 1967, Saunders, pp 1–9.
7. Epstein NE: Laminectomy for cervical myelopathy, *Spinal Cord* 41(6):317–327, 2003.

8. Kumar VG, Rea GL, Mervis LJ, et al: Cervical spondylotic myelopathy: functional and radiographic long-term outcome after laminectomy and posterior fusion, *Neurosurgery* 44(4):771–777, 1999; discussion, 777-778.
9. Miyazaki K, Tada K, Matsuda Y, et al: Posterior extensive simultaneous multi-segment decompression with posterolateral fusion for cervical myelopathy with cervical instability and kyphotic and/or S-shaped deformities, *Spine* 14:1160–1170, 1989.
10. Miyazaki K, Kirita Y: Extensive simultaneous multisegment laminectomy for myelopathy due to the ossification of the posterior longitudinal ligament in the cervical region, *Spine* 11:531–542, 1986. **A retrospective review showing good results with multilevel laminectomy in patients with cervical myelopathy owing to ossification of the posterior longitudinal ligament.**
11. Cusick JF, Pintar FA, Yoganandan N: Biomechanical alterations induced by multilevel cervical laminectomy, *Spine* 20:2392–2398, 1995.
12. Perez-Lopez C, Isla A, Alvarez F, et al: [Efficacy of arthrodesis in the posterior approach of cervical myelopathy: comparative study of a series of 36 cases], *Neurocirugia (Astur)* 12:316–324, 2001.
13. Hamanishi C, Tanaka S: Bilateral multilevel laminectomy with or without posterolateral fusion for cervical spondylotic myelopathy: relationship to type of onset and time until operation, *J Neurosurg* 85:447–451, 1996.
14. McAfee PC, Bohlman HH, Wilson WL: The triple wire fixation technique for stabilization of acute cervical fracture-dislocations: a biomechanical analysis, *Orthop Trans* 9:142, 1985.
15. Anderson PA, Henley MB, Grady MS, et al: Posterior cervical arthrodesis with AO reconstruction plates and bone graft, *Spine* 16(Suppl 3):S72–S79, 1991.
16. Ulrich C, Woersdoerfer O, Kalff R, et al: Biomechanics of fixation systems to the cervical spine, *Spine* 16(Suppl 3):S4–S9, 1991.
17. Jones EL, Heller JG, Silcox DH, et al: Cervical pedicle screws versus lateral mass screws. Anatomic feasibility and biomechanical comparison, *Spine* 22:977–982, 1997.
18. Kotani Y, Cunningham BW, Abumi K, et al: Biomechanical analysis of cervical stabilization systems. An assessment of transpedicular screw fixation in the cervical spine, *Spine* 19:2529–2539, 1994.
19. Oyama M, Hattori S, Moriwaki N: A new method of posterior decompression [in Japanese], *Chubuseisaisi* 16:792, 1973.
20. Hirabayashi K, Miyagawa J, Satomi K, et al: Operative results and postoperative progression of ossification among patients with ossification of cervical posterior longitudinal ligament, *Spine* 6:354–364, 1981.
21. Steinmetz MP, Resnick DK: Cervical laminoplasty [review], *Spine J* 6(Suppl 6):274S–281S, 2006.
22. Herkowitz H: Cervical laminaplasty: its role in the treatment of cervical radiculopathy, *J Spinal Disord* 1:179–188, 1988.
23. Shaffrey C, Wiggins GC, Piccirilli CB, et al: Modified open-door laminoplasty for treatment of neurological deficits in younger patients with congenital spinal stenosis: analysis of clinical and radiographic data, *J Neurosurg* 90(Suppl 2):170–177, 1999.
24. Gillett GR, Erasmus AM, Lind CR: CG-clip expansive open-door laminoplasty: a technical note, *Br J Neurosurg* 13(4):405–408, 1999.
25. Kurokawa T, Tsuyama N, Tanaka H: Enlargement of spinal canal by the sagittal splitting of the spinous process, *Bessatusu Seikeigeka* 2:234–240, 1982.
26. Hase H, Watanabe T, Hirasawa Y, et al: Bilateral open laminoplasty using ceramic laminas for cervical myelopathy, *Spine* 16:1269–1276, 1982.
27. Kawaguchi Y, Matsui H, Ishihara H, et al: Axial symptoms after en bloc cervical laminoplasty, *J Spinal Disord* 12:392–395, 1999.
28. Hosono N, Yonenobu K, Ono K: Neck and shoulder pain after laminoplasty: a noticeable complication, *Spine* 21:1969–1973, 1996.
29. Takemitsu M, Cheung KM, Wong YW, et al: C5 nerve root palsy after cervical laminoplasty and posterior fusion with instrumentation, *J Spinal Disord Tech* 21(4):267–272, 2008.
30. Tanaka N, Nakanishi K, Fujiwara Y, et al: Postoperative segmental C5 palsy after cervical laminoplasty may occur without intraoperative nerve injury: a prospective study with transcranial electric motor-evoked potentials, *Spine* 31(26):3013–3017, 2006.
31. Sakuura H, Hosono N, Mukai Y, et al: C5 palsy after decompression surgery for cervical myelopathy. Review of the literature, *Spine* 28:2447–2451, 2003.
32. Satomi K, Ogawa J, Ishii Y, et al: Short-term complications and long-term results of expansive open-door laminoplasty for cervical stenotic myelopathy, *Spine J* 1(1):26–30, 2001.
33. Chiba K, Ogawa Y, Ishii K, et al: Long-term results of expansive open-door laminoplasty for cervical myelopathy—average 14-year follow-up study, *Spine* 31(26):2998–3005, 2006.
34. Kawaguchi Y, Kanamori M, Ishihara H, et al: Minimum 10-year followup after en bloc cervical laminoplasty, *Clin Orthop Relat Res* 411:129–139, 2003.
35. Dickerman RD, Reynolds AS, Tackett J, et al: Dural laceration, *J Neurosurg Spine* 9(1):104, 2008; author reply, 104–105.
36. Shiraishi T: Skip laminectomy—a new treatment for cervical spondylotic myelopathy, preserving bilateral muscular attachments to the spinous processes: a preliminary report, *Spine J* 2(2):108–115, 2002.
37. Shiraishi T, Fukuda K, Yato Y, et al: Results of skip laminectomy—minimum 2-year follow-up study compared with open-door laminoplasty, *Spine* 28:2667–2672, 2003. **The results of using skip laminectomy and open-door laminoplasty to treat patients with CSM were compared to verify that skip laminectomy is less invasive to the posterior extensor mechanism of the cervical spine.**

38. Yukawa Y, Kato F, Ito K, et al: Laminoplasty and skip laminectomy for cervical compressive myelopathy: range of motion, postoperative neck pain, and surgical outcomes in a randomized prospective study, *Spine* 32(18):1980–1985, 2007. **In this prospective randomized clinical trial, outcomes for 41 patients were compared with CSM who underwent either a modified double-door laminoplasty (n = 21) or a skip laminectomy (n = 20). After at least 1 year of follow-up, no significant difference was noted between groups undergoing these two procedures in terms of clinical outcomes, cervical alignment, and cervical range of motion. No serious complications were noted in either group.**

39. Baisden J, Voo LM, Cusick JF, et al: Evaluation of cervical laminectomy and laminoplasty. A longitudinal study in the goat model, *Spine* 24(13):1283–1288, 1999; discussion, 1288–1289.

40. Subramaniam V, Chamberlain RH, Theodore N, et al: Biomechanical effects of laminoplasty versus laminectomy: stenosis and stability, *Spine* 34(16):E573–E578, 2009.

41. Hukuda S, Ogata M, Mochizuki T, et al: Laminectomy versus laminoplasty for cervical myelopathy: brief report, *J Bone Joint Surg Br* 70(2):325–326, 1988.

42. Nakano N, Nakano T, Nakano K: Comparison of the results of laminectomy and open-door laminoplasty for cervical spondylotic myeloradiculopathy and ossification of the posterior longitudinal ligament, *Spine* 13(7):792–794, 1988.

43. Herkowitz HN: A comparison of anterior cervical fusion, cervical laminectomy, and cervical laminoplasty for the surgical management of multiple level spondylotic radiculopathy, *Spine* 13(7):774–780, 1988. **A retrospective review comparing the results and complications of 45 patients with at least a 2-year follow-up who had undergone anterior fusion, cervical laminectomy, or cervical laminoplasty for the surgical management of multiple-level cervical radiculopathy owing to cervical spondylosis.**

44. Heller JG, Edwards CC 2nd, Murakami H, et al: Laminoplasty versus laminectomy and fusion for multilevel cervical myelopathy: an independent matched cohort analysis, *Spine* 26(12):1330–1336, 2001. **A comparison of the clinical and radiographic outcomes of multilevel corpectomy and laminoplasty using an independent matched-cohort analysis concluded that both multilevel corpectomy and laminoplasty reliably arrest myelopathic progression in multilevel cervical myelopathy and can lead to significant neurologic recovery and pain reduction in most patients.**

45. Nurick S: The natural history and the results of surgical treatment of the spinal cord disorder associated with cervical spondylosis, *Brain* 95:101–108, 1972.

46. Kaminsky SB, Clark CR, Traynelis VC: Operative treatment of cervical spondylotic myelopathy and radiculopathy. A comparison of laminectomy and laminoplasty at five year average follow-up, *Iowa Orthop J* 24:95–105, 2004.

47. Hardman J, Graf O, Kouloumberis PE, et al: Clinical and functional outcomes of laminoplasty and laminectomy, *Neurol Res* 32(4):416–420, 2010; Epub July 8, 2009.

48. Matsunaga S, Sakou T, Nakanisi K: Analysis of the cervical spine alignment following laminoplasty and laminectomy, *Spinal Cord* 37:20–24, 1999.

49. Otani K, Sato K, Yabuki S, et al: A segmental partial laminectomy for cervical spondylotic myelopathy: anatomical basis and clinical outcome in comparison with expansive open-door laminoplasty, *Spine* 34(3):268–273, 2009.

Chapter 7

Lumbar Degenerative Disk Disease: Fusion Versus Artificial Disk

Michael F. Duffy, Jack E. Zigler

The diagnosis and treatment of symptomatic lumbar intervertebral disk degeneration remains controversial in the medical literature. Although the pathoanatomy of the diseased intervertebral disk has been understood for quite a while, changes in clinical treatment have evolved slowly, and traditional treatment options, although numerous, have failed to provide a clear-cut gold standard with reproducible outcomes. The successful treatment of diskogenic back pain requires a systematic approach to diagnosis as well as a thorough understanding of the pain generator and the physiologic effects of various treatments.

Chronic low back pain has multiple possible causes. The spine is a dynamic structure, with several potential pain generators, including the facet joints, ligaments, muscles, and intervertebral disks. Because there is no single clinical test or physical examination finding to isolate the source of pain, the definitive pain generator remains unidentified in a significant proportion of patients. Furthermore, disk abnormalities are often accompanied by other painful spinal conditions, which makes diagnosis and treatment even more challenging. For diskogenic back pain to be primarily diagnosed, all other potential pain generators must be excluded based on imaging and failure of conservative treatments such as rest, medication, epidural steroids, and/or facet injections when indicated.

The concept that pain could arise from an intervertebral disk was slow to gain acceptance. Early thought was that nerve fibers did not penetrate the outer annulus. However, as scientific methods evolved, studies began to show that nerve fibers actually did penetrate into the disk and that ingrowth was potentially substantial.[1,2] These findings led to the postulate that diskogenic back pain might be a result of sensitization of these nerve fibers by nociceptive substances. Magnetic resonance imaging (MRI) has failed to definitively identify a symptomatic diseased intervertebral disk, which is evidenced by the fact that MRI shows disk abnormalities in 76% of patients without chronic low back pain.[3] This finding supports the need for provocative testing such as diskography to differentiate a diseased symptomatic disk from a degenerated, but asymptomatic, one. No clinical test is perfect, and diskography remains regionally controversial; however, it is the only provocative test that aids the practitioner in making a definitive diagnosis of diskogenic pain. Earlier human studies[4] had shown that after long-term (10-year) follow-up no changes were found in disks that had undergone diskography, but a more recent 10-year matched cohort study[5] has suggested that diskography of a control disk may be related to accelerated disk degeneration. The possibility of psychological confounders in this study may detract from the magnitude of this conclusion, yet it has raised new concerns about using a normal adjacent level as a control level in diskography.

Over the past two decades many options have been developed to treat painful disk degeneration, and varying clinical results have been reported. Inconsistencies in patient selection, study design, and methods of treatment have only added more uncertainty in this evolving field. Fusion has become a mainstay in treating functionally disabling diseased intervertebral disks. Cloward[6] first presented the technique of interbody fusion for diseased disks, in which removal of the painful disk was followed by fusion of the pain-generating segment. Interbody fusion has traditionally been done through an anterior or a posterior approach. With the anterior approach, there is greater access to the pain-generating disk and a more complete diskectomy is possible, but the potential for intraabdominal consequences such as vascular injury and sympathetic nerve injury (retrograde ejaculation in males) has deterred many surgeons and patients. The posterior approach is also not without its potential downsides—approach-related muscular damage, injury to nerve structures, and a less complete diskectomy. Studies[7,8] have shown that regardless of the approach used for fusion, well-selected patients with an identifiable diagnosis have similar fusion rates and clinical outcomes. The common theme of these various fusion techniques has been to rid the spine of the pain generator, create a biomechanically rigid environment, and promote fusion across a motion segment. A significant drawback of this classic treatment is the loss of motion. The advent of total disk replacement (TDR) offered a new alternative that aims to restore and maintain motion and function of the diseased segment. With this new surgical option comes increased scrutiny, just as with all advances in surgery. When Dr. John Charnley[9] first introduced the concept of joint replacement in 1961, fellow surgeons were skeptical of the advancement and were slow to adapt. Now, 50 years later, total hip arthroplasty is recognized as one of the most significant advancements in degenerative joint disease and is widely accepted and performed across the globe. Again, adoption of this technology was slow and not without significant criticism.

The history of disk arthroplasty began in the 1950s with insertion of metal spheres into the disk space after diskectomy by Fernström[10] (Figure 7-1). He reported his results in patients with herniated or degenerative disks treated with diskectomy and insertion of the sphere compared with 100 control patients who underwent diskectomy alone. His findings, although not statistically sound, showed that a substantially smaller number of patients reported back pain after the arthroplasty procedure than after the diskectomy alone (Table 7-1). His complication rate was reported as 1.4%.

The lumbar disk prosthesis continued to evolve during the 1970s as a nuclear implant, going from a metal sphere to a silicone rubber prosthesis to a polyurethane injectant. It was in 1984 that the modern lumbar disk arthroplasty implant began to be developed. Büttner-Janz and Schellnack designed a modular three-piece TDR device known as the SB Charité, and it was implanted in September 1984 at the

FIGURE 7-1 Radiograph depicting a Fernström ball within the L5-S1 disk space.

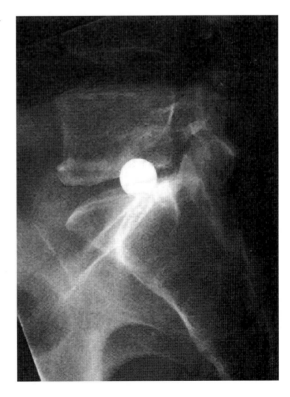

TABLE 7-1 Fernström's Results for the Percentage of Patients with Back Pain after Diskectomy Alone Versus Diskectomy and Placement of an Arthroplasty Device

	Patients Experiencing Back Pain (%)	
Treatment	**Degenerative Disk Group**	**Herniated Disk Group**
Diskectomy and arthroplasty	40	12
Diskectomy alone	88	60

From Fernström U: Arthroplasty with intercorporal endoprosthesis in herniated disc and in painful disc, *Acta Chir Scand Suppl* 357:154–159, 1966.

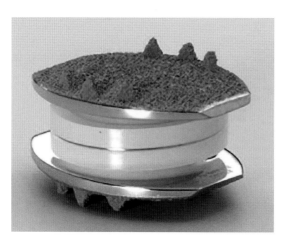

FIGURE 7-2 Third generation of the original SB Charité Artificial Disc, which is in use today.

Charité Hospital in Germany. The disk replacement underwent revision, but the third design of the Charité Artificial Disc (DePuy Spine, Raynham, Mass.) has been in worldwide use since 1987 (Figure 7-2). The ProDisc-L (Synthes Spine, West Chester, Pa.) was developed in France and first implanted by Thierry Marnay in March 1990. The Charité Artificial Disc was the first TDR device implanted in the United States and was used as part of a U.S. Food and Drug Administration (FDA) Investigational Device Exemption (IDE) study protocol in March 2000 at the Texas Back Institute; the first ProDisc-L used in the United States was implanted in October 2001 at the same institute. The Charité and the ProDisc-L are currently the only two FDA-approved devices in the United States for lumbar disk arthroplasty.

This chapter presents a case example of a patient with degenerative disk disease and discusses several different surgical treatment options. Both fusion and motion-preserving devices are considered for treatment. A detailed description of the fundamental technique and tips for the preferred treatment for this patient are provided. Based on discussion of the best evidence, several surgical options are considered so that the best surgical treatment choice for this particular case can be formulated and executed.

CASE PRESENTATION

A 38-year-old male professional athlete had a multiyear history of progressively worsening low back pain refractory to conservative treatment, including anti-inflammatory medications, muscle relaxants, physical therapy, and appropriate injections. His pain scale rating was 7 out of 10 and constant. The Oswestry Disability Index score was 56%. The patient's pain diagram portrayed 100% low back pain, without lower extremity complaints.

- PMH: Unremarkable

- PSH: Partial laminectomy and diskectomy at L4-5 performed 5 years earlier with complete relief of radicular symptoms.

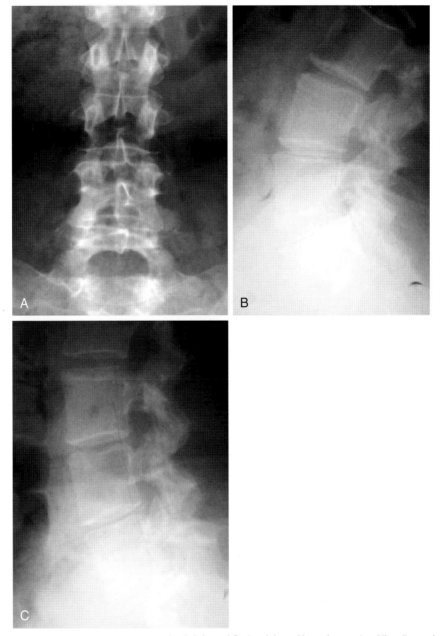

FIGURE 7-3 Preoperative anteroposterior (**A**), lateral flexion (**B**), and lateral extension (**C**) radiographs.

- Exam: The patient had significant muscle spasms with lumbar tenderness and decreased range of motion (ROM) in flexion. On manual motor testing, he had full muscle strength in the lower extremities and a negative result on the straight leg raise.

- Imaging: Plain radiographs (Figure 7-3) showed significant disk space narrowing at the L4-5 level without instability. Sagittal and axial MRI scans (Figures 7-4 and 7-5) revealed severe spondylosis and degeneration at the L4-5 level, with Modic changes within the end plates. The integrity of the left L4-5 facet joint was maintained after the initial laminectomy and diskectomy performed 5 years earlier. The diagnosis was postlaminectomy degenerative disk disease with functionally disabling mechanical low back pain, refractory to nonoperative treatment.

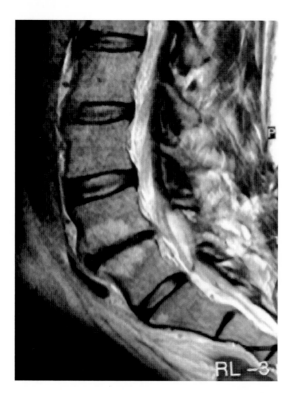

FIGURE 7-4 Preoperative MRI sagittal image showing significant Modic changes at the L4-5 end plates.

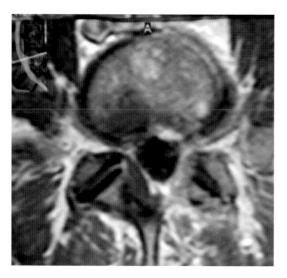

FIGURE 7-5 Preoperative MRI axial image. Note the integrity of the left facet joint.

SURGICAL OPTIONS

There are several surgical options for treating this patient. The common denominator of each option is to remove the pain generator—the diseased intervertebral disk. As for fusion options, the L4-5 disk could be addressed from an anterior approach (anterior lumbar interbody fusion), a direct lateral approach (far lateral interbody fusion), a posterolateral approach (transforaminal lumbar interbody fusion), or a posterior-only approach (posterior lumbar interbody fusion), all with the goal of achieving an interbody fusion. Pedicle screw instrumentation (or a side plate and screws in the case of the far lateral approach) with grafting material can be used in conjunction with any of these options to aid in obtaining posterolateral biologic

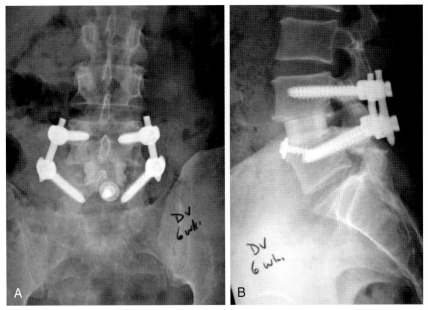

FIGURE 7-6 AP (**A**) and lateral (**B**) radiographs of an anterior-posterior fusion construct at L4-5 using the mini–open retroperitoneal approach to the anterior lumbar spine.

fusion. Other nonfusion options include the use of motion-preserving devices such as a TDR or dynamic stabilization system.

Anterior Lumbar Diskectomy and Interbody Fusion

Anterior lumbar diskectomy and interbody fusion is the most attractive option for the aforementioned case. The anterior approach allows for a more complete diskectomy than a posterior approach. Complete diskectomy has been shown to lead to a better ultimate fusion rate than a more partial, "reamed channel" diskectomy.[11] After the pain generator is addressed with a complete diskectomy, reconstruction with an anterior lumbar interbody fusion (ALIF) construct will restore disk height and indirectly distract the foramen. The anterior fusion can be used as a standalone construct in the properly selected patient or augmented with posterior instrumentation (Figure 7-6). For ALIF, there are many devices available, some with FDA approval as standalone devices. Newer polyetheretherketone (PEEK) devices are available as well, some with fixation techniques and 510k approval for standalone ALIF. The addition of posterior instrumentation increases biomechanical stability and reduces motion at the operative level, but clinical necessity and effect on fusion are still open to debate.[12,13] Whereas autograft was traditionally used within the cage, the advent of bone morphogenetic proteins (BMPs) has accelerated fusion time and rates in ALIF and is a preferred adjuvant for anterior fusions.[14] Many patients who have a low body mass index and no instability and who are adherent to prescribed medical regimens may be candidates for implantation of anterior standalone fusion devices with adjuvant BMP. In most other patients typical practice is to augment the anterior construct with percutaneous pedicle screw systems and posterolateral grafting using local bone and demineralized bone matrix. An anterior approach should be considered cautiously in patients with active disk space or systemic infection, significant vascular disease, or osteoporosis. The decision to use an anterior approach in most cases is individualized and is based on the experience and comfort level of the access surgeon and spine surgeon.

Tips from the Masters 7-1 • Participation of an experienced access surgeon is vital to accomplishing efficient and successful anterior lumbar surgery, while minimizing potential serious vascular complications.

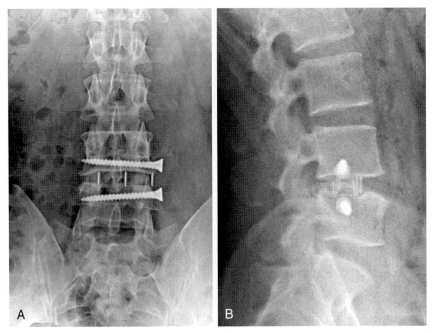

FIGURE 7-7 AP (**A**) and lateral (**B**) radiographs of the direct lateral fusion option at L4-5 level, with side fixation for added stability.

Absolute contraindications for an anterior approach are significantly calcified aorta or prior vascular reconstructive surgery. Relative contraindications are morbid obesity, previous intraabdominal or retroperitoneal surgery, history of severe pelvic inflammatory disease, and previous anterior spinal surgery.

Far Lateral or Trans-Psoas Approach

The far lateral or trans-psoas approach is another fusion option at the L4-5 and more cephalad levels (Figure 7-7). This recently popularized approach is attractive because it allows anterior access to the disk space without the need for an anterior access surgeon. Patient positioning is vital to the success and ease of the operation, and at the L4-5 level this is especially true due to the iliac crest overlap. Preoperative planning is key in determining if the crest is too high riding in relation to the L4-5 disk space. The dissection is directly lateral, centered over the disk space. After the external and internal oblique muscle layers are pierced through, the retroperitoneal dissection is completed bluntly down to the lateral border of the psoas muscle (Figure 7-8). Specialized dilators and retractors are then used to lessen the chance of neurologic injury as the approach extends through the psoas down to the disk space. After standard diskectomy and placement of the interbody lateral cage, use of a lateral plate or posterior pedicle screw construct is advisable; however, clinical and biomechanical literature evaluating these constructs is lacking. From an outcomes standpoint, the only direct lateral fusion study available is a short-term case series of patients undergoing lateral interbody fusion for degenerative scoliosis.[15] Knight and co-workers[16] presented perioperative data indicating that the procedure has an acceptable complication rate, comparable to that in historical controls. The incidence of major adverse events approached 9% and significant nerve irritation occurred in 3.4%. Recent cadaveric evidence has shown that use of this technique at L4-5 may result in a significant risk of iatrogenic injury to the lumbosacral plexus.[17] This anatomic study found that the lumbosacral plexus migrates anteriorly at each successive caudal disk space from L1 to L5, with L4-5 having the least amount of

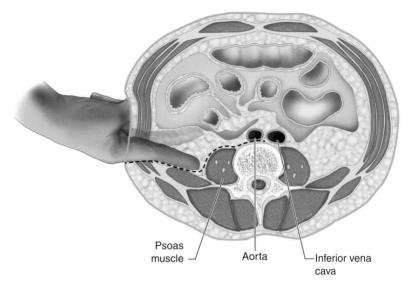

Psoas
muscle   Aorta   Inferior vena
cava

FIGURE 7-8 Retroperitoneal dissection for the direct lateral approach.

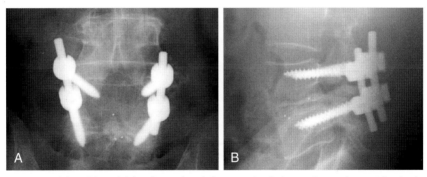

FIGURE 7-9 AP (**A**) and lateral (**B**) radiographs of the posterior fusion option at the L4-5 level using the posterior lumbar interbody fusion technique.

"safe zone" for a posteriorly positioned dilator or retractor. Regev and associates[18] also showed that the overlap of neural structures and retroperitoneal vascular structures increased from L1-2 to L4-5, with an 87% overlap at L4-5 (Tips from the Masters 7-2). This creates a very small safe operative window (as small as 13% of the disk space) for the trans-psoas approach at the L4-5 level.

Tips from the Masters 7-2 • The direct lateral approach is more difficult and carries a higher risk of neurovascular complications at the L4-5 level than at more cephalad levels.

Posterior Fusion (Transforaminal or Posterior Lumbar Interbody Fusion)

Posterior fusion, either transforaminal lumbar interbody fusion (TLIF) or posterior lumbar interbody fusion (PLIF), with or without interbody fixation (Figure 7-9), is also an option for the patient described in the Case Presentation. These procedures are attractive, particularly in cases in which an anterior approach is contraindicated. The downside of using a PLIF approach is the need to enter the spinal canal and retract the nerve roots and the thecal sac. The TLIF approach avoids the need for significant retraction on the thecal sac, but places the exiting nerve root in danger. Both posterior approaches obviate the need for an anterior access surgeon and also avoid the potential risks of vascular injury associated with the anterior approach.

Box 7-1 CONTRAINDICATIONS FOR TOTAL DISK REPLACEMENT

- Active systemic infection or infection localized to the site of implantation
- Osteopenia or osteoporosis defined as dual energy x-ray absorptiometry (DEXA)–measured bone density T-score of less than −1.0
- Bony lumbar spinal stenosis
- Allergy or sensitivity to implant materials (cobalt, chromium, molybdenum, polyethylene, titanium)
- Isolated radicular compression syndromes, especially due to disk herniation
- Pars defect
- Involved vertebral end plate dimensionally smaller that 34.5 mm in the medial-lateral and/ or 27 mm in the anterior-posterior direction
- Clinically compromised vertebral bodies at affected level due to current or past trauma
- Lytic spondylolisthesis or degenerative spondylolisthesis higher than Grade 1

Reported rates of postoperative neuralgia after posterior interbody fusion are near 7%[19] but are much lower in transforaminal approaches.[20]

Total Disk Replacement

The final surgical option for the particular case described earlier is motion preservation intervention—either TDR or use of a pedicle-based dynamic stabilization device. Currently available arthroplasty implants require an anterior approach, and their use is restricted by the contraindications for anterior lumbar surgery (see earlier) as well as those specific for TDR (Box 7-1).

Regarding posterior dynamic stabilizing devices, although multiple systems are commercially available, none of them has gained FDA approval for nonfusion stabilization of a degenerative motion segment. Although multiple biomechanical studies have supported the philosophy behind dynamic stabilization, there are no clinical studies indicating that it has a favorable effect on degenerative disk disease. In fact, the only clinical study to date examining the use of these systems in degenerative disk disease showed that the dynamic stabilization devices were associated with high rates of failure and low rates of clinical success within a 2-year follow-up period.[21]

FUNDAMENTAL TECHNIQUE

The patient underwent TDR at the L4-5 level without complications through a mini–open retroperitoneal approach (Figure 7-10). At 5 years of follow-up, the patient was free of back pain (visual analog scale [VAS] pain rating and Oswestry Disability Index score were at normal levels). He required no pain medication and was able to return to professional athletics.

For patients who have contraindications to TDR or who cannot obtain insurance authorization for the procedure, ALIF augmented by percutaneous posterior pedicle screw fixation would be the recommended procedure. At institutions with ready availability of excellent access surgeons, ALIF is the preferred procedure for reconstruction; posterior approaches (PLIF or TLIF) can be used when anterior surgery is contraindicated or when a concomitant decompression is required. The following sections offer a description of the anterior technique for approaching the spine, with specific considerations mentioned to aid the less experienced surgeon in successful insertion of a TDR prosthesis.

Patient Positioning

The patient is positioned supine on a regular operating room table. The iliac crest may be aligned with the break in the table to allow hyperextension of the lumbar region using the bed controls. Also, the plane of the left and right anterior superior iliac spines should be parallel to the floor. Use of a leveling bar can aid in

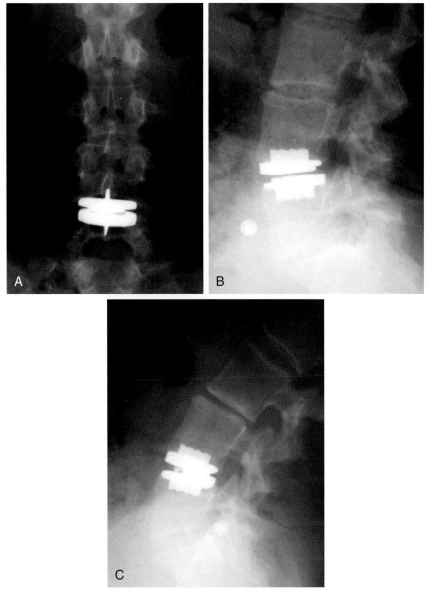

FIGURE 7-10 A, Immediately postoperative AP radiograph of L4-5 artificial disk replacement. **B** and **C,** Five-year follow-up AP and lateral flexion and extension radiographs. Note the visible motion maintained at the L4-5 artificial disk.

verification. The arms should be padded at the elbows and wrapped in front of the patient's chest in mummy fashion. The folded arms are then secured by taping to the bed. Both lower extremities should be in neutral position, with a pillow under the knees.

For anterior access, a paramedial, left-sided incision is preferred for a retroperitoneal approach. A good strategy is to use right-sided approaches for L5-S1 when the patient has subthreshold degenerated disks at L4-5 or L3-4, so that the left retroperitoneum remains available for surgery at a later time. The paramedial incision has been shown to have both a cosmetic and functional benefit compared with an anterolateral incision.[22] The incidence of retrograde ejaculation is tenfold lower when a retroperitoneal approach is used compared to when a transperitoneal approach is used.[23] Although access surgeons are commonly used in the United States, rates and types of complications are the same when a trained spine surgeon performs the approach procedure.[24] In a series of 1315 anterior access cases,

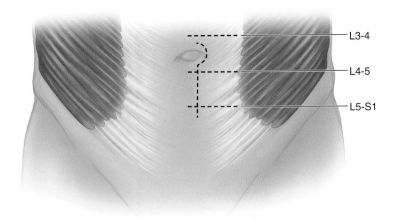

FIGURE 7-11 Illustration of the various incisions used for anterior mini–open retroperitoneal approach. The extensile, vertical incision should be reserved for more obese patients to gain exposure.

Brau and colleagues[25] reported a 0.45% incidence of iliac vein thrombosis and a 1.4% incidence of major vessel lacerations. Laparoscopic techniques have shown no functional advantage over the "mini-open" technique. In fact, use of a laparoscopic technique adds significant cost to the procedure.[26]

In smaller patients, the incision can usually be made horizontally for a one-level procedure. A 6- to 8-cm left-sided paramedial horizontal incision on the lower abdomen in line with the disk space is used. In more obese patients, a vertical incision should be used because it is more extensile (Figure 7-11). Based on the relation of the L4-5 disk space to the iliac crest on lateral radiographs, the incision may be situated either caudal or cephalad on the abdomen to the level of the crest. Some access surgeons like to verify the angle of the L5-S1 disk space using a lateral fluoroscopic image and radiopaque marker such as a pin, particularly early in their approach experience (Tips from the Masters 7-2).

After the skin incision is made, Bovie cauterization is used in the subcutaneous tissue layer to expose the anterior rectus fascia. The fascia is incised slightly obliquely and to a greater length than the skin incision to allow easier mobilization. The midline fascial raphe of the rectus is then identified, and the left rectus is mobilized to the left side with careful attention to avoid injury to the inferior epigastric vessels deep to the muscle. These vessels may need to be cauterized. Blunt finger dissection is then used to develop the retroperitoneal plane at the lateral edge of the fascial incision. The plane is bluntly dissected superficial to the peritoneum along the left abdominal wall around the sigmoid colon and taken posteriorly toward the psoas muscle (Figure 7-12). The entire peritoneal contents can be bluntly dissected and raised off the abdominal wall. A hand-held retractor can be useful. The ureter should be identified and retracted with the peritoneal contents, not dissected separate from the peritoneal sac. The genitofemoral nerve can usually be identified on the surface of the psoas muscle. Identification and ligation of the iliolumbar vein (or veins) is frequently necessary, because they may keep the iliac vein tethered anterior to the spine and inhibit proper mobilization of the great vessels. Once the peritoneum has been successfully mobilized, the vascular structures must be carefully dissected from the left anterolateral aspect of the spine to the right. Often there is inflammatory tissue anterior to the disk space, which makes mobilization of the vascular structures difficult. Identification and transection (between clips) of segmental vessels is sometimes necessary. Either table-held retractors or hand-held vein-type retractors can be used on each side of the spine to create a safe working area for the remainder of the procedure (Figure 7-13).

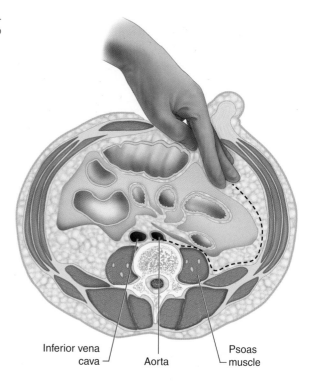

FIGURE 7-12 Retroperitoneal dissection for the mini-open approach to the anterior lumbar spine.

Inferior vena cava   Aorta   Psoas muscle

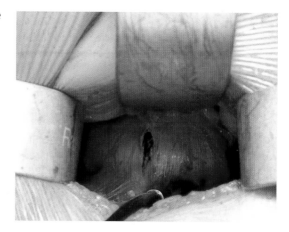

FIGURE 7-13 Completed approach to the disk space with retractors in place.

Identification of the Midline

Confirmation of the appropriate level and identification of the midline are crucial at this point of the procedure. A Z-shaped bent spinal needle, a specialized marker, or a 15-mm large-fragment screw can be placed into the disk space at the anticipated midline (the screw goes into the anterior bony cortex cephalad to the disk space). Lateral fluoroscopic images are used to verify the disk level, and an anteroposterior (AP) image, with the spine in neutral rotation, is used to show the relation of the needle or screw to the true midline. Neutral rotation should be verified by landmarks such as the symmetry of the pedicles, the position of the right and left vertebral body margins, and the location of the spinous process, in that order of reliability (Tips from the Masters 7-3). Rotation of the bed, rather than of the C-arm, may be necessary to give a true AP image. Cautery is generally used to mark the midline on the adjacent anterior vertebral bodies.

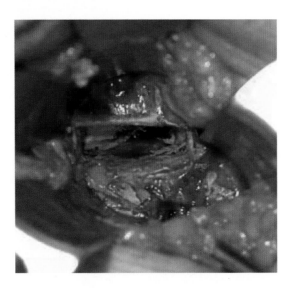

FIGURE 7-14 Clinical photograph of completed diskectomy.

Tips from the Masters 7-3 • Midline determination is vital for subsequent trialing and implantation of the TDR prosthesis.

Diskectomy and End-Plate Preparation

An anterior annulotomy is completed using a long-handled knife, centered on the midline mark, with the cutting always proceeding away from the retracted vessels. A sharp Cobb elevator is then used to carefully dissect the disk material off the superior and inferior end plates. The majority of the disk can then be excised using a pituitary rongeur. With severely collapsed disk spaces, small curettes may be needed to gain entry into the disk space. Larger curettes or ringed curettes are then used to débride the cartilaginous end plate. During end-plate preparation, careful attention should be used to avoid perforation of the end plate, which is especially important in arthroplasty cases (Tips from the Masters 7-4).

Tips from the Masters 7-4 • During end-plate preparation, it is critical to avoid perforation into cancellous bone, especially for TDRs. Also, special attention must be given to obtaining an adequate posterolateral corner diskectomy and end-plate preparation.

The entire disk space should be cleaned of all remaining disk material and end-plate cartilage; only the lateral annulus and the posterior longitudinal ligament should be left. Meticulous diskectomy in the posterolateral corners is more crucial for successful mobilization and implantation for arthroplasty than for fusion. The final diskectomy should be symmetrical and complete as far posterior as the posterior longitudinal ligament in all arthroplasty cases (Figure 7-14).

Remobilization

For successful arthroplasty, it is important to fully restore the disk height to re-create a mobile segment. Often the segment is significantly degenerated and collapsed, which makes it necessary to meticulously release all remaining constraining soft tissues. An angled curette placed within the disk space can be used to elevate the posterior longitudinal ligament from the posterior vertebral body of both the caudal and cephalad levels, which helps in remobilization. Lateral fluoroscopic images can be made with the curette in place to aid in accomplishing this dissection safely and successfully (Figure 7-15). Also, there is often a posterior lip of bone that may need to be removed to get the prosthesis as far posterior as possible. This too can be done

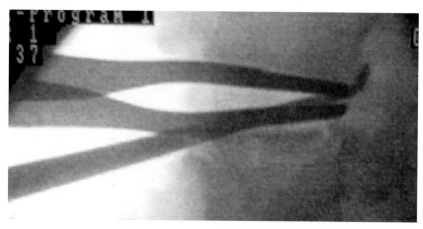

FIGURE 7-15 Release of the posterior longitudinal ligament with a curette dissecting along the posterior vertebral body.

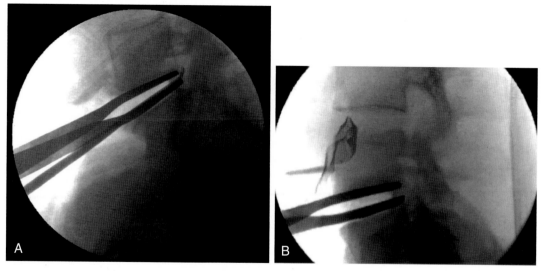

FIGURE 7-16 Intraoperative images showing use of disk space distractors to aid in remobilization. **A,** Initial insertion. **B,** After distraction.

with a curette or a Kerrison rongeur. In very collapsed disk spaces, the posterior longitudinal ligament may need to be resected.

Tips from the Masters 7-5 • Remobilization is an important step in the procedure and directly affects the function of the TDR device.

Specialized distractors may also be used to aid in remobilization of the degenerative segment (Tips from the Masters 7-5). Care must be taken to insert the distractors properly, placing them as far posterior in the disk space as possible, resting on the cortical ring, to avoid perforation of the end plate (Figure 7-16).

Trialing

After remobilization of the spinal segment, trial implants can be inserted into the disk space. For the ProDisc-L, it is best always to start with a 10-mm trial implant and increase the size depending on the resistance felt and the relative disk height of the adjacent levels as seen on lateral fluoroscopic images. The trial implants should be centered on the previously marked midline on the vertebral bodies. Having the operating bed break at the level of the operated disk space can aid in placing the trial implant

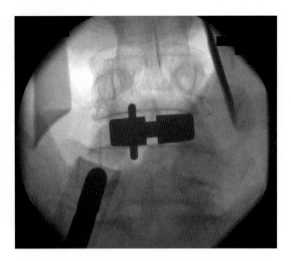

FIGURE 7-17 Trial implant in place. Notice that the notch in the center of the trial device lines up with the spinous processes and that the lateral disk space remaining is equal on the left and right.

TABLE 7-2   Different Size Combinations of the ProDisc-L and Charité Artificial Disk Replacements

ProDisc-L	Charité
Medium or large footprint	Anteroposterior length of 25-31 mm; width of 31.5-42 mm
Superior end-plate angulation of 6° or 11°	End-plate angulation of 0°, 5°, 7.5°, or 10°
Ultra-high-molecular-weight polyethylene insert height of 10 mm, 12 mm, or 14 mm	Core height of 7.5-10.5 mm

by putting the torso into extension and thereby opening the anterior disk space. Once a trial implant of the appropriate size is placed, an AP image is taken to verify the position of the implant in the midline (Figure 7-17). Careful attention should be paid to implant rotation as well. If the trial implant is translated off center, further diskectomy or annulotomy may be required to balance the disk and allow the implant to center.

Device Preparation

For arthroplasty, the two FDA-approved devices at this time are the ProDisc-L and the Charité. The size of the device for implantation should be decided from the fit of the trial component. Both devices are available in several different variations and combinations of width, depth, and height (Table 7-2). The Charité device has spikes on the end-plate surface for initial stabilization. It requires no further preparation. The ProDisc-L device is a keeled device and requires preparation of the vertebral bodies for the keels. This is accomplished by using the trial implant as a cutting jig and using the appropriately sized chisel that slides over the trial implant insertion stem. If the table has been broken for disk space access, the bed should be returned to a neutral position before the keel channels are cut. After keel preparation, the keel tract should be débrided of any remaining cancellous bone debris and the disk space cleared of any remaining debris.

Device Insertion

Steady, deliberate mallet blows should be applied to the insertion device for both the ProDisc-L and the Charité implants. Ancillary personnel in the operating room should visually aid the surgeon in keeping the device handle perpendicular to the floor. Lateral fluoroscopic images should be made frequently to verify the trajectory angle as well as the depth. Ideally, the device should be inserted as far posterior as possible (see Figure 7-10). For the ProDisc-L, the polyethylene portion of the bearing surface is inserted last, between the two end plates. It is crucial to verify proper insertion and locking of the polyethylene component. Recently, the manufacturer

FIGURE 7-18 Final intraoperative AP fluoroscopic image showing correct placement of the device. Again, note that the keel lines up with the spinous processes and that the lateral disk space remaining is equal on the left and right.

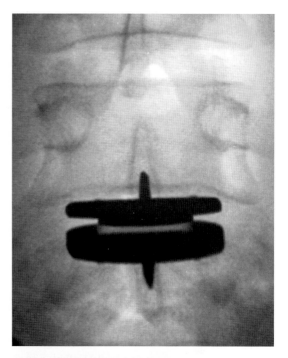

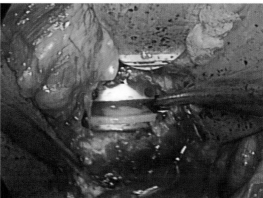

FIGURE 7-19 Intraoperative clinical photograph showing correct device placement. Notice that for this particular semiconstrained device, there is no gapping or separation at the juncture of the polyethylene and the inferior end plate of the device. When an unconstrained device is used, the surgeon must check that the polyethylene core is properly engaged by the end plates.

has added a radiopaque marker within the anterior aspect of the polyethylene that aids identification of the anterior aspect of the component on lateral fluoroscopic images, but it should *not* be used as an aid in determining locking of the polyethylene component. This must be done by visual and tactile confirmation by the operating surgeon. Final AP fluoroscopic images should be made to verify the position of the prosthesis within the center of the disk space, using the appropriate anatomic landmarks previously described (Figure 7-18).

Finally, the device and disk space should be inspected visually to verify that there is no significant debris within the bearing surfaces and to confirm that the TDR device is still properly assembled after insertion (Figure 7-19).

DISCUSSION OF BEST EVIDENCE

Although the literature is replete with case reports, case series, and retrospective studies, the current trend in validating treatment options in spinal surgery is to use studies with the highest level of evidence possible. To make evidence-based decisions regarding treatment options, it is necessary to concentrate on Level I evidence. Sackett[27] first described a grading system to classify clinical research studies, and the *Journal of Bone and Joint Surgery, American Volume,* modified the grading system in 2003.[28] This system has been applied to all *Journal of Bone and Joint Surgery* studies since then. Many other journals have followed this trend. In the journal *Spine,* approximately 16% of studies published are considered to provide the highest level of evidence—level I.[29] A Level I study is defined as a well-designed randomized controlled trial with standardized randomization and follow-up of more than 80% of patients. Systematic reviews of randomized controlled trials are also considered Level I studies. The FDA IDE studies of arthroplasty versus fusion fit the respective criteria for a Level I study.

In determining whether fusion or TDR should be performed, several areas need to be considered to formulate an evidence-based conclusion. First and foremost, is an intervention even warranted in cases of degenerative disk disease? Has the patient failed to benefit from an adequate course of nonoperative treatment and is the patient functionally disabled due to a clearly defined pain generator within the disk? What advantages does one surgical treatment offer over the other in terms of complications related to the intervention, cost-effectiveness, longevity of the implant, and adjacent-segment considerations?

Operative versus Nonoperative Treatment

Historically, determining the appropriate treatment of degenerative disk disease has presented a difficult situation for the patient and the spinal surgeon. What constitutes adequate nonoperative treatment is widely debated and is the topic of several-day–long scientific meetings. Long-term data on spinal fusion operations have classically failed to show consistent outcomes, and outcomes have not improved with fusion rates. Unfortunately, many of these studies have historically combined patients with various diagnoses and have failed to specifically identify patients with truly diskogenic back pain. Very few studies specifically deal with symptomatic degenerative disk disease in patients who had positive diskogram findings.[30-32] When patients were appropriately selected based on provocative diskographic results, these studies showed a 65% to 85% success rate after fusion.

In regard to operative versus nonoperative intervention, there does appear to be a statistically significant trend favoring operative treatment after adequate conservative treatment. The 2001 Volvo clinical study award was given to a **randomized controlled multicenter study** comparing surgical and nonsurgical interventions for chronic low back pain with evidence of disk degeneration on radiographic studies.[33] The surgical group consisted of 222 patients treated with different types of fusion techniques; the nonsurgical group was comprised of 72 patients managed with intensive conservative treatment. Patient ages ranged from 25 to 65 years and follow-up was a minimum of 24 months. At follow-up, the surgical group showed statistically better results with regard to back pain, Oswestry Disability Index score, patient satisfaction, and rate of return to work. Although there was a 17% complication rate in the surgical group, the study concluded that the surgical intervention, regardless of fusion technique, was superior to nonsurgical treatment in this patient population.

Carreon and colleagues[8] conducted a systematic **review of the literature** concerning operative versus nonoperative treatment of chronic low back pain. Using only well-designed prospective randomized trials, they concluded that patients with a specific diagnosis and surgical indication (spondylolisthesis or degenerative disk disease) had a better outcome with fusion than with nonsurgical treatments. Another systematic review showed significant flaws in the study design of qualified Level I studies with regard to treatment options for chronic low back pain, noting that these studies had shortcomings, including high crossover rates, low follow-up rates, and insufficient power.[34] Ultimately, there are no well-designed Level I studies comparing nonsurgical treatment with fusion in which patients with positive findings on diskography are randomly assigned into treatment groups; however, based on the best available evidence, it seems that surgical intervention imparts a statistically significant outcomes advantage over nonsurgical treatment in appropriately selected patients.

Disk Replacement versus Fusion

In regard to TDR, the only existing long-term series are European studies. David[35] reported greater than an 80% excellent or good long-term (more than 10 years) clinical success rate after TDR using the Charité device. This study found that 90% of prostheses were still mobile at a mean of 13.2 years of follow-up. The reoperation rate for TDR patients was 7.5%, and the rate of adjacent-level degeneration was found to be 2.8%. Almost 90% of the patients returned to work after TDR. As for complications, David reported a 4.6% rate of facet arthrosis, a 2.8% rate of subsidence, and less than a 2% rate of core subluxation. Lemaire and co-workers[36] showed similar long-term success rates using the Charité device at a mean 10.3 years of follow-up, with only 10% of patients having a poor clinical outcome. This study reported a subsidence rate of 2%, with a 5% rate of revision to a fusion. The Lemaire study also found that about 90% of eligible patients returned to their previous work status. Both the aforementioned European studies demonstrated a successful long-term clinical outcome, but both studies lack comparison to a control group and thus are deemed Level III studies.

Prospective randomized clinical trials comparing TDR to fusion have come from the FDA-regulated studies. At the time of this writing, results of two of these Level I trials have been published.[37,38] In the Charité Artificial Disc study, single-level TDR at L5-S1 or L4-5 was compared with anterior fusion with standalone Bagby and Kuslich (BAK) cages (Spine-Tech, Inc., Minneapolis) and autograft.[37] In the ProDisc-L study, TDR was compared with combined anterior-posterior fusion for single-level involvement at L5-S1, L4-5, or L3-4.[38] In both trials, TDR produced results at least similar to those of fusion and superior to fusion results on some measures. The longest follow-up for FDA-regulated trials is 5 years. The Charité study reported that at 5-year follow-up, lumbar TDR produced similar outcomes overall compared with the fusion procedure. Improvements in Oswestry Disability Index, VAS, and Short Form 36 (SF-36) Health Survey scores were similar in both groups.[39] The TDR group showed less long-term disability and higher rates of full-time employment than the fusion group ($P < .05$). Additional index-level surgery was needed in 7.7% of TDR patients versus 16.3% of fusion patients. Adjacent-level range of motion (ROM) and index-level ROM were not statistically different from the 2-year data.[40] There were no differences in TDR function and outcomes compared with fusion regardless of whether TDR was carried out at the L4-5 level or at the L5-S1 level.

Adjacent-Level Disease

In a **literature review** (Level III study), Park and associates[41] reported a wide variation in rates of adjacent-segment degeneration (ASD) after lumbar fusion, ranging from 5% to 100%. The classic article on ASD by Ghiselli and colleagues[42] reported the rate of symptomatic ASD after fusion to be 16% at 5 years and 36.1% at 10 years. Although this was also a Level III study, it provides a historic control for the expected rate of ASD. Furthermore, the only published prospective study of ASD, which was categorized as a Level II study owing to loss of patients to follow-up, shows a comparable 10-year rate of ASD of 38%.[43]

With regard to ASD after TDR, clinical data are still being collected and analyzed. Long-term European studies have shown ASD to be less than 3% at 13 years of follow-up.[35] Studies in the United States have not reported long-term clinical data as of yet. The hypothesis is that TDR, by maintaining motion at the index level, should lessen the burden on adjacent levels to restore total lumbar motion. A recent **cadaveric study**[44] specifically investigated adjacent-level kinematics and intradisk pressures in the intact spine compared with those in an L4-5 TDR-instrumented spine and a salvage fusion of the L4-5 TDR (addition of pedicle screws). After TDR, the motion at the adjacent level was either maintained or slightly decreased in comparison with the intact spine. With the simulated fusion at the L4-5 level, there was a significant decrease in motion at the operative level and a compensatory increase in adjacent-level motion in flexion only. The intradisk pressure of the adjacent level was increased in lateral bending, but not with flexion. A finite element analysis also showed a compensatory increase in adjacent-level annular stress and ROM after a fusion procedure (PLIF with pedicle screws), whereas the TDR model showed hypermobility at the index level but maintained motion and normal facet contact stresses at both adjacent levels.[45] These biomechanical studies support the notion that TDR has positive effects on the adjacent level compared with what occurs in the setting of fusion and resultant loss of motion at the index level. These in vitro findings have yet to be validated clinically in a Level I study; however, when the rate of adjacent-level disease found in David's TDR study (2.8%)[35] is compared with the historical rate of adjacent disease in the patient undergoing fusion (36% at 10-year follow-up),[42] there is an obvious demonstrable clinical advantage of the TDR procedure in reducing degenerative changes at the adjacent level.

Complications

Both fusion and arthroplasty have their respective complications. The anterior approach itself carries the potential for vascular complications, retrograde ejaculation, hernia formation, sympathetic nerve disruption, and bowel injuries (although the latter is rare). When access is performed by experienced surgeons, the overall rate of serious vascular complications with an anterior approach is less than 2%.[25] With TDR, device failure is also an inherent concern. In the European long-term studies,[35] there was a 4.7% rate of device-related complications, with three instances of subsidence and two occurrences of core subluxation. In the FDA IDE **prospective randomized clinical trial** comparative studies,[37] the Charité trial reported that complication rates were similar for the TDR group and the fusion group at 2-year follow-up. The 5-year data for this trial showed a higher rate of additional index-level surgery in the fusion group than in the TDR group (16.3% vs. 7.7%), which indicates a higher rate of complicated outcomes in the fusion group.[39] The ProDisc-L FDA trial actually showed a 0% rate of serious complications in the TDR group and a statistically superior neurologic outcome in this group compared with the fusion group.[38]

Posterior fusion using interbody devices also has associated complications, with the rate of neurologic injury reported to be as high as 7%.[19] Although no Level I studies exist comparing TLIF or PLIF with TDR, when fusion in general is compared with TDR, it is evident that the rate of complications in patients undergoing TDR is the same as or better than the rate in patients undergoing fusion, especially with regard to the need for additional surgical intervention at the index level.

Financial Considerations

In this society focused on evidence-based medicine, there is also a push toward cost-effectiveness of surgical interventions. For degenerative disk disease, there are no prospective studies investigating the financial implications of nonoperative versus operative intervention; however, multiple studies have investigated the cost differences between fusion and TDR in **retrospective reviews.** Examining solely hospital charges, Patel and colleagues[46] compared the costs for single-level TLIF, anterior-posterior fusion, anterior standalone fusion, and TDR. No fusion procedures used BMPs, which would have added significantly to the hospital charges in the fusion cases. Patel and colleagues found that TLIF, anterior fusion, and TDR incurred similar costs, whereas AP fusion was significantly more expensive. Levine and associates[47] also showed that for single-level degenerative disk disease, circumferential fusion was significantly more expensive than TDR ($46,280 vs. $35,593). Taking into consideration both the direct medical costs of the index procedure and costs incurred in the first 2 years postoperatively, Guyer and co-workers[48] showed that TDR was no more expensive than fusion procedures. Based on these retrospective economic evaluations, the choice between fusion and TDR has no significant economic repercussions in terms of direct medical costs.

COMMENTARY

The advent of TDR marks a movement toward motion-preserving technology in treatment of the spine, analogous to the situation in the 1960s and 1970s when peripheral joint arthroplasty supplanted fusion in the treatment of functionally disabling degenerative joint disease of the hip and knee. Preservation of motion is intuitively desirable. TDR has been shown to maintain motion at the index level and lessen the stress at adjacent-level disks[44]; this forms the biomechanical foundation from which TDR has evolved. In the laboratory, based on cadaveric preparations as well as computer models using finite element analysis, TDR has been shown to protect the adjacent-level disk better than fusion. This finding is clinically mirrored in long-term data from Level III studies in Europe showing a rate of degeneration in adjacent levels of less than 3%,[35] compared with long-term data for fusions that report adjacent-level disease rates nearing 40% at 10 years.[43,49]

As with any new technology, ongoing scrutiny is mandatory. Postmarket surveillance has been required by the FDA for both the ProDisc-L and Charité single-level devices. A mechanism for extremely high capture of real-life complication rates is thereby in place.

A thorough review has been presented of the surgical options and evidence-based decision making that justify the opinion that motion preservation is equal if not superior to fusion for the particular patient described in the Case Presentation. Medium-term follow-up is now available in Level I studies that support this view. It should be stressed that appropriate patient selection and meticulous surgical technique are paramount in obtaining successful clinical outcomes. TDR would also be a viable option at the L3-4 level and the L5-S1 level. Since March 2000, the surgical group at the Texas Back Institute has implanted over 1000 lumbar TDR devices from L3 to S1. Their unpublished data show a revision rate of less than 2% for all TDR devices implanted, whereas the rate of reoperation in fusion patients nears 17% in the 5-year data from the FDA IDE.[39] Based on this experience, and on the available best evidence as discussed in this chapter, TDR appears to be equivalent and possibly superior to fusion with regard to clinical outcomes, radiographically determined success, complication profiles, and cost-effectiveness. With secondary findings of earlier and more frequent return to work and decreased medication usage in the arthroplasty patient cohorts, indirect costs for arthroplasty may prove to be significantly better in the intermediate stages. If a decrease in adjacent-level disease is demonstrated in coming years, resulting in a less frequent need for transition-level reoperation (the holy grail of arthroplasty), the choice of arthroplasty may be overwhelmingly favored.

REFERENCES

1. Coppes MH, Marani E, Thomeer RT, et al: Innervation of "painful" lumbar discs, *Spine* 22:2342–2349, 1997.
2. Freemont AJ, Peacock TE, Goupille P, et al: Nerve ingrowth into diseased intervertebral disc in chronic back pain, *Lancet* 350:178–181, 1997.
3. Boos N, Rieder R, Schade V, et al: 1995 Volvo Award in clinical sciences. The diagnostic accuracy of magnetic resonance imaging, work perception, and psychosocial factors in identifying symptomatic disc herniations, *Spine* 20:2613–2625, 1995.
4. Flanagan MN, Chung BU: Roentgenographic changes in 188 patients 10-20 years after discography and chemonucleolysis, *Spine* 11:444–448, 1986.
5. Carragee EJ, Don AS, Hurwitz EL, et al: 2009 ISSLS prize winner: Does discography cause accelerated progression of degeneration changes in the lumbar disc: a ten-year matched cohort study, *Spine* 34:2338–2345, 2009.
6. Cloward RB: *New treatment of ruptured intervertebral discs*, May 1945, Paper presented at the annual meeting of the Hawaii Territorial Medical Association.
7. Fritzell P, Hagg O, Wessberg P, et al: Chronic low back pain and fusion: a comparison of three surgical techniques: a prospective multicenter randomized study from the Swedish Lumbar Spine Study Group, *Spine* 27:1131–1141, 2002.
8. Carreon LY, Glassman SD, Howard J: Fusion and nonsurgical treatment for symptomatic lumbar degenerative disease: a systematic review of Oswestry Disability Index and MOS Short Form-36 outcomes, *Spine J* 8:747–755, 2008.

9. Charnley J: Arthroplasty of the hip. A new operation, *Lancet* 1:1129–1132, 1961.
10. Fernström U: Arthroplasty with intercorporal endoprosthesis in herniated disc and in painful disc, *Acta Chir Scand Suppl* 357:154–159, 1966.
11. McAfee PC, Lee GA, Fedder IL, et al: Anterior BAK instrumentation and fusion: complete versus partial discectomy, *Clin Orthop Relat Res* (394):55–63, Jan 2002.
12. Gerber M, Crawford NR, Chamberlain RH, et al: Biomechanical assessment of anterior lumbar interbody fusion with an anterior lumbosacral fixation screw-plate: comparison to stand-alone anterior lumbar interbody fusion and anterior lumbar interbody fusion with pedicle screws in an unstable human cadaver model, *Spine* 31:762–768, 2006.
13. Tzermiadianos MN, Mekhail A, Voronov LI, et al: Enhancing the stability of anterior lumbar interbody fusion: a biomechanical comparison of anterior plate versus posterior transpedicular instrumentation, *Spine* 33:E38–E43, 2008.
14. Burkus JK, Gornet MF, Dickman CA, et al: Anterior lumbar interbody fusion using rhBMP-2 with tapered interbody cages, *J Spinal Disord Tech* 15:337–349, 2002.
15. Anand N, Baron EM, Thaiyananthan G, et al: Minimally invasive multilevel percutaneous correction and fusion for adult lumbar degenerative scoliosis: a technique and feasibility study, *J Spinal Disord Tech* 21:459–467, 2008.
16. Knight RQ, Schwaegler P, Hanscom D, et al: Direct lateral lumbar interbody fusion for degenerative conditions: early complication profile, *J Spinal Disord Tech* 22:34–37, 2009.
17. Benglis DM, Vanni S, Levi AD: An anatomical study of the lumbosacral plexus as related to the minimally invasive transpsoas approach to the lumbar spine, *J Neurosurg Spine* 10:139–144, 2009.
18. Regev GJ, Chen L, Dhawan M, et al: Morphometric analysis of the ventral nerve roots and retroperitoneal vessels with respect to the minimally invasive lateral approach in normal and deformed spines, *Spine* 34:1330–1335, 2009.
19. Krishna M, Pollock RD, Bhatia C: Incidence, etiology, classification, and management of neuralgia after posterior lumbar interbody fusion surgery in 226 patients, *Spine J* 8:374–379, 2008.
20. Humphreys SC, Hodges SD, Patwardhan AG, et al: Comparison of posterior and transforaminal approaches to lumbar interbody fusion, *Spine* 26:567–571, 2001.
21. Grob D, Benini A, Junge A, et al: Clinical experience with the Dynesys semirigid fixation system for the lumbar spine: surgical and patient-oriented outcome in 50 cases after an average of 2 years, *Spine* 30:324–331, 2005.
22. Jagannathan J, Chankaew E, Urban P, et al: Cosmetic and functional outcomes following paramedian and anterolateral retroperitoneal access in anterior lumbar spine surgery, *J Neurosurg Spine* 9:454–465, 2008.
23. Sasso RC, Kenneth Burkus J, LeHuec JC: Retrograde ejaculation after anterior lumbar interbody fusion: transperitoneal versus retroperitoneal exposure, *Spine* 28:1023–1026, 2003.
24. Jarrett CD, Heller JG, Tsai L: Anterior exposure of the lumbar spine with and without an "access surgeon": morbidity analysis of 265 consecutive cases, *J Spinal Disord Tech* 22:559–564, 2009.
25. Brau SA, Delamarter RB, Schiffman ML, et al: Vascular injury during anterior lumbar surgery, *Spine J* 4:409–412, 2004.
26. Rodriguez HE, Connolly MM, Dracopoulos H, et al: Anterior access to the lumbar spine: laparoscopic versus open, *Am Surg* 68:978–982, 2002.
27. Sackett DL: Rules of evidence and clinical recommendations on the use of antithrombotic agents, *Chest* 89:2S–3S, 1986.
28. Wright JG, Swiontkowski MF, Heckman JD: Introducing levels of evidence to the journal, *J Bone Joint Surg Am* 85-A:1–3, 2003.
29. Wupperman R, Davis R, Obremskey WT: Level of evidence in *Spine* compared to other orthopedic journals, *Spine* 32:388–393, 2007.
30. Blumenthal SL, Baker J, Dossett A, et al: The role of anterior lumbar fusion for internal disc disruption, *Spine* 13:566–569, 1988.
31. Newman MH, Grinstead GL: Anterior lumbar interbody fusion for internal disc disruption, *Spine* 17:831–833, 1992.
32. Linson MA, Williams H: Anterior and combined anteroposterior fusion for lumbar disc pain. A preliminary study, *Spine* 16:143–145, 1991.
33. Fritzell P, Hagg O, Wessberg P, et al: 2001 Volvo Award Winner in Clinical Studies: Lumbar fusion versus nonsurgical treatment for chronic low back pain: a multicenter randomized controlled trial from the Swedish Lumbar Spine Study Group, *Spine* 26:2521–2532, 2001. **This study is a randomized controlled trial with 2 years of follow-up comparing the outcomes in patients with chronic low back pain and disk degeneration treated by surgical and nonsurgical means. Patients were randomly chosen to receive either surgical or nonsurgical treatment. A total of 222 patients were randomly assigned to undergo one of three different fusion procedures, and the remaining 72 received various physical therapy treatments. Intergroup differences in disability scores, back pain ratings, rate of return to work, and self-ratings of improvement all reached statistical significance in favor of surgical intervention.**
34. Mirza SK, Deyo RA: Systematic review of randomized trials comparing lumbar fusion surgery to nonoperative care for treatment of chronic back pain, *Spine* 32:816–823, 2007.
35. David T: Long-term results of one-level lumbar arthroplasty: minimum 10-year follow-up of the CHARITE artificial disc in 106 patients, *Spine* 32:661–666, 2007. **A Level III study of total disk arthroplasty with long-term follow-up. Eighty percent of patients reported excellent or good clinical results after TDR using the Charité implants at a mean of 13.2 years of follow-up. Ninety percent of prostheses were still mobile. The reoperation rate for TDR patients was 7.5%, and the rate of adjacent-level**

degeneration was found to be 2.8%. Almost 90% of the patients returned to work after TDR. Complication rate was 4.6%, with subsidence occurring in 2.8% of patients and core subluxation in fewer than 2%.

36. Lemaire JP, Carrier H, Sariali el H, et al: Clinical and radiological outcomes with the Charité artificial disc: a 10-year minimum follow-up, *J Spinal Disord Tech* 18:353–359, 2005.

37. Blumenthal S, McAfee PC, Guyer RD, et al: A prospective, randomized, multicenter Food and Drug Administration investigational device exemptions study of lumbar total disc replacement with the CHARITE artificial disc versus lumbar fusion. Part I: evaluation of clinical outcomes, *Spine* 30: 1565–1575, 2005. A Level I study comparing TDR with the Charité Artificial Disc to anterior lumbar interbody fusion for the treatment of single-level degenerative disk disease from L4 to S1. Three hundred four patients were enrolled in the study and were randomly assigned in a 2:1 ratio to either the TDR or the fusion procedure. Minimum follow-up was 24 months. Patients in both groups showed significant improvement following surgery, but the artificial disk group experienced faster recovery and lower levels of disability. At the 24-month follow-up, a significantly greater percentage of patients in the TDR group than in the fusion group were satisfied with the outcome (*P* < .05). The hospital stay was significantly shorter in the TDR group (*P* <.05); complication rates were similar in the two groups.

38. Zigler J, Delamarter R, Spivak JM, et al: Results of the prospective, randomized, multicenter Food and Drug Administration investigational device exemption study of the ProDisc-L total disc replacement versus circumferential fusion for the treatment of 1-level degenerative disc disease, *Spine* 32: 1155–1162, 2007. A Level I study comparing lumbar TDR using the ProDisc-L device with circumferential spinal fusion for the treatment of diskogenic pain at a single level from L3 to S1 in 286 patients. At 24 months, 91.8% of patients undergoing TDR and 84.5% of patients undergoing fusion had improvement in Oswestry Disability Index scores from preoperative levels, and overall neurologic success in the TDR group was superior to that in the fusion group (91.2% in the TDR group vs. 81.4% in the fusion group; *P* = .0341). The VAS pain assessment showed statistically significant improvement from preoperative levels regardless of treatment (*P* < .0001), with a statistically significant difference favoring TDR over fusion (*P* = .015). Radiographically determined ROM was maintained within a normal functional range in 93.7% of patients undergoing TDR and averaged 7.7 degrees.

39. Guyer RD, McAfee PC, Banco RJ, et al: Prospective, randomized, multicenter Food and Drug Administration investigational device exemption study of lumbar total disc replacement with the CHARITE artificial disc versus lumbar fusion: five-year follow-up, *Spine J* 9:374–386, 2009. Analysis of follow-up data for patients enrolled in the randomized controlled Charité IDE trial, with 160 patients completing the 5-year follow-up. Overall success was 57.8% in the group undergoing TDR using the Charité device group versus 51.2% in the group undergoing fusion using the BAK cage and iliac crest autograft (*P* = .0359). No statistical differences were found in clinical outcomes between the two groups. In patient satisfaction surveys, 78% of TDR patients were satisfied versus 72% of fusion patients. A total of 65.6% of patients in the TDR group were employed full time versus 46.5% of patients in the fusion group (*P* = .0403). Additional index-level surgery was performed in 7.7% of TDR patients and 16.3% of fusion patients. At the 5-year follow-up, the mean ROM at the index level was 6.0 degrees for TDR patients and 1.0 degrees for fusion patients.

40. McAfee PC, Cunningham B, Holsapple G, et al: A prospective, randomized, multicenter Food and Drug Administration investigational device exemption study of lumbar total disc replacement with the CHARITE artificial disc versus lumbar fusion. Part II: evaluation of radiographic outcomes and correlation of surgical technique accuracy with clinical outcomes, *Spine* 30:1576–1583, 2005. A Level I study with 24-month follow-up in which a total of 304 patients were randomly assigned in a 2:1 ratio to undergo TDR using the Charité Artificial Disc or anterior fusion using a BAK cage and iliac crest bone graft. Patients in the TDR group had a 13.6% mean increase in ROM, and those in the fusion group had an 82.5% decrease at 24 months postoperatively compared with baseline. There was significantly less subsidence in the TDR group than in the fusion group (*P* < .05). Flexion-extension range of motion and prosthesis function improved with the surgical technical accuracy of placement as determined radiographically (*P* = 0.003), which was found to be ideal in 83% of implants.

41. Park P, Garton HJ, Gala VC, et al: Adjacent segment disease after lumbar or lumbosacral fusion: review of the literature, *Spine* 29:1938–1944, 2004.

42. Ghiselli G, Wang JC, Bhatia NN, et al: Adjacent segment degeneration in the lumbar spine, *J Bone Joint Surg Am* 86-A:1497–1503, 2004. A long-term analysis with survivorship curves investigating the rate of degeneration in adjacent segments after lumbar fusion. Two hundred fifty patients underwent posterior lumbar fusion and were followed for a mean of 6.7 years. Radiographic analysis of the adjacent disk space for evidence of degeneration was performed. The disease-free prediction based on survivorship statistics was 83.5% and 63.9% at 5 and 10 years, respectively. These data indicate that the rate of adjacent-segment degeneration would be greater than 35% at 10-year follow-up after a lumbar fusion.

43. Ekman P, Moller H, Shalabi A, et al: A prospective randomised study on the long-term effect of lumbar fusion on adjacent disc degeneration, *Eur Spine J* 18(8):1175–1186, 2009.

44. Ingalhalikar AV, Reddy CG, Lim TH, et al: Effect of lumbar total disc arthroplasty on the segmental motion and intradiscal pressure at the adjacent level: an in vitro biomechanical study: presented at the 2008 Joint Spine Section Meeting Laboratory investigation, *J Neurosurg Spine* 11:715–723, 2009. Ten human cadaveric spines (L2 to S1) were potted and treated with a Maverick ball-and-socket artificial disk at the L4-5 level. Motion at both the implanted level and immediately adjacent levels was measured, and intradisk pressure at the L3-4 adjacent level was also measured. After addition of pedicle screws and rods at the L4-5 level, the segments were retested. The artificial disk was found to maintain

or reduce adjacent-level motion and intradisk pressure, compared with the intact spine. The addition of pedicle screws significantly increased motion at adjacent levels in flexion and significantly increased intradisk pressure in lateral bending.

45. Chen SH, Zhong ZC, Chen CS, et al: Biomechanical comparison between lumbar disc arthroplasty and fusion, *Med Eng Phys* 31:244–253, 2009.
46. Patel VV, Estes S, Lindley EM, et al: Lumbar spinal fusion versus anterior lumbar disc replacement: the financial implications, *J Spinal Disord Tech* 21:473–476, 2008.
47. Levin DA, Bendo JA, Quirno M, et al: Comparative charge analysis of one- and two-level lumbar total disc arthroplasty versus circumferential lumbar fusion, *Spine* 32:2905–2909, 2007.
48. Guyer RD, Tromanhauser SG, Regan JJ: An economic model of one-level lumbar arthroplasty versus fusion, *Spine J* 7:558–562, 2007.
49. Ekman P, Moller H, Shalabi A, et al: A prospective randomised study on the long-term effect of lumbar fusion on adjacent disc degeneration, *Eur Spine J* 18:1175–1186, 2009.

Chapter 8

Degenerative Spondylolisthesis with Radicular Pain: Decompression-Only Versus Decompression and Fusion

Tuan V. Nguyen, Robert A. McGuire, Jr.

Descriptions of deformity of the lumbosacral spine comprising slipped vertebrae or defects of the pars interarticularis were first reported in 1782 by Herbiniaux.[1] Since that time, multiple classifications have been proposed to describe spondylolisthesis in terms of pathology related to the pars interarticularis and/or facet anatomy. Degenerative spondylolisthesis has been included in the most commonly used classification scheme used today. Other types include congenital, isthmic, traumatic, pathologic, and postsurgical.[2]

Degenerative spondylolisthesis is most commonly seen in middle-aged women at L4-5, less commonly at L3-4, and rarely at L5-S1. Synovial surfaces of the superior and inferior facets at these levels are biomechanically important because they resist rotation along the coronal plane and anterior slippage along the sagittal plane. The degenerative cascade results in damage to the facet joint and hypermobility, which contributes to spondylolisthesis. Concomitant hypertrophy of the ligamentum flavum and facet joint below an intact posterior neural arch that has slipped forward produces spinal stenosis and resulting clinical neurogenic claudication as the neural elements are compromised. The cause of symptoms is lateral recess stenosis from slippage of the inferior facet forward and central stenosis from disk herniation.

In the process of neural element decompression, the spondylolisthesis can be exacerbated. The management of this disease process in grade I spondylolisthesis is discussed in this chapter, with an emphasis on best evidence.

CASE PRESENTATION

A 72-year-old white woman had a 4-year history of progressive low back pain and neurogenic claudication symptoms.

- PMH: Unremarkable
- PSH: Unremarkable
- Exam: Well-developed, well-nourished elderly woman, ambulatory with cane assistance, antalgic gait, normal muscle bulk and tone, motor strength 5/5 in all extremities, normal results on sensory examination, deep tendon reflexes symmetric bilaterally.
- Imaging: Preoperative radiographs showed grade I spondylolisthesis at L3-4 (Figure 8-1, *A* and *B*). Magnetic resonance imaging (MRI) of the lumbar spine revealed degenerative Modic end-plate changes at L5-S1; lumbar stenosis at L3-5 secondary to facet arthropathy greater at L3-4 than at L4-5; and a hypertrophic ligamentum flavum. The spondylolisthesis at L3-4 and disk herniation at this level contributed to central and lateral recess stenosis (Figure 8-1, *C* through *E*) (Tips from the Masters 8-1).

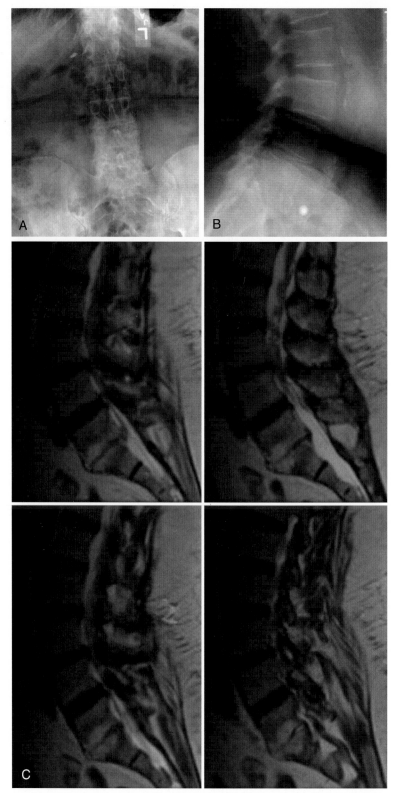

FIGURE 8-1 Preoperative images showing grade I spondylolisthesis at L3-4. **A,** Anteroposterior radiograph of lumbar spine. **B,** Sagittal radiograph of lumbar spine. **C,** T2-weighted sagittal MRI images of the lumbar spine.

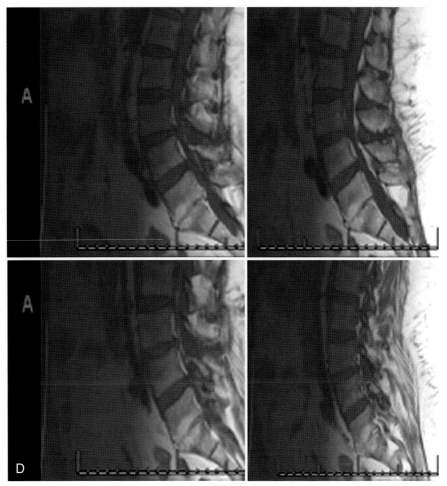

FIGURE 8-1, cont'd D, T1-weighted sagittal MRI images of the lumbar spine.

Tips from the Masters 8-1 • Look for a high-intensity area within the facet joint complex preoperatively on axial T1-weighted MRI images.

TREATMENT OPTIONS

Observation

Referral to a nutritionist for dietary management to achieve weight loss can be recommended for overweight or obese patients. Physical therapy with instruction in core stabilization exercises, appropriate lifting mechanics, and functional aerobics including water therapy can be instituted. The use of nonsteroidal antiinflammatory medications can be considered if there are no medical contraindications. Referral to a pain management clinic for consideration of epidural steroid injections may also be offered.

Laminectomy Decompression at L3 through L5

Laminectomy decompression at L3 through L5 can relieve neural compression and improve the claudication symptoms. The technique consists of medial facetectomies, which decompress the lateral recess. The MRI scan for the patient

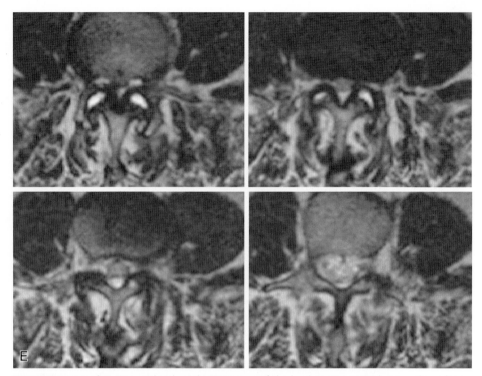

FIGURE 8-1, cont'd **E,** T2-weighted axial MRI images of the lumbar spine. MRI images show degenerative Modic end-plate changes at L5-S1; lumbar stenosis at L3-5 secondary to facet arthropathy that is greater at L3-4 than at L4-5; and a hypertrophic ligamentum flavum. The spondylolisthesis at L3-4 and disk herniation at this level contribute to central and lateral recess stenosis. Note the hyperintense signal within the facet joints bilaterally, which can indicate instability.

described in the Case Presentation revealed high-intensity signals within the facet joint, which raises the concern of instability. Caution should be used in recommending decompression only under these circumstances in patients with significant back pain.

Decompression and Fusion without Instrumentation

Decompression and fusion without instrumentation involves a posterolateral fusion of the transverse processes with local autograft, allograft bone, and demineralized bone matrix. The use of synthetic extenders with bone marrow aspirate has also been shown to lead to good fusion.

Decompression and Fusion with Instrumentation

If decompression and fusion with instrumentation is elected, inclusion of L2 or S1 should be considered. The quality of bone should also be taken into account with long constructs such as these which require that either a laterally directed sacral alar screw or an iliac screw be used to increase the stability of the construct. The use of titanium polyaxial screws and rods are recommended for improved MRI compatibility, more appropriate material elastic modulus, and ease of instrument insertion.

The patient underwent decompression and instrumented fusion from L2 through L5 because of the multiple levels of unstable spondylolisthesis and stenosis (Figure 8-2). Because the L5-S1 segment was transitional and already fused, there was no need to instrument to S1.

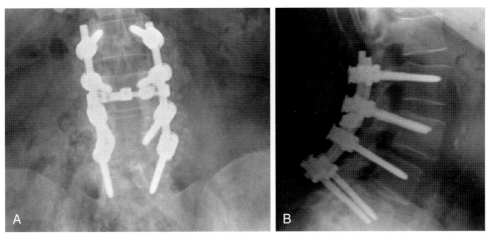

FIGURE 8-2 Postoperative images showing placement of instrumentation. **A,** AP radiograph of lumbar spine. **B,** Lateral radiograph of lumbar spine.

FUNDAMENTAL TECHNIQUE

After induction of general anesthesia, a gravity-draining Foley catheter is placed and a preoperative antibiotic (usually cefazolin) is given. The patient is turned prone onto an Andrews table, and all pressure points of the face, torso, and extremities are carefully padded. The patient is converted to a kneeling position, and care is taken to make sure the belly hangs free to limit pressure on the inferior vena cava, which aids in minimizing blood loss. Standard landmarks of the iliac crest and palpation up from the sacrum are used to delineate L2 through S1 with a marking pen. Taking radiographs at this time with a needle in place between spinous processes can help in centralizing the incision. The skin is cleansed and draped in sterile fashion. After the skin incision is made, Bovie electrocautery is used to dissect the paraspinal muscles subperiosteally so that the facet capsules and transverse processes are exposed bilaterally at each level. Care is taken not to violate facet capsules that do not need to be fused. Using standard landmarks, pilot holes are drilled, and the pedicles of L2 through S1 are probed and circumferential bone is confirmed with a ball-tip probe. These holes are covered with thrombin-soaked absorbable gelatin sponges. From the preoperative images, it is clear that the neurogenic claudication symptoms in the patient described in the Case Presentation were related primarily to the significant stenosis at L3-4 and less so to that at L4-5. In such cases, bilateral laminectomies from L3 through L5 are performed with decompression centrally and along the lateral recesses at L3-4. Ideally, leaving at least 5 mm and, if possible, 7 mm of the pars interarticularis is recommended to avoid postoperative pars fracture when the patient is upright. When undercutting to achieve a medial facetectomy, an attempt should be made to ensure that 50% of a functional facet joint complex remains, inclusive of a functioning superior facet and inferior facet. A Woodson dental instrument is used to palpate after decompression to ensure that adequate bilateral foraminotomies have been performed. A high-speed drill bur is used to decorticate the transverse processes bilaterally and the facet complexes. Locally harvested bone autograft from the spinous processes, lamina, and facets is morselized and placed in the lateral gutters to achieve posterolateral arthrodesis. Part of the pain experienced by the patient described in the Case Presentation was related to hypermobility at L3 through L5, and posterior instrumentation with a pedicle screw and rod construct provides immediate fixation and symptomatic improvement (Tips from the

Masters 8-2). A cross-link can be added to increase the overall rigidity and resist rotational forces.

Tips from the Masters 8-2 • Check standing neutral and flexion-extension radiographs preoperatively to assess for hypermobility. This can be confirmed intraoperatively with distraction on the spinous processes at L2-3 with a towel clamp, and a decision to change pedicle screw and rod instrumentation to include L2 can be made.

DISCUSSION OF BEST EVIDENCE

Studies comparing conservative treatment, laminectomy, and fusion with or without instrumentation for degenerative grade I spondylolisthesis are discussed. Investigations of the use of posterior spinous process devices are excluded. Whenever possible degenerative spondylolisthesis should be considered separately from stable lumbosacral spinal stenosis.[3]

The results of surgical intervention versus conservative treatment were evaluated by Matsudaira and colleagues[4] in a **retrospective study** involving 55 patients. At 2 years of follow-up they found that 19 patients who underwent laminectomy alone and 20 patients who underwent laminectomy with posterior instrumentation had better Japanese Orthopaedic Association (JOA) scores than 16 medically treated patients. There were no significant differences in clinical outcomes between the laminectomy and fusion groups, but both surgical arms had better outcomes than the medical therapy group. Progression of slip increased in the medical treatment and primary laminectomy groups. Weinstein and associates[5] evaluated results for an experimental cohort randomly assigned to a treatment method and an observational cohort selecting treatment in consultation with their physicians (304 and 303 patients, respectively). They found that patients with degenerative spondylolisthesis and spinal stenosis treated surgically with decompressive laminectomy with or without fusion had significantly greater improvement in pain and function during a 2-year period than patients treated nonsurgically. Weinstein and colleagues[6] later reported an "as treated" analysis of these same cohorts at 4-year follow-up. The advantages of surgery over nonsurgical care were maintained, with reduced bodily pain and increased physical function in the surgically treated group.

Fischgrund and co-workers[7] evaluated the role of instrumentation along with laminectomy in a **prospective randomized trial** involving 76 patients, although only 89% were available for 2-year follow-up. They concluded that instrumentation with posterolateral fusion increased the likelihood of arthrodesis compared with no instrumentation, but there was no significant difference in clinical outcome with the two procedures. In a **retrospective study** Kimura and colleagues[8] looked at results for 28 patients who underwent decompression and fusion without instrumentation and 29 who underwent decompression and instrumented fusion, with a 6-year follow-up for the noninstrumented group and a 3-year follow-up for the instrumented group. They found no significant benefit for instrumentation. A systematic review by Martin and associates[9] of studies with a minimum follow-up of 1 year concluded that fusion leads to better clinical outcomes than decompression alone. The addition of instrumentation results in better fusion rates and less pseudoarthrosis, but no significant differences in clinical outcome were seen for instrumented and noninstrumented fusion.

A **prospective study** by Herkowitz and Kurz[10] compared outcomes in 25 patients treated with decompression and 25 patients undergoing decompression with fusion. At 3-year follow-up the group undergoing decompression with fusion had significantly more improvement of low back pain and leg pain than the group treated with decompression alone. In the most recent of several **retrospective studies,** Ghogawala and associates[11] looked at results for 20 patients undergoing laminectomy and 14 undergoing laminectomy with posterior instrumented fusion. At 6- and 12-month follow-up they found an 83% fusion rate in the latter group. Oswestry Disability Index (ODI) scores improved by 27.5 points in the decompression and fusion group and 13.6 points in the decompression only group. Scores on the Short Form 36 (SF-36) Health Survey also showed improved functional outcome in the patients undergoing decompression and fusion. Lombardi and colleagues[12] retrospectively looked at data for 47 patients, including 6 undergoing wide laminectomy, 20 undergoing standard laminectomy with preserved facets, and 21 undergoing standard laminectomy and fusion. Mean follow-up was 2.7 years. The authors concluded that decompression with transverse process fusion was superior to decompression alone. Postacchini and Cinotti[13] retrospectively reviewed results for 8 patients treated with bilateral laminectomy and 10 patients treated with laminectomy with fusion after a mean follow-up of 8.6 years. Satisfactory results were achieved in 80% of the group undergoing fusion compared with 33% of the group undergoing decompression only. There were 16 patients with degenerative spondylolisthesis; 10 of the 16 had concomitant fusion. The authors concluded that decompression with fusion provided satisfactory long-term results. An earlier study by Postacchini and colleagues[14] retrospectively evaluated results for 32 patients after a mean 2.8-year follow-up. Fifteen had decompression alone, and 17 underwent laminectomy and fusion. The authors concluded that the addition of instrumentation led to good to excellent outcomes (100% for the instrumented group vs. 67% for the noninstrumented group). In a **prospective study** Bridwell and co-workers[15] compared results in 44 patients, only 43 of whom were available for 2-year follow-up. Nine patients had laminectomy only; the rest underwent fusion with or without instrumentation. Patients undergoing fusion with instrumentation (24 patients) were found to have a higher fusion rate and a lower proportion of slippage than patients undergoing fusion without instrumentation (10 patients). In addition, patients with stable spondylolisthesis had longer walking distances.

Controversy exists regarding whether posterior lumbar interbody fusion (PLIF) improves fusion rates or provides beneficial clinical outcomes beyond that provided by posterior instrumentation and onlay arthrodesis. In a **retrospective analysis** Rousseau and associates[16] looked at outcome data for 24 patients undergoing decompression and posterior fusion. Eight of the 24 also had PLIF. Mean follow-up was 2.8 years, with 75% of patients followed for longer than 2 years. The authors concluded that the addition of PLIF adds marginal benefit to posterior decompression and fusion alone. In another **retrospective study** Yone and colleagues[17] evaluated results for 7 elderly patients undergoing laminectomy and 10 undergoing laminectomy and instrumented fusion, and found that decompression plus fusion was better than decompression alone in individuals older than 60 years of age. Gibson and Waddell's[18] **meta-analysis** and systematic review of 31 randomized controlled trials revealed that instrumentation improved fusion rates, but clinical outcomes were only marginally better with instrumentation, and instrumentation was associated with a higher risk of complications. Mardjetko and colleagues[19] performed a **meta-analysis** of studies encompassing 889 patients: 216 treated with laminectomy, 500 undergoing laminectomy with noninstrumented fusion, 101 undergoing laminectomy with posterior instrumented fusion, and 72 treated with anterior fusion. The authors found that the addition of fusion with or without instrumentation yielded better clinical outcomes than decompression alone; however, the use of instrumentation did not improve clinical outcomes or fusion rates compared with uninstrumented fusion. The Spine Patient Outcomes Research Trial (SPORT) also evaluated in situ fusion, pedicular fusion, and 360-degree fusion and found no significant differences among any of the fusion techniques in outcome at 4 years.[20]

Booth and co-workers,[21] studying the results of decompression and instrumented posterior fusion for the treatment of degenerative spondylolisthesis, identified 41 patients who were followed for 5 to 10.7 years. Clinical outcome measures were available for 36 patients. Eighty-three percent reported high satisfaction with the procedure, 86% had reduced back and leg pain, and 46% had increased function. Kornblum and associates[22] evaluated results for 47 patients undergoing a noninstrumented fusion procedure and found that 22 of 47 patients achieved a solid fusion. The authors found that patients with solid fusion had statistically better clinical outcomes than those with a pseudoarthrosis as determined from responses on the Swiss Spinal Stenosis Questionnaire at 5 to 14 years. Abdu and colleagues[20] analyzed data for 380 surgical patients enrolled in SPORT, of whom 21% underwent posterolateral noninstrumented fusion, 56% were treated with pedicle screw instrumentation and fusion, 17% received pedicle screws and an interbody device, and 6% underwent decompression alone. At 4-year follow-up, there was no consistent difference among the three fusion groups in clinical outcome.

COMMENTARY

Controversy remains as to whether decompression alone, noninstrumented fusion, or instrumented fusion provides more long-lasting benefits for patients. Results of short- and long-term studies show a trend toward superior clinical results for decompression alone compared with the natural history of degenerative spondylolisthesis. If the spine is unstable when viewed on dynamic radiographs or intraoperatively, then fusion is likely a prudent adjunct to the decompression. In those patients with significant instability, decompression with the addition of instrumentation assists in achieving solid fusion and likely reducing the pain associated with abnormal segmental motion. The studies reviewed earlier are highly heterogeneous; some report results in terms of commonly used standardized clinical outcome measures, but in others standardized outcome measures are not used. Many investigations provide only rudimentary grading of patient satisfaction, which makes it difficult to compare findings across studies. Ultimately, the decision to fuse or not to fuse should be individualized for each patient, based on preoperative radiographs and MRI images in conjunction with intraoperative observation of abnormal motion and overall bone quality.

REFERENCES

1. Herbiniaux G: *Traite sur divers accouchements laborieux et sur les polypes de la matrice*, Brussells, 1782, JL Boubers. First report of slipped vertebrae or defects of the pars interarticularis.
2. Wiltse LL, Newman PH, McNab I: Classification of spondylolysis and spondylolisthesis, *Clin Orthop Rel Res* 117:23–29, 1976.
3. Pearson A, Blood E, Lurie J, et al: Degenerative spondylolisthesis versus spinal stenosis: does a slip matter? Comparison of baseline characteristics and outcomes (SPORT), *Spine* 35(3):298–305, 2010. "As treated" analysis of SPORT data for patients with degenerative spondylolisthesis and patients with spinal stenosis revealed that after surgery spondylolisthesis patients were more likely to achieve fusion than lumbar stenosis patients. Outcome measures of bodily pain, physical function, and ODI score were all better in the spondylolisthesis patients undergoing surgery. Nonsurgical outcomes were similar in both cohorts.
4. Matsudaira K, Yamazaki T, Seichi A, et al: Spinal stenosis in grade I degenerative lumbar spondylolisthesis: a comparative study of outcomes following laminoplasty and laminectomy with instrumented spinal fusion, *J Orthop Sci* 10(3):270–276, 2005. Japanese comparative study with 2-year follow-up including 16 patients treated conservatively, 18 undergoing lumbar laminoplasty, and 19 undergoing laminectomy with instrumented fusion. Surgery was shown to be superior to conservative therapy, but no clinical difference was seen between laminoplasty and laminectomy combined with instrumented fusion.
5. Weinstein JN, Lurie JD, Tosteson TD, et al: Surgical versus nonsurgical treatment for lumbar degenerative spondylolisthesis, *N Engl J Med* 356(22):2257–2270, 2007. Prospective randomized multicenter trial included a randomized cohort of 304 patients and an observational cohort of 303 patients. Crossover in the randomized cohort was about 40% in each direction, and 17% in the observational cohort crossed over to surgery. "As treated" analysis showed that patients with degenerative spondylolisthesis treated surgically were substantially better after 2 years of follow-up.
6. Weinstein JN, Lurie JD, Tosteson TD, et al: Surgical compared with nonoperative treatment for lumbar degenerative spondylolisthesis. Four-year results in the Spine Patient Outcomes Research Trial (SPORT) randomized and observational cohorts, *J Bone Joint Surg Am* 91(6):1295–1304, 2009. Same cohorts as in the previous study were followed out to 4 years. "Intention to treat" analysis was limited due to crossover to nonassigned group. "As treated" analysis showed that improvements in bodily pain, physical function, and ODI scores were maintained at 4 years.

7. Fischgrund JS, Mackay M, Herkowitz HN, et al: 1997 Volvo Award winner in clinical studies. Degenerative lumbar spondylolisthesis with spinal stenosis: a prospective, randomized study comparing decompressive laminectomy and arthrodesis with and without spinal instrumentation, *Spine* 22(24):2807–2812, 1997. In this prospective study 76 patients were randomly assigned to undergo posterior decompression and arthrodesis with or without instrumentation; 67 patients were available for follow-up at 2 years. Excellent or good clinical outcomes were found in 85% of patients in the noninstrumented group and in 76% of patients in the instrumented group. Successful fusion occurred in 45% and 82%, respectively, but clinical outcome did not correlate with successful arthrodesis.

8. Kimura I, Shingu H, Murata M, et al: Lumbar posterolateral fusion alone or with transpedicular instrumentation in L4-L5 degenerative spondylolisthesis, *J Spinal Disord* 14(4):301–310, 2001. Japanese retrospective analysis of outcomes in 57 patients with L4-L5 degenerative spondylolisthesis who underwent decompression with noninstrumented and instrumented fusion and were followed for 2 years. Fusion rates were 82.8% and 92.8% in the noninstrumented and instrumented fusion groups, respectively, and rates of satisfactory outcome were 72.4% and 82.1%; these differences were found to be nonsignificant.

9. Martin CR, Gruszczynski AT, Braunsfurth HA, et al: The surgical management of degenerative lumbar spondylolisthesis: a systematic review, *Spine* 32(16):1791–1798, 2007. Thirteen randomized controlled and comparative observational studies were included in this review. The authors concluded that spinal fusion may lead to a better clinical outcome than decompression alone. However, no conclusions could be drawn about the clinical benefit of instrumenting a spinal fusion.

10. Herkowitz HN, Kurz LT: Degenerative lumbar spondylolisthesis with spinal stenosis. A prospective study comparing decompression with decompression and intertransverse process arthrodesis, *J Bone Joint Surg Am* 73(6):802–808, 1991. Thirty-six women and 14 men with degenerative lumbar spondylolisthesis were randomly assigned to undergo decompression alone or decompression with transverse process arthrodesis (25 patients in each group). At follow-up of 2.4 to 4 years, the group treated with arthrodesis was found to have greater relief of back and leg pain.

11. Ghogawala Z, Benzel EC, Amin-Hanjani S, et al: Prospective outcomes evaluation after decompression with or without instrumented fusion for lumbar stenosis and degenerative grade I spondylolisthesis, *J Neurosurg Spine* 1(3):267–272, 2004. Prospective study of 20 patients who underwent laminectomy alone and 14 patients who had laminectomy with instrumented fusion. At 1 year, ODI score had improved by 27.5 in the instrumented group and 13.6 in the laminectomy alone group. SF-36 scores corroborated this finding. The authors concluded that surgery improves outcomes as evaluated by standardized measuring scales and that fusion leads to greater clinical improvement.

12. Lombardi JS, Wiltse LL, Reynolds J, et al: Treatment of degenerative spondylolisthesis, *Spine* 10(9):821–827, 1985. Retrospective analysis of data for 47 patients undergoing surgical treatment of spondylolisthesis who were followed for 2 to 7 years. Good or excellent results were achieved in only 33% of the patients undergoing wide laminectomy and facetectomy; in contrast, 88% of those undergoing laminectomy with preservation of facet had good or excellent results, and adding transverse process fusion increased the proportion to 90%.

13. Postacchini F, Cinotti G: Bone regrowth after surgical decompression for lumbar spinal stenosis, *J Bone Joint Surg Br* 74(6):862–869, 1992. Retrospective review of outcomes for 40 patients treated surgically for lumbar stenosis with an average follow-up of 8.6 years. Of the 16 patients with degenerative spondylolisthesis treated with laminectomy or laminotomy, 10 had concomitant fusion. Bone regrowth was more severe in those who did not undergo concomitant fusion, and this correlated with less satisfactory clinical results.

14. Postacchini F, Cinotti G, Perugia D: Degenerative lumbar spondylolisthesis. II. Surgical treatment, *Ital J Orthop Traumatol* 17(4):467–477, 1991. Italian retrospective review analyzing treatment results for 32 patients with degenerative spondylolisthesis undergoing unilateral laminotomy, bilateral laminotomy with or without transverse process fusion, bilateral laminectomy with or without spinal fusion, and laminectomy with spinal fusion and interspinous wiring. Satisfactory results were achieved in 84%, and 76% of patients showed progression of spondylolisthesis. The authors recommended no fusion when spondylolisthesis is mild and there is no significant hypermobility on lateral flexion-extension radiographs.

15. Bridwell KH, Sedgewick TA, O'Brien MF, et al: The role of fusion and instrumentation in the treatment of degenerative spondylolisthesis with spinal stenosis, *J Spinal Disord* 6(6):461–472, 1993. Prospective nonrandomized study encompassing 44 patients, of whom 43 were followed for 2 years or longer. Nine patients were treated with decompression surgery without fusion, 19 patients underwent transverse process fusion with autogenous bone graft, and 24 patients had transverse process fusion with the addition of instrumentation. Instrumentation enhanced the chances for successful fusion and was associated with reduced progression of spondylolisthesis. Nonprogression of spondylolisthesis correlated with better clinical outcomes.

16. Rousseau MA, Lazennec JY, Bass EC, et al: Predictors of outcomes after posterior decompression and fusion in degenerative spondylolisthesis, *Eur Spine J* 14(1):55–60, 2005. French retrospective review examining results for 24 patients undergoing surgery for lumbar spondylolisthesis, of whom 8 were lost to follow-up after a minimum of 0.87 years. Beaujon functional score was improved and fusion was seen in all cases. The authors concluded that the addition of an interbody device leads to higher scores than decompression with pedicle screw fusion.

17. Yone K, Sakou T, Kawauchi Y, et al: Indication of fusion for lumbar spinal stenosis in elderly patients and its significance, *Spine* 21(2):242–248, 1996. Japanese study evaluating outcomes for 34 elderly patients with spinal stenosis, of whom 17 were considered to have instability as determined by Posner's method. Ten of these 17 patients with instability underwent decompression and fusion, whereas 7 underwent decompression alone. The patients who did not show instability had decompression only.

Patients with instability who underwent only decompression had the worst JOA scores, and patients undergoing fusion had the best outcomes.

18. Gibson JN, Waddell G: Surgery for degenerative lumbar spondylosis, *Cochrane Database Syst Rev* (4):CD001352, 2005. Meta-analysis of 31 randomized trials examining treatment of lumbar spondylosis. Seven of these trials evaluated surgical treatment of spondylolisthesis with spinal stenosis, but the methodologies were too heterogeneous to allow good comparison. The authors found that the use of instrumentation is associated with higher fusion rates, but clinical outcomes are only marginally better than with noninstrumented fusion procedures.

19. Mardjetko SM, Connolly PJ, Shott S: Degenerative lumbar spondylolisthesis. A meta-analysis of literature 1970-1993, *Spine* 19(Suppl 20):S2256–S2265, 1994. The 889 patients encompassed by this meta-analysis included 216 treated with laminectomy, 500 undergoing laminectomy with noninstrumented fusion, 101 undergoing laminectomy with posterior instrumented fusion, and 72 treated with anterior fusion. The authors found that the addition of fusion with or without instrumentation led to better clinical outcomes than decompression alone; however, the use of instrumentation did not improve clinical outcomes or fusion rates compared with uninstrumented fusion.

20. Abdu WA, Lurie JD, Spratt KF, et al: Degenerative spondylolisthesis: does fusion method influence outcome? Four-year results of the Spine Patient Outcomes Research Trial, *Spine* 34(21):2351–2360, 2009. This SPORT subgroup analysis compares results for 380 spondylolisthesis patients undergoing laminectomy only, noninstrumented fusion, fusion with pedicle screw instrumentation, or fusion with pedicle screws plus interbody device for a 360-degree fusion. An "as treated" analysis of both randomized and observational cohorts revealed no consistent differences in outcomes for any of the fusion methods at 4 years.

21. Booth KC, Bridwell KH, Eisenberg BA, et al: Minimum 5-year results of degenerative spondylolisthesis treated with decompression and instrumented posterior fusion, *Spine* 24(16):1721–1727, 1999. Nonrandomized prospective study involving 49 patients who were treated with decompression and autologous posterior and posterolateral fusion with pedicle screw instrumentation and were followed for 5 to 10.7 years. Eight patients died and 41 patients were included in the sample. Of 36 patients who returned an outcome questionnaire and had current radiographs, 83% reported high satisfaction with the procedure, 86% had reduced back and leg pain, and 46% had increased function. Radiographic transitions were found to be common, but only 5 of the 12 patients affected were symptomatic.

22. Kornblum MB, Fischgrund JS, Herkowitz HN, et al: Degenerative lumbar spondylolisthesis with spinal stenosis: a prospective long-term study comparing fusion and pseudoarthrosis, *Spine* 29(7):726–733; discussion, 733–724, 2004. Prospective randomized study involving 47 patients with single-level lumbar spondylolisthesis who were followed for 5 to 14 years. Good or excellent clinical outcomes were more frequently achieved among patients with a solid arthrodesis (86%) than among patients with a pseudoarthrosis (56%), and the solid fusion group also experienced significantly greater improvement in back and leg pain.

Chapter 9

Asymptomatic Intradural Schwannoma: Surgery Versus Radiosurgery Versus Observation

Christopher E. Mandigo, Paul C. McCormick

Solitary nerve sheath tumors are the most commonly occurring intradural spinal tumors in adults. They represent approximately 10% to 30% of all primary spinal tumors depending on the patient series.[1-4] They typically occur in the fourth and fifth decades of life and affect women and men equally.[1-7] A small percentage of patients with this tumor have neurofibromatosis type 1 (NF-1) or NF-2. These tumors are thought to originate from the Schwann cell and are almost uniformly benign. A subset of patients with NF-2 may have malignant schwannomas.

The growth of these tumors is usually very slow and is typically concentric along the spinal nerve. The tumors can demonstrate various configurations depending on their anatomic location. They can be spherical or hourglass shaped secondary to growth constriction at the neural foramen or dural aperture. Approximately 80% to 90% of these tumors are intradural and 10% to 20% are dumbbell shaped with foraminal or extraforaminal components. Approximately 10% of all tumors arise from extradural components of the nerve and have proximal growth within or into the foramen. The majority of these tumors arise from the sensory root.

Increasingly, asymptomatic patients are diagnosed with incidental spinal tumors. Management considerations for these patients can be complex and depend on many factors, such as patient age and comorbid conditions, size and location of the tumor, and patient preference. This chapter discusses some of the management considerations for a patient with a schwannoma.

CASE PRESENTATION

A healthy 35-year-old woman was referred for evaluation of severe right-sided leg pain of 9 weeks' duration.

- PMH: Unremarkable
- PSH: Unremarkable
- Exam: The pain was in a typical S1 nerve root distribution. Neurologic examination revealed a positive finding on right straight leg raising at 20 degrees, numbness on the lateral aspect of the right foot, 4/5 strength in plantar flexion and ankle external rotation, and an absent right Achilles reflex.
- Imaging: Magnetic resonance imaging (MRI) revealed a large extruded right L5-S1 disk fragment with caudal migration and severe compression of the right S1 nerve root (Figure 9-1, *A* and *B*). An intradural abnormality was identified at the level of the L3 vertebral body on the initial MRI, so contrast-enhanced MRI was performed. This revealed a small, well-defined, uniformly enhancing intradural mass on the left side of the spinal canal (Figure 9-1, *C* and *D*) consistent with the diagnosis of nerve sheath tumor. The patient had no signs or symptoms related to this tumor.

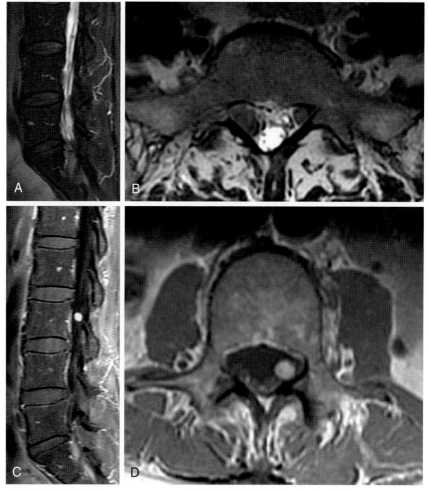

FIGURE 9-1 T1-weighted sagittal (**A**) and axial (**B**) MRI scans of the lumbosacral spine show a right-sided L5-S1 herniated disk with caudal migration and compression of the right S1 nerve root. T1-weighted contrast-enhanced sagittal (**C**) and axial (**D**) MRI scans show a uniformly enhancing mass at the level of the L3 vertebral body.

MANAGEMENT CONSIDERATIONS

Any decision making and management planning should first and foremost be predicated on the nature of the condition that is potentially to be treated. Most importantly, the specific pathologic diagnosis and natural history should be considered. Obviously, the consequences of the different management strategies, including no treatment, must also be considered, as should the patient's preference. For the patient described in the Case Presentation, the diagnosis of an L5-S1 disk herniation was made with a high degree of confidence based on the clinical presentation and the MRI scan appearance. What is not as certain is the individual natural history for this patient in terms of the probability of improvement without surgical intervention, both for the relief of pain and for the recovery of neurologic function. Although nonoperative management could result in improvement, there is also a possibility of worsened neurologic function as well as a concern that the longer the S1 nerve root remains compressed, the less likely that improvement will occur after successful surgical removal. On the other hand, although microdiskectomy is highly effective in relieving the pain from nerve root compression, it can be associated with complications, and there is no guarantee of return of neurologic function.

The management considerations for the intradural mass at the L3 level are quite different for several reasons. First, the specific pathologic diagnosis is less certain.

Although a benign nerve sheath tumor is likely based on location and appearance, the correct diagnosis cannot be known for sure. Moreover, even if one could be assured that this was a schwannoma, the natural history in terms of biology and growth rate can vary considerably. Finally, unlike the disk herniation, this lesion is asymptomatic, and the risks associated with surgical resection are higher.

Due to the uncertainties of this case there are a number of options that can reasonably be considered. Because of the persistence of severe pain for over 2 months and the presence of objective neurologic deficit from the L5-S1 disk herniation, microdiskectomy is probably the preferred option. Continued nonoperative management remains a rational option, but just as the surgeon must discuss the risks and complications of surgical intervention, the potential implications of nonoperative management must also be considered. Ultimately, the patient must make a decision under conditions of uncertainty, so it is the responsibility of the surgeon to ensure that the patient has as much information as possible to choose the most rational option for him or her.

The benefit of surgical treatment for the intradural mass is primarily prophylactic, since the patient is currently asymptomatic. Surgical resection would also provide a precise histopathologic diagnosis. Presumably, the tumor will never be smaller and the risk of surgery will never be lower than at the present time. On the other hand, surgery does carry some risk for either neurologic deficit or lower back dysfunction that could be permanent.

In the patient described here, the tumor is relatively small, is not associated with any significant mass effect, and is below the level of the spinal cord. It is also more laterally situated, although not dura based, which strongly supports the diagnosis of a Schwann cell tumor arising from a root of the cauda equina. Although the specific root of origin with respect to level and dorsal or ventral root cannot be known for certain, dorsal root schwannomas are more common than ventral root tumors (there are more fascicles in the dorsal root); however, dorsal root tumors are more likely to present with radicular pain. Based on the lateral location, the nerve root level of origin is most probably L4 or L5, due to the somatotopic organization of the cauda equina. In either case, therefore, this tumor arises from a critical lumbar nerve root. Resection of a critical root of origin may be associated with a neurologic deficit, so this must be considered.

In the end, the recommendation for this patient was surgical microdiskectomy for removal of the extruded right L5-S1 disk fragment, but no treatment of the incidental cauda equina lesion. It was certainly an option to remove the tumor following microdiskectomy, but it was felt that this was a significantly different additional procedure (different level, intradural) that would have added measurable risk to an otherwise extremely safe microdiskectomy. Periodic clinical and radiographic surveillance of the tumor was recommended. Repeat MRI at 3 months postoperatively was recommended to ensure that this was not a biologically aggressive tumor. If no growth was apparent, then MRI would be performed annually. If the patient became symptomatic or the tumor showed significant growth, then surgery would be recommended. In many cases little or no growth is apparent after even several years. Furthermore, experience indicates that this tumor could more than double in size without risking neurologic deficit or adding to the risk or technical complexity of tumor resection. There are numerous exceptions to this expectant management strategy. For example, due to the often slow growth rate of these tumors, they can have considerable size and mass effect on the spinal cord or cauda equina at presentation. One patient recently had an incidental tumor at the T3 level with significant spinal cord compression at presentation (Figure 9-2). In these cases resection is typically recommended due to the concern for potentially rapid neurologic deterioration or an increasingly more technically challenging surgical resection. On the other hand, early surgery is also recommended for even small, centrally located asymptomatic cauda equina tumors. Although such lesions may be schwannomas from sacral nerve roots, they may also represent filum terminale myxopapillary ependymomas. These latter unencapsulated tumors may exhibit dissemination via the cerebrospinal fluid (CSF) or sheetlike extension along the roots of the cauda equina that precludes safe total resection. Early surgery in these situations seems prudent.

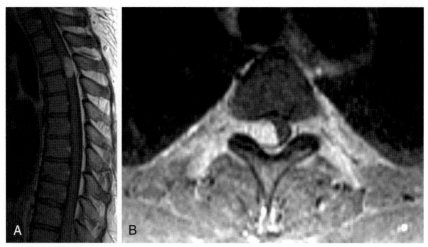

FIGURE 9-2 T1-weighted sagittal (**A**) and axial (**B**) MRI scans of the thoracic spine show a large, uniformly enhancing tumor at the T3-4 level producing significant compression of the spinal cord.

An alternative treatment is focused radiotherapy or stereotactic radiosurgery. Various modalities have been described, including proton beam radiosurgery, linear accelerator radiosurgery (CyberKnife, Accuray Corp., Sunnyvale, Calif.; Synergy system, Elekta AB, Stockholm, Sweden; Novalis system, Brainlab AG, Feldkirchen, Germany), and intensity-modulated radiation therapy (IMRT). Although most reports on spinal radiosurgery involve treatment of malignant primary and metastatic disease of the vertebral spine, there is accumulating experience with radiosurgery for benign intradural spinal lesions.[8-12] Benefits of such treatment include the possibility for long-term tumor control without the associated risks of open surgery. Limitations of this strategy are numerous. First, as with nonoperative management, no tissue is obtained to verify the histologic characteristics of the tumor. Second, since these tumors are slow growing, it may be difficult to accurately assess the effectiveness of the treatment in individual cases. Third, there is a risk of radiation injury, particularly at spinal cord levels.[9] In addition, subsequent operative intervention may be compromised by prior radiosurgery. In the end, for reasonably healthy patients with a single intradural spinal lesion surgery is such a highly effective and safe treatment that radiosurgery is generally not considered as a primary treatment modality. Patients with significant comorbid conditions, recurrent or residual tumors, or multiple lesions, particularly patients with von Hippel–Lindau disease or neurofibromatosis, are currently the most likely to be considered for radiosurgery as a primary or adjunctive treatment option. This is an evolving technology, however, and treatment considerations are likely to change in the future.

SURGICAL CONSIDERATIONS

Understanding the anatomic relationships of these tumors is essential to successful surgery. The optimal goal of surgery is gross total resection with preservation of nerve function. Complete visualization of these tumors usually can be achieved with posterior or posterolateral approaches to the spine. Microsurgery is invaluable for opening of the dura and arachnoid layers covering the tumor and for debulking and dissection of the tumor capsule. Use of intraoperative neurophysiologic monitoring is a useful tool to determine if there is functional nerve worth preserving within the tumor.

SURGICAL OPTIONS

Schwannomas may be completely resected from a variety of approaches depending on location. Often with dumbbell tumors there are advantageous changes within the surrounding bony anatomy of the spinal column from the slow-growing tumor that may aid in the dissection. Often, the bony elements of the foramen are attenuated, expanded, or nonexistent. The need for stabilization and bony fusion depends on the degree of preexisting biomechanical instability secondary to tumor-related changes and the amount of bone and ligament that must be removed for adequate tumor exposure and excision.

Expected rates of neurologic improvement after surgical resection range from 80% to 95% of patients based on large surgical series.[5-7] A secondary goal of surgery is to preserve the function of the involved nerve root. Preservation of nerve function may not require anatomic preservation of the affected nerve root. Some degree of anatomic preservation is usually possible with small, intradural tumors, but complete removal of larger tumors may require sacrifice of rootlets or the entire nerve. Dorsal nerve roots can be cut during surgery for these tumors with minimal adverse effect. Hypesthesia has been documented in a small percentage of patients.[5-7,13-16] Enhanced motor weakness usually is not a complication of surgery, even in situations in which the ventral nerve root is sacrificed, because the affected nerve roots are often nonfunctional before surgery. Motor weakness occurred in approximately 10% to 33% of patients who underwent sectioning of the affected nerve in functional nerve roots (C5 through T1 and L1 through S1). The mechanism of this phenomenon is unclear. Presumably, gradual functional denervation of the involved nerve root allows reinnervation to occur by means of sprouting at the anterior horn cell or muscle end-plate level. The delicate intradural nerve fascicles of the entire motor or sensory root of tumor origin usually disappear into the substance of the tumor, because they do not have a well-developed interfascicular connective tissue matrix. A thin arachnoid layer separately ensheathes the motor and sensory roots. Although this sheath might allow anatomic preservation of the corresponding motor root for intradural sensory root tumors, or vice versa, sacrifice of the entire motor and sensory root is required if the tumor extends through the root sleeve, distal to the dorsal root ganglion[17] (Tips from the Masters 9-1).

Tips from the Masters 9-1 • Paired intradural dorsal and ventral nerve roots are often contained within a common arachnoid sheath, particularly laterally, and in the cauda equina. Although the root of origin is usually not functional, the paired root generally is. The paired root may be tightly applied to the surface of the tumor capsule, but it can be safely dissected from the tumor surface, especially at critical cervical (C5 through C8) and lumbosacral (L2 through S1) levels.

Posterior Approach

The posterior approach is appropriate for tumors that are completely intradural. A simple laminectomy covering the rostrocaudal extent of the tumor is necessary to define normal spinal cord anatomy. Microscopic dissection of the dura and arachnoid planes is recommended.[18] Internal debulking is often necessary before dissection of the tumor capsule. Triggered electromyography is useful to differentiate tumor capsule from functional nerve root tissue to aid in resection. Stabilization is not necessary for simple laminectomies. Laminoplasty has been advocated by some, but no long-term data exist to demonstrate improved outcome. The extent of safe tumor resection is likely the most important variable in determining a positive outcome.

Posterolateral Approach

Tumors with foraminal and extraforaminal components require complete exposure by removal of the bony elements involved and/or adequate soft tissue dissection. Posterior laminectomy with a unilateral facetectomy allows for single-stage resection. For cervical tumors, the vertebral artery is usually displaced anteromedially and can be dissected from the surface of the tumor easily. This approach can permit exposure up to 4 cm from the lateral dural edge and the lateral third of the vertebral body in the cervical spine. Tumor extension beyond these boundaries makes an anterolateral approach necessary. Thoracic and lumbar tumors may require a lateral extracavitary approach. Indications for this approach include very large dumbbell tumors, upper thoracic paraspinal tumors, and extensive anterior and posterior paraspinal tumors with spinal canal and vertebral column involvement. This approach can provide exposure of intradural structures as well as extensive access to the anterior and posterior paraspinal region, ventral spinal canal, and vertebral body.[19,20] After the tumor is adequately visualized, dural and arachnoid opening is best performed with the aid of an operative microscope. Tumors with intradural and extradural components may require a T-shaped dural opening, with one limb along the nerve root sleeve. Stabilization with metallic instrumentation for bony fusion is usually necessary after tumor resection if a full laminectomy and unilateral facetectomy are performed.

Anterolateral Approach

The anterolateral approach is typically reserved for cervical tumors that have a large extraforaminal component.[21-23] When tumors are adherent to the vertebral artery or brachial plexus in this situation, a small residual may be left behind. Complete resection can be achieved in most patients. Intraoperative stimulation can be used to help decide whether the root can be divided without producing a postoperative deficit. The anterolateral approach requires experience with the anterior cervical approach beyond the routine exposure for treatment of degenerative disease. The dissection is a modification of the approach described originally by Verbiest. A complete understanding of the relationship of the vertebral artery, the nerve root, the transverse process, the prevertebral muscles, and the sympathetic chain is necessary to avoid injury and complications.

FUNDAMENTAL TECHNIQUE

Surgical Technique—Posterior

After routine induction, endotracheal anesthesia, and placement of the appropriate venous and arterial lines, the patient is placed in the prone position. For lesions located rostral to the T6 level, a Mayfield head holder is used, and the arms are tucked at the side. The head is placed on a padded headrest for tumors caudal to the T6 level, and the shoulders are abducted and the elbows flexed to no more than 90 degrees. Perioperative intravenous antibiotics and corticosteroids are administered. The dosage of corticosteroids and duration of treatment vary, but typically 10 mg dexamethasone (Decadron) is given every 4 hours during surgery, and the dose is then tapered off over 5 to 7 days. Both somatosensory and motor evoked potentials are often monitored throughout the procedure, and intraoperative stimulation can be a useful tool during tumor dissection, debulking, and removal. The skin incision is planned by using fluoroscopy or plain radiography to localize the operative levels. It is important to reconcile tumor level as identified by preoperative imaging studies, usually MRI, with level determined by intraoperative localization methods (i.e., plain radiographs or fluoroscopy), especially for thoracic tumors. The surgical field is prepared and draped in a standard fashion.

Completely intradural tumors can be approached with laminectomies or hemilaminectomies alone. Adequate bony exposure should reveal the entire margin of the tumor. Tumors with foraminal or extraforaminal components require some degree of lateral exposure. The techniques for resection of these dumbbell tumors have been described in detail in the literature, and the general approach varies according to the spinal level. The lateral extracavitary approach can be used for large dumbbell tumors in the thoracolumbar spine, whereas posterolateral and anterolateral approaches are used in the cervical spine.[15,18]

Cervical Spine—Posterolateral

For the cervical spine, a midline incision can be used. Subperiosteal exposure of the posterior spinal elements can be limited to the affected side, unless the tumor extends to the midline or bilateral fixation and fusion are planned. The entire facet joint of the affected level is exposed. A table-mounted retractor can be used to maintain the exposure. The contralateral extent of the laminectomy is determined by the size of the intradural component; it should permit complete visualization of the tumor margins and the interface of the tumor and spinal cord. The intradural tumor component is removed first. For large intradural tumors, a longitudinal paramedial durotomy that is gently curved laterally at either end is used. For small, laterally placed intradural tumors, a transverse dural incision in line with the dural root sleeve might be used. The intradural portion of the tumor is removed using standard microsurgical techniques. Although preservation of the motor root and some sensory fascicles is usually possible with dorsal root intradural nerve sheath tumors, sacrifice of the entire spinal nerve will usually be required if the tumor extends into the nerve root sleeve beyond the dorsal root ganglion. After intradural tumor removal, the dural incision is extended laterally over the nerve root sleeve. An intrafascicular tumor dissection is performed if root preservation is possible. If sacrifice of the nerve root is required or has already been performed, the lateral dural incision should extend around the dural root sleeve to disarticulate it from the dural tube. The dural root sleeve cuff and attached distal dorsal and ventral nerve root stumps are displaced laterally, and the dural tube is reconstructed so as to be watertight, with a fascial graft if necessary, to prevent intradural blood contamination during the often bloody subsequent extraforaminal dissection.

Removal of the foraminal and extraforaminal tumor components depends upon their size and relationship to the nerve root and nerve root sleeve. Small tumors might be totally confined within the nerve root sheath. If the nerve has previously been sacrificed proximally, the dissection might proceed on the surface of the expanded root sleeve to define the tumor margins. Dissection of this plane might be bloody because of the extensive venous plexus that surrounds the nerve root and vertebral artery. Alternatively, the nerve sheath might be opened to allow either an intrafascicular tumor removal, with or without nerve root preservation, or internal decompression for larger tumors. Preservation of the involved nerve root is often possible if there is no intradural tumor component.

The tumor is followed distally along the nerve root to its lateral margin. Detachment of the levator scapulae and posterior and middle scalene muscle attachments from the posterior tubercles of the transverse processes allows exposure to extend 3.5 to 4 cm from the lateral dural margin. Small dorsal rami can be divided. Although the dorsal scapular nerve and long thoracic nerve might occasionally be encountered, brachial plexus trunk formation does not occur until at least 5 cm from the lateral dural margin. The rostral and caudal tumor margins are then defined. Internal decompression might be required to provide adequate visualization of the ventral tumor margins. The vertebral artery is consistently displaced ventromedially and separated from the tumor capsule or nerve sheath, the periosteum, and a perivertebral venous plexus. If the dissection remains on the tumor surface, the tumor is easily dissected from the vertebral artery.

Stabilization, if necessary, is performed after tumor removal. Onlay dural substitutes, such as DuraGen (Integra LifeSciences Corporation, Plainsboro, N.J.), with or without a sealant such as DuraSeal (Confluent Surgical, Waltham, Mass.), can be used to cover the dura. The deep muscles are reapproximated with a running absorbable monofilament suture. Absorbable braided suture is used to close the deep fascia and subcutaneous tissue, and a running nonlocked nylon suture is used for the skin closure. The patient is maintained on bed rest for 36 hours after surgery, and then mobilization is begun. If fusion has been performed, use of a hard cervical orthosis is required for 8 to 12 weeks.

Thoracolumbar Spine—Posterolateral

Adequate exposure can be achieved with a midline incision that extends enough rostrocaudally to allow lateral retraction toward the affected side. This may be most appropriate for completely intradural tumors or those with foraminal involvement without much extension into the extraforaminal space. The techniques involved for tumors that can be approached with a midline incision in the thoracolumbar spine are very similar to those described earlier for the cervical spine. For tumors with large paraspinal components, the lateral extracavitary approach can be used. This is described in detail here.

After the patient is turned to the prone position onto an appropriate table, a smaller bolster is placed on the side opposite the operative approach. The table is initially rotated toward the operative side to establish a true prone position. This maximizes the operative table rotation of the patient into a three-quarter prone position when anterior compartment visualization is needed. A hockey stick incision with the midline long limb centered over the abnormality and the short limb gently curving 8 to 10 cm toward the operative side is planned. The midline portion of the incision is continued down through the subcutaneous tissue to the spinous processes. A routine subperiosteal elevation of the paraspinal muscles is performed bilaterally if posterior spinal exposure is required for laminectomy and/or posterior instrumentation. Adequate caudal midline spinal exposure, particularly for the placement of spinal instrumentation, must be assured at this point, because further caudal exposure is limited once the lateral limb of the incision has been opened.

After the midline soft tissue dissection is complete, the lateral limb of the skin incision is opened. This incision is continued down to the longitudinally oriented paraspinal muscles (i.e., erector spinae). In the thoracic region, portions of the trapezius muscle, the rhomboids, and the upper latissimus dorsi muscles are transversely incised in line with the skin incision, whereas only the thin thoracodorsal fascia is incised in the lumbar region. The myocutaneous flap is elevated to expose the longitudinally oriented paraspinal muscle mass. The lateral margin of this muscle mass is identified and medially elevated to expose the ribs in the thoracic region and the quadratus lumborum and psoas muscles at lumbar levels. The paraspinal muscle dissection continues over the facet joints to join the midline dissection. This allows the surgeon to simultaneously or alternatively work on either side of the now completely mobilized paraspinal muscle mass.

The lateral extracavitary approach may be modified according to the exposure requirements and surgical objective. Paraspinal tumors, for example, do not require intraspinal or posterior spinal exposure. In patients with these tumors, no midline subperiosteal dissection is performed. Instead, the midline incision is continued down only to the tip of the spinous processes. The midline insertion of the scapular muscles or thoracodorsal fascia is detached and laterally continued to elevate the superficial flap. Detachment of the lateral margin of the paraspinal muscle insertion from the iliac crest and resection of a posterosuperior iliac crest segment facilitate ventral exposure at lower lumbar levels (i.e., below L4). The sequence of the lateral extracavitary approach may also be varied as necessary according to the surgical strategy or tumor characteristics. Decompression of the spinal canal, for example, may proceed before the paraspinal exposure, or vice versa.

Complete dissection of the lateral spinal elements (facet joints, pedicle, transverse process, and ribs) one level above and below the pathologic segment is required to achieve adequate ventral exposure. The ventral and lateral surfaces of the ribs are subperiosteally exposed with Cobb elevators down to their vertebral body articulations. The intertransverse process ligament, psoas muscle, and diaphragm attachments (at upper lumbar levels) are released from the transverse process to the lateral pedicle margin at lumbar levels. The transverse processes at these levels are removed, as is a 6- to 8-cm segment of rib at the pathologic thoracic level. Removal of a shorter proximal rib segment (i.e., 3 to 4 cm) at adjacent thoracic levels provides adequate ventral spinal exposure while diminishing postoperative flail chest deformity. The segmental nerves at and one level above the pathologic level are identified. The intercostal neurovascular bundle lies deep to the intercostal muscles and is imbedded within the endothoracic fascia. The nerve is dissected free from the neurovascular bundle and elevated off the underlying fascia. The thoracic nerve roots are divided, and the proximal nerve stumps are elevated medially toward the foramen. Lumbar nerves are more difficult to identify, because they directly course through the psoas muscle. These nerves hinder ventral exposure, because they cross the surgical field and, unlike thoracic nerves, cannot be sacrificed and dorsally displaced. Dissection of lumbar nerves over several centimeters allows for adequate nerve mobilization and prevents a postoperative stretch palsy. Vessel loop retraction of these nerves may improve ventral visualization. Initial exposure of the anterior thoracic paraspinal region is achieved by blunt ventral displacement of the pleura, once the intercostal nerves have been freed from its surface. Depression of the psoas muscle and/or diaphragm after lumbar nerve dissection provides anterior lumbar paraspinal exposure. Continued anterior compartment dissection is dictated by tumor characteristics. Paraspinal tumor components will be encountered before identification of the pedicle or lateral vertebral margin. Most tumors are closely located to the spine, and their margins can easily be separated from the surrounding pleura and endothoracic fascia in the thoracic spine. Table-mounted blade retractors and packing sponges maintain lung retraction, and the dissection remains entirely extrapleural for this area of the spine. The operating table is rotated away from the surgeon to improve ventral visualization. The pleura, diaphragm, and/or psoas muscle are bluntly dissected ventrally off the lateral vertebral body with Cobb elevators. Sharp dissection may be required at the disk space. Any remaining rib head is removed from the vertebral body articulation. Dorsal segmental and foraminal branches from the intercostal or lumbar vessels, including the ascending lumbar vein, are cauterized and divided. Proximal dissection of the segmental nerves identifies the foramen. The margins of the pedicle are sharply defined with curettes. The pedicle is resected with Kerrison rongeurs and/or a high-speed drill. Partial resection of the superior facet joint and contiguous lateral vertebral elements exposes the lateral dural margin, which facilitates dissection and improves ventral canal visualization. Mobilization of the segmental nerves continues to the lateral dural margin. This requires a section of proximal dorsal and autonomic rami and an often bloody dissection of an extensive perineural venous plexus. Once the lateral dural margin has been exposed, resection of the vertebral body and ventral spinal canal decompression may commence. Incision and evacuation of the disk precedes vertebral body resection, which is performed with rongeurs, curettes, and/or a high-speed drill. Ventral canal tumor and/or retropulsed bone fragments are quickly delivered down into the corpectomy defect with reverse-angle curettes to minimize epidural bleeding. This bleeding is controlled with absorbable gelatin sponges and cautery. Spinal stabilization with an anterior interbody strut graft and/or posterior fixation, if necessary, can be performed once tumor resection and hemostasis have been achieved. Divided thoracic nerve roots are clipped proximal to the dorsal root ganglion to prevent a painful postoperative neuralgia.

En bloc marginal resection of paraspinal and/or unilateral vertebral element or rib head neoplasms requires circumferential exposure of the tumor margins, ideally with a cuff of surrounding normal tissue. Development and disarticulation of the remaining medial vertebral element tumor attachment is achieved with osteotomes and rongeurs. Occasionally, a spinal nerve may need to be included in the resected specimen.

The pleura are inspected for tears or an air leak. Most small tears can be repaired and do not require use of a chest tube if no air leak or lung collapse is detected. This is preferable if the CSF space has been entered, to prevent a CSF-pleural fistula. The remainder of the wound is closed in layers.

DISCUSSION OF BEST EVIDENCE

Accumulated clinical evidence over the past several decades has identified intradural spinal nerve sheath tumors as well-encapsulated benign tumors with a relatively slow, but individually variable, growth rate. Numerous uncontrolled **retrospective trials**[5-7,13-16] have established surgical resection as a safe and highly effective primary treatment that provides long-term control or cure with preservation or even improvement of neurologic function. It is currently the treatment of choice for the majority of patients who harbor this tumor.

Less evidence is available for radiosurgery. Current evidence suggests that long-term tumor control may be achieved in some patients, but this effect is specifically unpredictable.[8-12] Currently, high-risk patients, patients with multiple tumors, or those with recurrent or residual tumors may represent the best candidates for radiosurgery.

Evidence in support of nonoperative management of asymptomatic intradural spinal nerve sheath tumors is largely anecdotal and based on observation of the often extremely slow growth rate of many of these tumors. Since surgery is associated with some risk, it is reasonable to offer some period of nonoperative management or at least to discuss the option with the patient.

COMMENTARY

"Surgery can't make a normal patient better" is an aphorism well known to most surgeons. Spinal neurosurgeons also generally adhere to the adage to "treat the patient, not the imaging." Although the wisdom contained in these phrases is self-evident, it is also true that they overly simplify the numerous relevant factors that must be considered when determining the appropriate management options for each patient. Often, the consequences of specific management recommendations—whether surgery, radiotherapy, or nonoperative observation—cannot be predicted at the individual level. One simply cannot know, in any particular case, whether a patient will have an adverse response to surgery such as a nerve root or spinal cord deficit, wound infection, CSF leak, or chronic neck or back pain. Furthermore, whether a specific tumor will respond to focused radiotherapy or will show an adverse effect cannot be predicted. In the absence of serial imaging, the biology and growth rate of the tumor cannot be known, and without a tissue sample one cannot be certain of the tumor histologic type or grade. Under such circumstances, there may be more than one rational treatment option. It is important, therefore, that the surgeon discuss these issues in detail with the patient so that the patient can make an informed decision. From a surgeon's perspective, it is important to consider the consequences of a wrong decision and to imagine the worst in relation to each management option. For example, if nonoperative management is recommended, what if the tumor type is more aggressive than initially assumed? This is why early follow-up imaging is done within narrow time frames in these patients and why early surgery is recommended for even small midline cauda equina tumors or tumors producing significant mass effect. On the other hand, consider the patient described in the Case Presentation, who has a small nerve sheath tumor at the L3 level. If early surgery were undertaken, she does risk permanent lumbar motor root deficit of moderate morbidity. In many instances serial follow-up imaging will show little or no growth for several years. Thus, not performing surgery allows such a patient to remain neurologically normal for many years before undertaking the risks of surgery. If substantial growth is identified early on serial MRI scans, then both the patient and the surgeon clearly know that surgery should be undertaken despite the fact that the tumor may still be asymptomatic. Both patient and surgeon are better able to accept the small but possibly significant consequences of surgery under these circumstances.

REFERENCES

1. Helseth A, Mork SJ: Primary intraspinal neoplasms in Norway, 1955 to 1986. A population-based survey of 467 patients, *J Neurosurg* 71(6):842–845, 1989.
2. Preston-Martin S: Descriptive epidemiology of primary tumors of the spinal cord and spinal meninges in Los Angeles County, 1972-1985, *Neuroepidemiology* 9(2):106–111, 1990.
3. Schellinger K, Propp J, et al: Descriptive epidemiology of primary spinal cord tumors, *J Neurooncol* 87(2):173–179, 2008. Incidence of spinal cord tumors was estimated from cases diagnosed between 1998 and 2002 in 16 CBTRUS collaborating state cancer registries. Of the spinal cord tumors identified (n = 3,226), 24% were nerve sheath tumors.
4. Engelhard H, Villano J, et al: Clinical presentation, histology, and treatment in 430 patients with primary tumors of the spinal cord, spinal meninges, or cauda equina, *J Neurosurg Spine* 13(1):67–77, 2010. Patients diagnosed with primary CNS neoplasms during the year 2000 were identified within a prospectively collected database in a Patient Care Evaluation Study conducted by the Commission on Cancer of the American College of Surgeons. Patients with primary intraspinal tumors represented 4.5% of the CNS tumor group, and had a mean age of 49.3 years. Pain was the most common presenting symptom, while the most common tumor types were meningioma (24.4%), ependymoma (23.7%), and schwannoma (21.2%). Resection, surgical biopsy, or both were performed in 89.3% of cases. Complications were low, but included neurological worsening (2.2%) and infection (1.6%).
5. Conti P, Pansini G, et al: Spinal neurinomas: retrospective analysis and long-term outcome of 179 consecutively operated cases and review of the literature, *Surg Neurol* 61(1):34–43, 2004; discussion 44.

Results of 179 surgically treated spinal neurinomas in 152 patients. All patients had follow-up for longer than 5 years. The most common symptom was segmental pain. Total removal of the lesion was possible in the first operation for 174 neurinomas. Neurologic recovery noted in 108 patients.

6. Jinnai T, Koyama T: Clinical characteristics of spinal nerve sheath tumors: analysis of 149 cases, *Neurosurgery* 56(3):510–515, 2005; discussion 510-515. **Retrospective review of 149 patients with spinal nerve sheath tumors treated between 1980 and 2001. One hundred seventy-six resected tumors were classified into five groups according to the relationship to the dura mater and/or the intervertebral foramen. A relationship between likelihood of intradural versus combined intradural/extradural or extradural tumors was discovered. Cervical tumors are more often have an extradural component compared to the thoracolumbar nerves. Different growth patterns may be explained by the anatomic features of the spinal nerve roots, which have a longer intradural component at the more caudal portion of the spinal axis.**

7. Matti T, Matti J, Risto J, et al: Long-term outcome after removal of spinal schwannoma: a clinico-pathological study of 187 cases, *Journal of Neurosurgery* 83(4):621–626, 1995. **Median follow-up of 12.9 years with 187 patients treated with surgery. Safe in the short term with some mild symptoms in 80% in late follow-up and 20% more serious complications.**

8. Ryu S, Chang S, Kim D, et al: Image-guided hypo-fractionated stereotactic radiosurgery to spinal lesions, *Neurosurgery* 49(4):838–846, 2001.

9. Dodd R, Ryu M, Kamnerdsupaphon P, et al: CyberKnife radiosurgery for benign intradural extramedullary spinal tumors, *Neurosurgery* 58(4):674–685, 2006. **Report on 24-month follow-up of 30 spinal schwannomas treated with Cyberknife radiosurgery.**

10. Gerszten P, Burton S, Ozhasoglu C, et al: Radiosurgery for benign intradural spinal tumors, *Neurosurgery* 62(4):887–896, 2008. **Seventy-six tumors treated with radiosurgery, follow-up 8 to 71 months. Nineteen tumors had undergone surgical resection. All had radiographic control, but there were three cases of radiation-induced spinal cord toxicity. Long-term pain improvement was seen in 73% of cases.**

11. Sachdev S, Dodd R, Chang SD, et al: Stereotactic radiosurgery yields long-term control for benign intradural, extramedullary spinal tumors, *Neurosurgery* 69(3):533–539, 2011. **Report on 103 tumors in 87 patients, treated with cyberknife radiosurgery. Follow-up over 6 to 87 months with 86% of schwannomas symptomatically stable at last follow-up.**

12. Chang U, Rhee CH, Youn SM, et al: Radiosurgery using the Cyberknife for benign spinal tumors: Korea Cancer Center Hospital experience, *J Neurooncol* 101(1):91–99, 2011. **Report on 30 tumors in 20 patients. Follow-up of 12 to 84 months with more than 90% symptomatic control or relief.**

13. George B, Lot G: Neurinomas of the first two cervical nerve roots: a series of 42 cases, *J Neurosurg* 82(6):917–923, 1995.

14. Kim P, Ebersold M, et al: Surgery of spinal nerve schwannoma. Risk of neurological deficit after resection of involved root, *J Neurosurg* 71(6):810–814, 1989. **Thirty-one patients underwent sacrifice of a root critical for the function of the upper (C5-T1, 14 cases) or the lower extremities (L3-S1, 17 cases). Only seven patients (23%) developed detectable motor or sensory deficits postoperatively. All deficits were no more than partial loss of strength or sensation. These results indicate that the spinal roots giving origin to schwannoma are frequently nonfunctional at the time of surgery, and risks of causing disabling neurological deficit after sacrificing these roots are small.**

15. Lot G, George B: Cervical neuromas with extradural components: surgical management in a series of 57 patients, *Neurosurgery* 41(4):813–820, 1997; discussion 820-812.

16. Schultheiss R, Gullotta G: Resection of relevant nerve roots in surgery of spinal neurinomas without persisting neurological deficit, *Acta Neurochir (Wien)* 122(1-2):91–96, 1993.

17. McCormick P: Anatomic principles of intradural spinal surgery, *Clin Neurosurg* 41:204–223, 1994.

18. McCormick P: Surgical management of dumbbell tumors of the cervical spine, *Neurosurgery* 38(2):294–300, 1996.

19. Larson S, Holst R, et al: Lateral extracavitary approach to traumatic lesions of the thoracic and lumbar spine, *J Neurosurg* 45(6):628–637, 1976.

20. McCormick P: Surgical management of dumbbell and paraspinal tumors of the thoracic and lumbar spine, *Neurosurgery* 38(1):67–74, 1996; discussion 74-75.

21. George B, Zerah M, et al: Oblique transcorporeal approach to anteriorly located lesions in the cervical spinal canal, *Acta Neurochir (Wien)* 121(3-4):187–190, 1993.

22. Hakuba A, Komiyama M, et al: Transuncodiscal approach to dumbbell tumors of the cervical spinal canal, *J Neurosurg* 61(6):1100–1106, 1984.

23. Verbiest H: A lateral approach to the cervical spine: technique and indications, *J Neurosurg* 28(3):191–203, 1968.

Chapter 10 Pseudotumor: Transoral Versus Posterior Fusion

Daniel M. Sciubba, Ali Bydon, Jean-Paul Wolinsky, Ziya L. Gokaslan

Atlantoaxial arthritis is not as common as arthritis of the subaxial spine, but when it occurs, it can be associated with severe pain and myelopathy. Most commonly occurring in the setting of rheumatoid arthritis, a pannus of the C1-2 joint can also result from atlantoaxial osteoarthritis or healing following trauma to the C1-2 junction. When degenerative in nature, the pannus has also been termed pseudotumor or articular, ganglion, synovial, or juxtafacet cyst.[1] The classic presentation is mechanical suboccipital pain and/or myelopathy from ventral spinal cord compression at the craniocervical junction.

The diagnosis of C1-2 pseudotumor is best made based on a thorough medical history in combination with the findings of various imaging modalities. Magnetic resonance imaging (MRI) is ideal for evaluation of spinal cord pathology and is thus essential in the workup to determine the location and severity of spinal cord or brainstem compression. In conjunction, computed tomography (CT) is used to evaluate at least three important aspects of the bony anatomy. First, the degree of bony erosion must be assessed to determine the extent of atlantodental arthritis and lateral mass arthritis. This is especially relevant when basilar invagination has occurred secondary to cranial settling and "pistoning" of the dens upward as the C1-2 joint subluxes and rotates. Second, the pannus should be evaluated for calcification to provide a sense of overall rigidity of the mass. Third, if surgery is to be planned, bony anatomy must be clarified for purposes of both decompression and instrumentation. A final important imaging modality is flexion-extension radiography to determine motion and thus instability at the C1-2 joint. Classically, motion is examined most closely by assessing the atlantodental interval; however, in the setting of a previous trauma, motion at the base of the odontoid should also be examined. Unfortunately, differentiating a degenerative pannus or rheumatoid pannus from older healing C2 fractures, calcium pyrophosphate deposition, metastatic lesions, primary bone tumors (chordomas), primary cartilaginous tumors (chondromas, chondrosarcomas), or meningiomas can be difficult using imaging studies alone.[1]

Surgical decompression is the definitive treatment for a degenerative pannus leading to myelopathy. Historically, transoral decompression combined with posterior stabilization has been most commonly used. However, posterior-only approaches have been used to avoid the morbidity associated with the transoral route. In such cases, the hope is that progression of myelopathy can be halted with stabilization, and in cases of a noncalcified pannus, the mass may resolve following the procedure. The controversy regarding which approach is preferable is the subject of this chapter. A case of a C1-2 pannus is first presented. Surgical options are then discussed, and a literature review is provided to support the best approach.

CASE PRESENTATION

A 77-year-old woman came for treatment of neck pain after experiencing a series of falls over the previous 2 years. After the falls she did not initially seek treatment for the neck pain. However, the neck pain became progressively severe. In addition, she began to complain of increased clumsiness of gait. She went to her

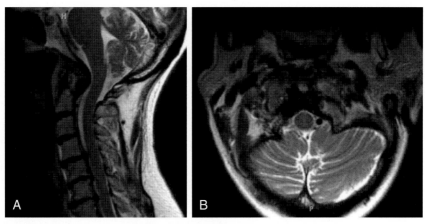

FIGURE 10-1 T2-weighted sagittal (**A**) and axial (**B**) MRI scans of the cervical spine showing a C1-2 pannus from nonhealed type II odontoid fracture.

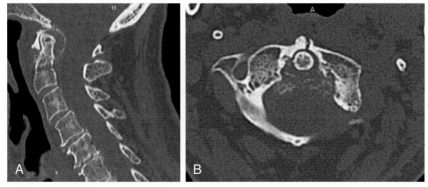

FIGURE 10-2 Sagittal (**A**) and axial (**B**) CT images of the cervical spine showing an old type II odontoid fracture and a calcified pannus around the C1-2 joint. On the axial view, an old fracture in the anterior C1 tubercle can also be seen.

primary care physician, who ordered an MRI scan and sent her for neurosurgical consultation.

- PMH: Unremarkable

- PSH: Unremarkable

- Exam: The patient reported no problems with fine motor movement of her hands, and no bowel or bladder symptoms. She also did not complain of any cranial nerve dysfunction (difficulty swallowing, coughing, gagging, impaired lingual articulation, etc.) or of the Lhermitte phenomenon. She also had no history of rheumatoid arthritis. On physical examination, the patient's neck was supple, and she did not guard against movements in any degrees of motion. Her strength was 5/5 in all muscle groups of the upper and lower extremities. She had an antalgic gait that she attributed to long-standing left hip arthritis, but otherwise showed no ataxia or spasticity in walking. Reflexes were 1+ throughout. She had no Hoffman sign, Babinski reflex, or clonus. Sensation was grossly intact to light touch and pinprick.

- Imaging: An MRI scan of the cervical spine revealed a pannus at the C1-2 joint leading to some distortion of the anterior thecal sac (Figure 10-1). No signal change was present in the spinal cord or lower brainstem. CT images of the cervical spine revealed the presence of an old type II odontoid fracture, anterior tubercle of C1 fracture, and calcified pannus around the C1-2 joint (Figure 10-2). Flexion-extension radiographs were taken, but did not show any gross movement of the odontoid process or change in the atlantodental interval (Figure 10-3).

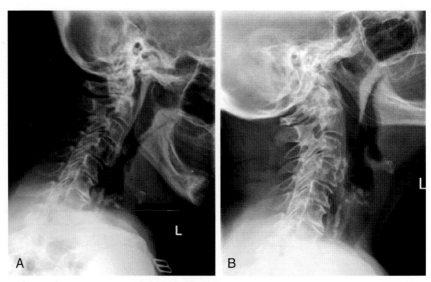

FIGURE 10-3 Flexion and extension lateral radiographs show no gross movement of the odontoid process or change in the atlantodental interval.

SURGICAL OPTIONS AND FUNDAMENTAL TECHNIQUES

Transoral-Transpharyngeal Decompression Plus Posterior Stabilization

In cases demonstrating clear anterior spinal cord compression that is irreducible, direct ventral decompression of the spinal cord is indicated. This approach provides access to the lower clivus, foramen magnum, anterior arch of C1, underlying odontoid process of C2, and down to the C3 vertebral body in some patients. Since first described in 1917 by Kanavel,[2] transoral approaches have been used extensively to address a wide range of pathologic entities.

Contraindications to this approach include surgeon unfamiliarity with the procedure, limited patient mouth opening, and extensive pathology that extends beyond the access of a standard transoral approach (e.g., large tumors, basilar invagination). Such situations may warrant extended transoral approaches involving maxillary or mandibular osteotomies.

The technique involves supine positioning followed by orotracheal intubation. Initial direct palpation of the posterior oropharynx allows identification of the anterior arch of C1 and the body of C2. The oral cavity is cleansed with chlorhexidine gluconate oral solution, intravenous antibiotics are provided, and the face is draped to allow access to the mouth and the nasal cavity. A self-retaining oral retractor (classically a Crockard retractor) is placed over the teeth and expanded to keep the mouth open. Self-retaining retractors are then attached to the retractor to keep the tongue depressed. If required for improved visualization, the soft palate can be divided in its midline. To avoid postoperative swallowing and phonation problems that may arise after palatal splitting, some authors suggest securing the uvula to a red rubber catheter that can be placed through the nares and out the pharynx and secured to retract the soft palate.

The posterior pharyngeal mucosa is infiltrated with local anesthetic and epinephrine, and a midline posterior incision is made from the clivus to the upper border of the third cervical vertebra (Tips from the Masters 10-1). The pharyngeal mucosa, pharyngeal constrictor musculature, and longus colli and longus capitis musculature are then elevated as a single myomucosal flap from the underlying anterior longitudinal ligament. Resection of the pannus is done piecemeal with curettes, rongeurs, and high-speed drilling. Some surgeons advocate maintaining the C1 anterior arch and pulling the resected odontoid and pannus tissue out from underneath it (Tips from the Masters 10-2). This maneuver maintains the integrity of the C1 ring. Access to the pannus may be challenging, however, and thus resection of the anterior C1 ring may be required. Resection of the hypertrophied tectorial membrane is also often required to truly decompress the dura. Unfortunately, this maneuver may be associated with a cerebrospinal fluid (CSF) leak, and the anterior dura may be exceptionally difficult to repair primarily. Dural graft onlays may be used with fibrin glues in conjunction with a lumbar drain to help with healing.

Tips from the Masters 10-1 • Unipolar cautery should be used carefully laterally, because the carotid arteries are close as they enter the skull base.

Tips from the Masters 10-2 • Removing the anterior C1 arch and removing the odontoid from the top down is suggested. This will avoid a "floating" odontoid process, which may be difficult to secure and remove.

Watertight closure of the posterior pharynx should be attempted in all cases, especially if CSF is encountered. It should be closed in two layers (pharyngeal musculature and pharyngeal mucosa), and the soft palate (if sectioned) should then be carefully approximated in three layers (nasal mucosa, muscularis, and oral mucosa), all with interrupted absorbable sutures. Postoperative stabilization is carried out as soon as possible.

More recent modifications of the standard transoral approach include use of image guidance via stereotactic navigation, intraoperative MRI, and endoscopy to improve the view without performing additional osteotomies. Specifically, the ability to visualize the lower and middle clivus is limited with the transoral approach, and full soft palate splitting, hard palate splitting, or extended maxillotomy procedures may be required. Such procedures may lengthen operating time, prolong recovery, and increase patient morbidity, and a 30-degree endoscope may be used to avoid these additional procedures.[3]

Transcervical Decompression Plus Posterior Stabilization (Transcervical Endoscopic Odontoidectomy)

In an attempt to limit the approach-related morbidity of the transoral route (infection from oral flora, meningitis, need for oral rest for pharyngeal healing, etc.), Wolinsky and colleagues[4] developed a minimally invasive method of performing an odontoidectomy via a standard anterior cervical approach. Based on a traditional Smith-Robinson anterior cervical approach, the surgical corridor follows the trajectory of a transodontoid screw, which allows exposure from the midcervical spine (C4) to the inferior clivus. In this way, the approach and anatomy are familiar to spine surgeons, and the oral cavity is completely isolated from the surgical field. However, surgery must be done via a tubular retractor, and thus navigation and endoscopy are recommended (Tips from the Masters 10-3). In addition, as with transodontoid screw placement, an ideal trajectory may not be achieved in patients who are obese, barrel-chested, or severely kyphotic.

Tips from the Masters 10-3 • Visualization is key because drilling of the odontoid is being done down a narrower tube. Thus, the endoscope should be rigidly fixed and routinely cleaned.

The technique involves supine positioning of the patient with the head fixed to the bed via a halo or Mayfield clamp. Using isocentric fluoroscopy, a CT-like image is acquired, which allows registration of preoperative images with the current position in the operating room. A standard Smith-Robinson approach to the cervical spine is then pereformed.[5] Blunt dissection along the anterior spine proceeds rostrally until the anterior tubercle of C1 is identified. A beveled tubular retractor is then inserted and rigidly secured to the bed so that it is docked in the midline, with the rostral tip of the retractor on the C1 tubercle and the caudal aspect over the C2-3 disk. A 30-degree endoscope is then placed down the retractor so that the

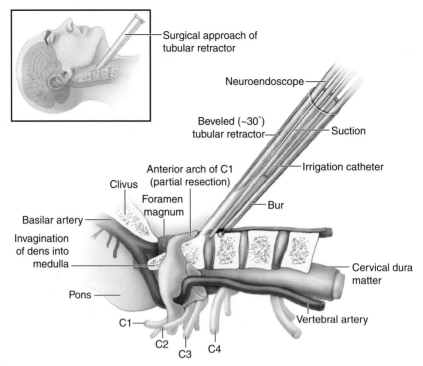

Surgical approach of
tubular retractor

Neuroendoscope

Beveled (~30°)
tubular retractor

Suction

Irrigation catheter

Anterior arch of C1
(partial resection)

Clivus

Foramen
magnum

Bur

Basilar artery

Invagination
of dens into
medulla

Cervical dura
matter

Pons

C1

Vertebral artery

C2
C3
C4

FIGURE 10-4 Illustration of the transcervical endoscopic odontoidectomy as described by Wolinsky and co-workers.[4]

endoscope lies in the superior aspect of the retractor field. At this point, endoscopic visualization of anatomic landmarks is correlated with the frameless stereotactic system (Tips from the Masters 10-4).

Tips from the Masters 10-4 • Confirmation of anatomy should be done routinely, ideally with intraoperative CT or isocentric C-arms, to actively assess the amount of bony compression remaining.

Described by Wolinsky and colleagues[4] for the treatment of basilar invagination, this technique provides good radiographic and neurologic results in both adults and children (Figure 10-4).[6] Following such decompression, the incision is closed in a standard, multilayered fashion as would be done for a Smith-Robinson cervical exposure. The halo ring is secured to the halo vest with the neck now placed in a neutral position, and the patient is repositioned for a posterior cervical or occipital cervical fusion. Postoperatively, the patient is left intubated overnight. After extubation, the patient can resume oral intake.

Posterior Fixation Alone

There are multiple techniques by which to secure C1 to C2 posteriorly. Although the vast array of techniques is beyond the scope of this chapter, it is worth mentioning the evolution in operative fixation techniques. Early on, methods described by Brooks, Gallie, and Sonntag utilized wiring techniques in conjunction with structural autograft. It was recommended that all patients wear a halo orthosis following such treatments. Since that time, C1-2 transarticular screws have been used, which has been associated with a large improvement in rigidity and subsequent bony union (Tips from the Masters 10-5).[7] However, one major anatomic limitation to the use of transarticular screws is the presence of a small C2 pars interarticularis. In such cases, safe passage of a screw without injury to the vertebral artery may not be possible. For this reason, others have developed techniques by which C1 and C2 can be rigidly be fixated. Harms and Melcher[8] described the placement

FIGURE 10-5 Intraoperative lateral radiograph taken after placement of C1 lateral mass screws and C2 pedicle screws and rod fixation.

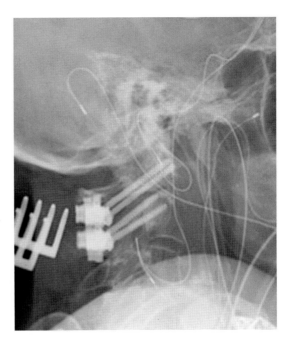

of C1 lateral mass screws and C2 pars interarticularis screws connected by rods. Theoretically, the chance of vertebral artery injury may be decreased with such techniques (Tips from the Masters 10-6). Others since have also described various techniques of C2 fixation, including the use of C2 pedicle screws and C2 laminar screws.[9,10]

Tips from the Masters 10-5 • C1 screws should be bicortical. Gentle tapping and palpation must be done to avoid inadvertent injury to the carotid artery anterior to the spine.

Tips from the Masters 10-6 • C2 pedicle screws can be placed safely only after preoperative MRI or CT scans confirm the absence of large or aberrantly located vertebral arteries.

Regardless of the technique used for fixation, basic guidelines apply to posterior stabilization. First, fixation must be rigid, because the pannus represents instability. If the pannus is soft, it may regress over time with such fixation, although this may take months to years. Second, in cases of obvious gross instability, subluxation can be corrected posteriorly, which thus indirectly decompresses the spinal canal. O'Brien and co-workers[11] described intraoperative reduction of C1-2 subluxation via manipulation of posterior instrumentation in C1 and C2. Third, all anterior decompressive procedures require posterior fixation. Thus, after an anterior approach, the spine should be assumed to be extremely unstable, due to resection of the atlantodental articulation. In such cases patients require rigid external immobilization until posterior instrumentation can be implanted.

The patient was offered surgical treatment for her condition via a posterior route. She consented to the operation and underwent a C1-2 instrumented fusion with use of allograft. C1 lateral mass screws and C2 pedicle screws were placed and fixed via small rods in the standard fashion as described by Harms and Melcher[8] (Figure 10-5). Ideal placement of the hardware was then confirmed postoperatively with a CT scan (Figure 10-6). The patient did well during and after surgery. Follow-up over the last 2 years has shown durable relief of her neck pain and no signs of myelopathy. Recent MRI done 18 months after surgery shows a stable construct and absence of spinal cord or lower brainstem compression (Figure 10-7).

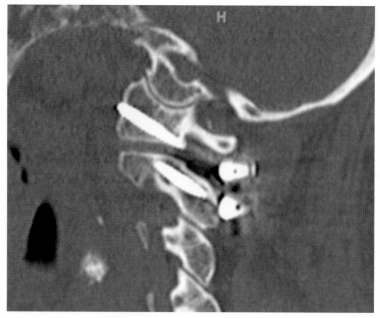

FIGURE 10-6 Sagittally reconstructed CT scan showing placement of the C1 lateral mass and C2 pedicle screws.

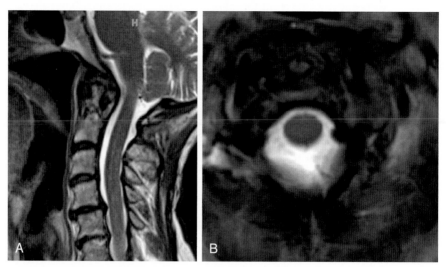

FIGURE 10-7 T2-weighted sagittal (**A**) and axial (**B**) MRI scans of the cervical spine showing stability of a C2 pannus and absence of spinal cord and lower brainstem compression.

DISCUSSION OF BEST EVIDENCE

Arthritis of the atlantodental joint leading to a pannus is most commonly caused by rheumatoid arthritis. Degenerative osteoarthritis is a less common cause and, in general, less progressive. As a result, most attention in the literature has been given to pannus associated with rheumatoid arthritis, and it is on the findings of these studies that most of the recommendations are based. In treating a patient with a pannus, the patient must first be evaluated fully via history taking, physical examination, and radiography.

Based on history, potential risk factors for progression of a rheumatoid pannus have been identified.[12] Nonradiographic risk factors include male gender, rheumatoid factor seropositivity, and the prolonged use of corticosteroids for treatment of rheumatologic disease.[13] Based on clinical progression of neurologic dysfunction, Ranawat and colleagues[14] classified patients into three categories to define the extent of myelopathy and plan treatment. Class I patients have no neurologic dysfunction. Class II patients have subjective weakness with hyperreflexia and dysesthesias. Class III patients have objective weakness and long-tract signs. These patients were further subcategorized into class IIIA patients, who are ambulatory, and class IIIB patients, who are no longer ambulatory. Higher classifications are associated with worse neurologic outcomes with or without surgical intervention.

Radiographic measurements have been traditionally based on plain radiographs and have included measurements such as the anterior atlantodental interval, the posterior atlantodental interval, and superior migration of the dens past the McGregor line (the line connecting the hard palate to the occiput). However, Riew and associates recently found that no single test reliably assessed C1-2 deformity associated with rheumatoid arthritis and concluded that a number of measurements should be considered together to evaluate patients.[15] With the more common use of MRI, space around the spinal cord can be evaluated directly and not indirectly from plain radiographs. It is therefore now generally agreed that 13 mm of space is needed at the C1-2 junction in the adult patient to allow the spinal cord to be free from compression.[16]

Once the patient is evaluated clinically and radiographically, options for treatment can be provided to the patient. Currently, there is no randomized controlled trial comparing the results of conservative versus surgical management. In addition, there is no study comparing anterior with posterior approaches. The main evidence for state-of-the-art treatment of C1-2 pannus is provided by retrospective case series. Although such studies may not provide the most rigorous scientific data, they form the basis for the current approach to this condition. Inherent in the decision making process is a fundamental assumption regarding patients with pannus. Namely, patients with severe neurologic deficits have less potential for neurologic improvement with surgical intervention than patients with a less advanced condition.[14] This assumption has not only been supported by the work of Ranawat and colleagues, but Reiter and Boden[13] have shown that earlier surgical intervention in patients with milder myelopathy often leads to a more satisfactory outcome.

In terms of an algorithmic approach to this condition, the most agreed-upon indication for surgical intervention is the presence of a neurologic deficit in the setting of instability. Not only is such an indication the basis for any possible spinal surgery, but there are few other situations involving a degenerative spine in which conservative management has the potential for such drastic negative consequences. For instance, the reported mortality for patients with cervical myelopathy from rheumatoid arthritis at 1 year if left untreated can reach 50%, as shown by Kraus and co-workers.[17] On the other hand, the treatment of asymptomatic patients with radiographically demonstrated instability has been controversial over the past several decades. However, with the more consistent use of MRI in such patients, most would agree that evidence of cord compression, even if asymptomatic, mandates surgery. Casey and associates[18] argue that if the space available for the cord is less than 13 mm, a posterior cervical fusion should be considered. Such stabilization will prevent pannus progression, and in cases of a noncalcified mass, the pannus may regress over time.

In those patients with spinal cord compression, with or without neurologic deficit, many argue that reduction should be attempted.[12] If reduction can be obtained with the use of cervical traction, then surgical methods can be used to accomplish stabilization in the reduced state.[12] Alternatively, intraoperative reduction can be attempted using posterior cervical instrumentation without the use of traction.[11] If reduction cannot be obtained, but posterior decompression is expected to provide adequate room for the spinal cord, a C1 laminectomy can be performed, followed by an occipitocervical fusion. If myelopathy worsens postoperatively after the use of such techniques, persistent anterior compression at the cervicomedullary junction may require an anterior odontoid resection. However, initial anterior approaches should be considered at the outset in cases of severe anterior compression or cranial settling with basilar invagination that may not respond to traction and/or posterior stabilization alone. Based on their experience, Finn and co-workers[1] contend that it is best to decompress the neural elements anteriorly at the outset in such patients. They argue that it provides the best neural decompression and chance for neurologic recovery, and it may allow easier and more optimal atlantoaxial reduction before posterior fusion. This experience may be due in part to the fact that the pannus often prevents optimal posterior atlantoaxial reduction. Because of approach-related morbidity, however, most would argue that the transoral approach is indicated in patients with irreducible ventral compression at the cervicomedullary junction, as suggested in a **retrospective study.**[19] In neurologically intact patients who do not meet the criteria stated earlier, conservative management may be considered, but careful follow-up must be maintained to detect new evidence of myelopathy.

The patient described in the Case Presentation underwent surgery based on two main considerations in this algorithm. First, she had decreased spinal canal diameter with distortion of the spinal cord. Second, she had mechanical pain unresponsive to conservative management. She was not placed in traction because in this case C1-2 did not show gross instability that required reduction. In addition, it was felt that the anterior compression did not require an anterior decompressive procedure both because of the absence of significant ventral compression on radiographs and because of the absence of myelopathy.

The Ranawat classification has been considered a simple but reliable tool for predicting neurologic recovery after stabilization. Casey and colleagues[18] showed that the majority of patients improve by at least one Ranawat class after surgical intervention. Patients with pure atlantoaxial instability also fare better than patients with basilar invagination. Finally, the prognosis has been shown to be poorer in patients with a subaxial canal diameter of less than 14 mm than in patients with a large canal diameter.[12] Postoperatively, progression of myelopathy has been reported in 4% to 8% of cases in a **retrospective study** by Boden and co-workers.[20] Potential causes of delayed worsening include the natural history of myelopathy in the setting of prior spinal cord damage, persistent compression, and nonunion, the latter of which can occur in up to 50% of cases involving a rheumatoid spine.[16]

The transoral approach is a well-established procedure for treatment of anterior compression at the craniovertebral junction, and it has gained great acceptance due in part to the work of Menezes and colleagues.[21] Nonetheless, there is substantial potential morbidity associated with this approach, including the need for prolonged tube feeding, the need for tracheostomy, soft palate and pharyngeal wound dehiscence, and CSF fistulas.[19] Furthermore, following anterior decompression, the patient is often in overtly unstable condition until the posterior fusion is completed. For this reason, patients must be firmly immobilized after anterior decompression until posterior fixation is accomplished. At a time when posterior stabilization of C1-2 was less safe and more cumbersome, Menezes and co-workers[21] reported that roughly 75% of patients undergoing a transoral decompression required dorsal fixation after odontoidectomy. According to a **retrospective review** by Menezes and Van Gilder,[22] when osteoarthritis was present in the atlantoaxial joints, posterior fixation often was not required. However, given the efficiency and safety with which posterior instrumentation can be placed, and the likelihood that such arthritis would create pain for the patient, posterior stabilization after an anterior decompression is always recommended.

COMMENTARY

C1-2 instability can lead to pain and neurologic dysfunction from spinal cord or brainstem compression. For those patients with pain alone, conservative management should be considered. However, in the presence of persistent pain, pannus enlargement, or instability on dynamic imaging, posterior fixation should be considered. In patients with spinal cord compression with or without neurologic dysfunction, surgery is indicated. If the compression is reducible, posterior fixation is the treatment of choice. If the compression is not reducible, two broad options exist: posterior decompression and posterior fusion, and anterior decompression and posterior fusion. As has been suggested earlier, the pannus may regress over time after posterior stabilization alone. However, this change may take months, and thus persistent anterior compression may require a subsequent anterior approach, such as a transoral approach. An anterior approach as the initial procedure may achieve a more optimal decompression of anterior lesions, but should only be carried out by surgeons experienced in this approach because of associated complications. For this reason, the patient must also be clearly warned of the potential approach-related morbidity. However, in light of recent advancements such as the transcervical odontoidectomy, in which the C1-2 pannus may be resected via a more classic anterior cervical approach, anterior approaches to the craniovertebral junction may carry less morbidity and thus may be used for severe pathologic conditions such as marked basilar invagination.

REFERENCES

1. Finn M, Fassett DR, Apfelbaum RI: Surgical treatment of nonrheumatoid atlantoaxial degenerative arthritis producing pain and myelopathy, *Spine* 32(26):3067–3073, 2007. **This article describes the surgical experience of Dr. Apfelbaum, who is one of the most experienced surgeons in dealing with C1-2 pathology. In the article, the authors not only review their experience retrospectively, but also provide a working algorithm for dealing with nonrheumatoid atlantoaxial degenerative arthritis. It is a great read for both the beginner and the expert.**
2. Kanavel AB: Bullet located between the atlas and the base of the skull: technique of removal through the mouth, *Surg Clin Chicago* 1:361–366, 1917.
3. Frempong-Boadu AK, Faunce WA, Fessler RG: Endoscopically assisted transoral-transpharyngeal approach to the craniovertebral junction, *Neurosurgery* 51(Suppl 5):S60–S66, 2002.
4. Wolinsky JP, Sciubba DM, Suk I, et al: Endoscopic image-guided odontoidectomy for decompression of basilar invagination via a standard anterior cervical approach. Technical note, *J Neurosurg Spine* 6(2):184–191, 2007.
5. Robinson RA, Southwick WO: Surgical approaches to the cervical spine, *Instr Course Lect* 17:299–330, 1960.
6. McGirt MJ, Attenello FJ, Sciubba DM, et al: Endoscopic transcervical odontoidectomy for pediatric basilar invagination and cranial settling. Report of 4 cases, *J Neurosurg Pediatr* 1(4):337–342, 2008.
7. Magerl F, Seemann P-S: Stable posterior fusion of the atlas and axis by transarticular screw fixation. In Kehr P, Weidner A, editors: *Cervical spine*, Vienna, 1985, Springer-Verlag.
8. Harms J, Melcher RP: Posterior C1-C2 fusion with polyaxial screw and rod fixation, *Spine* 26(22):2467–2471, 2001.
9. Sciubba DM, Noggle JC, Vellimana AK, et al: Radiographic and clinical evaluation of free-hand placement of C-2 pedicle screws. Clinical article, *J Neurosurg Spine* 11(1):15–22, 2009.
10. Sciubba DM, Noggle JC, Vellimana AK, et al: Laminar screw fixation of the axis, *J Neurosurg Spine* 8(4):327–334, 2008.
11. O'Brien JR, Gokaslan ZL, Riley LH 3rd, et al: Open reduction of C1-C2 subluxation with the use of C1 lateral mass and C2 translaminar screws, *Neurosurgery* 63(1 Suppl 1):ONS95–98; discussion, ONS98-99, 2008.
12. Nguyen HV, Ludwig SC, Silber J, et al: Rheumatoid arthritis of the cervical spine, *Spine J* 4(3):329–334, 2004.
13. Reiter MF, Boden SD: Inflammatory disorders of the cervical spine, *Spine* 23(24):2755–2766, 1998.
14. Ranawat CS, O'Leary P, Pellicci P, et al: Cervical spine fusion in rheumatoid arthritis, *J Bone Joint Surg Am* 61(7):1003–1010, 1979.
15. Riew KD, Hillibrand AS, Palumbo MA, et al: Diagnosing basilar invagination in the rheumatoid patient. The reliability of radiographic criteria, *J Bone Joint Surg Am* 83-A(2):194–200, 2001.
16. Papadopoulos SM, Dickman CA, Sonntag VK: Atlantoaxial stabilization in rheumatoid arthritis, *J Neurosurg* 74(1):1–7, 1991.
17. Kraus DR, Peppelman WC, Agarwal AK, et al: Incidence of subaxial subluxation in patients with generalized rheumatoid arthritis who have had previous occipital cervical fusions, *Spine* 16(Suppl 10):S486–S489, 1991.
18. Casey AT, Crockard HA, Stevens J: Vertical translocation. Part II. Outcomes after surgical treatment of rheumatoid cervical myelopathy, *J Neurosurg* 87(6):863–869, 1997. **Dr. Crockard is one of the leading craniocervical surgeons in the world. In this article he and coauthors review his surgical outcomes for rheumatoid cervical myelopathy, underlining for the reader the outcomes that may be expected in this challenging group of patients..**
19. Landeiro JA, Boechat S, Christoph Dhe H, et al: Transoral approach to the craniovertebral junction, *Arq Neuropsiquiat* 65(4B):1166–1171, 2007. **This is a great technical review on the anatomic approach to the craniocervical junction. The transoral approach can be a daunting one even for the experienced spinal surgeon, and this article underlines some of the important aspects of the approach.**

20. Boden SD, Dodge LD, Bohlman HH, et al: Rheumatoid arthritis of the cervical spine. A long-term analysis with predictors of paralysis and recovery, *J Bone Joint Surg Am* 75(9):1282–1297, 1993.
21. Menezes AH, VanGilder JC, Graf CJ, et al: Craniocervical abnormalities. A comprehensive surgical approach, *J Neurosurg* 53(4):444–455, 1980. **Dr. Menezes is one of the most experienced craniocervical surgeons and treats some of the most challenging pathologic conditions. This article underlines some of the ways in which he reviews and approaches such complex problems at the craniocervical junction.**
22. Menezes AH, VanGilder JC: Transoral-transpharyngeal approach to the anterior craniocervical junction. Ten-year experience with 72 patients, *J Neurosurg* 69(6):895–903, 1988. **A follow-up article to the previous one by the same authors, this article specifically reviews the transoral approach to the craniocervical junction. Drawing on his vast clinical experience, Dr. Menezes sheds light upon the array of pathologic conditions that can be encountered at this area and describes his results.**

Chapter 11 Odontoid Fracture in the Elderly: Odontoid Screws Versus Posterior Fusion

Harvey E. Smith, Scott D. Daffner, Alexander R. Vaccaro

Type II odontoid fracture is the most common cervical spine fracture in the elderly, and the incidence of this injury is increasing.[1] The odontoid peg is central to the stability of the upper cervical spine—the posterior ring of C1 articulates with the anterior odontoid process, and axial rotation at this joint accounts for approximately 60 degrees of rotation.[2] Stability is afforded via ligamentous constraint: The transverse ligament inserts posteriorly on the odontoid, preventing anterior-posterior translation of C1 relative to C2. Consequently, a fracture of the odontoid process may allow the translation of the occiput-C1-odontoid complex relative to the body of C2.

The management of type II odontoid fractures in the elderly is controversial for several reasons. Odontoid fractures in the elderly are associated with significant morbidity, irrespective of the type of management chosen. In the octogenarian population acute inpatient mortality may exceed 10%, regardless of management option.[3] There is consensus that in the elderly patient with a displaced fracture the most likely outcome of nonoperative management (either with cervical orthosis or halothoracic vest bracing) is a nonunion. In addition, there is growing consensus that in elderly patients halothoracic vest immobilization is associated with significant morbidity.[4]

Nonoperative treatment of a displaced type II odontoid fracture is associated with a nonunion rate that approaches 80% in the elderly.[5,6] An unstable nonunion has an associated risk of catastrophic neurologic injury with subsequent falls, as well as a well-documented risk of late-onset progressive myelopathy.[7] The goal of surgical management is to restore stability to the upper cervical spine, either through direct osseous union of the odontoid fracture or through posterior fusion of the ring of C1 to the posterior elements of C2.

CASE PRESENTATION

An 82-year-old woman fell from standing and came to a regional level I trauma spinal cord injury referral center.

- PMH: Unremarkable
- PSH: Unremarkable
- Exam: The patient was neurologically intact, with normal reflexes. Head trauma was present with ecchymosis and a scalp hematoma over the right occiput. There was no tenderness to palpation along the posterior spinal elements.
- Imaging: Initial anteroposterior (AP), lateral, and open-mouth odontoid images demonstrated a type II odontoid fracture. AP and lateral radiographs of the thoracic and lumbar spine were negative for fracture. Due to the displaced odontoid fracture, a computed tomography (CT) scan of the cervical spine, as well as a magnetic resonance imaging (MRI) scan of the cervical spine with magnetic resonance angiography, were obtained. The CT scan (Figure 11-1) demonstrated a posteriorly displaced odontoid fracture with comminution at the fracture site.

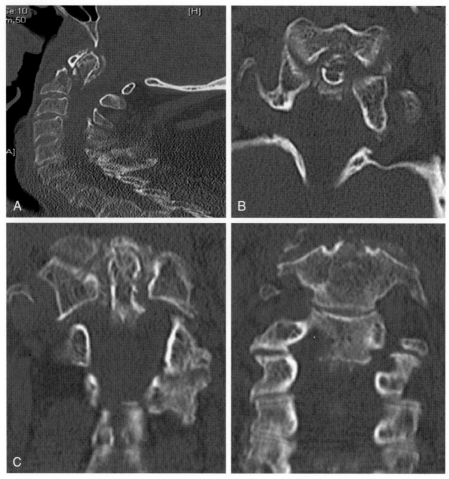

FIGURE 11-1 Sagittally reconstructed CT scan (**A**) demonstrates a posteriorly displaced type II odontoid fracture with fracture comminution. The axial (**B**) and coronal (**C**) images illustrate the posterior translation of the C1-odontoid complex relative to the body of C2.

SURGICAL OPTIONS

The surgical management options for a type II odontoid fracture can be divided into two subsets: anterior approach and fixation with the goal of direct osteosynthesis, and posterior approach and fusion of the C1-C2 complex.

Anterior Odontoid Screw

Direct union of an odontoid fracture through placement of anterior odontoid screws[8] is attractive mainly because it avoids the morbidity of the posterior approach and maintains axial rotation of the C1-C2 articulation. Apfelbaum and colleagues[9] reported on a large cohort of 147 patients who underwent anterior screw fixation and demonstrated it to be an effective technique irrespective of age, but they found that outcomes were worse for fractures with an anterior-oblique orientation and for fractures treated longer than 18 months after injury. To achieve direct osteosynthesis, however, one must obtain a complete reduction of the fracture or be able to achieve reduction of the fracture in the operating room. Similar results have been found with single- and multiple-screw fixaion.[10] A partially threaded screw should be used (or the proximal fragment overdrilled by 1 mm), and the threads must be advanced completely across the fracture site. In addition, the transverse ligament must be carefully assessed for injury, because injury to this ligament is a contraindication to anterior odontoid screw fixation. Direct repair of the fracture will not restore C1-C2 stability in the setting of an incompetent ligament.

The presence of osteoporosis raises concern for increased risk of instrumentation failure with anterior fixation, as reported by Andersson and associates.[11] However, Borm and co-workers[12] reported on a cohort of elderly patients treated successfully with anterior odontoid fixation, and Harrop and colleagues[13] found that age per se was not a contraindication, but that the presence of osteoporosis carries a risk of instrumentation failure. Direct comparison between outcomes for anterior odontoid screw fixation and posterior C1-C2 fusion in a retrospective review involving an elderly cohort suggested better overall results with the posterior procedure when fusion rate and rate of reoperation were considered.[14] A retrospective study of data for a cohort of elderly patients who underwent surgery for acute type II odontoid fractures found a significantly higher incidence of postoperative pneumonia, dysphagia, and vocal cord problems in the patients undergoing anterior screw fixation (compared with those treated using various posterior techniques).[1] In patients with good bone quality and appropriate fracture orientation, anterior odontoid screw fixation has been demonstrated to be associated with a fusion rate of approximately 90%, but the use of the technique in the elderly and/or patients with osteoporosis remains controversial.

Posterior C1-C2 Fusion

Posterior C1-C2 fusion may be achieved via posterior wiring and bone grafting (Brooks or Gallie technique), placement of posterior C1-C2 transarticular screws (Magerl[15]), posterior C1 lateral mass–C2 pars instrumentation and fusion (popularized by Harms and Melcher[16]), and placement of posterior C1 lateral mass–C2 laminar screws. The use of transarticular screws and C1 lateral mass–C2 pars/laminar screws[17] has largely supplanted sublaminar wiring.[1] Advantages of a posterior fusion procedure include the ability to restore stability in the setting of transverse ligament injury as well as in the setting of an irreducible fracture. With the increasing biomechanical stability afforded by later-generation posterior constructs there has been a concomitant decrease in the use of postoperative halo vest immobilization.[1,18] Relative risks of a posterior C1-C2 procedure are the morbidity of the posterior approach, risk of brisk bleeding from the venous plexus, risk of injury to the vertebral artery, as well as risk of injury to the carotid artery or esophagus with anterior perforation of a C1 lateral mass screw.

The patient described in the Case Presentation is an octogenarian who incurred her injury in a fall from standing. As with most such fractures, the patient is neurologically intact. The fracture is posteriorly displaced and angulated. Because posterior displacement and patient age are significant risk factors for nonunion, the options in this case are to provide surgical management or to accept a likely nonunion with use of a cervical orthosis. Preoperative reduction of such a fracture has been demonstrated to be associated with significant risk of airway compromise.[19] In addition, if the surgeon is unable to achieve an anatomic reduction in the operating room, any planned anterior procedure would need to be aborted and changed to a posterior procedure.

The long-term morbidity of a nonunion is unclear. Some literature contends that a fibrous nonunion may be an acceptable outcome,[20,21] and this may be the case in an elderly patient with significant comorbid medical conditions that result in a predominantly sedentary lifestyle. However, for an independent, active elderly patient, a nonunion likely portends worse outcomes. A displaced fracture that has not healed leaves the upper cervical spine at significant risk in the event of a subsequent fall. Furthermore, although the incidence of late-onset myelopathy is not established, the report by Crockard and colleagues[7] suggests that it is in the setting of a displaced fracture with subsequent nonunion that late-onset myelopathy is most likely to occur. Interestingly, Crockard's group found that in the cohort with nonunion the transverse ligament was frequently interposed in the fracture site. Consequently, for an active elderly patient such as the one described in the Case Presentation, surgical management is a reasonable option. Which option is the best for any given patient

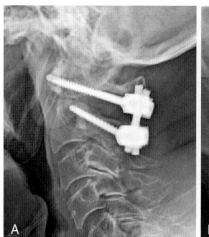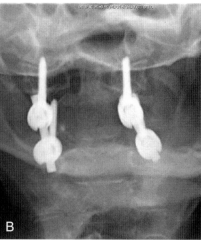

FIGURE 11-2 Postoperative lateral (**A**) and AP (**B**) radiographs demonstrating fracture reduction with C1 lateral mass and C2 pars instrumentation.

is a complex question and ultimately must be decided by the patient and physician based on patient-specific factors.

If surgical management is undertaken in the patient in the Case Presentation, a posterior C1-C2 fusion may be more desirable than anterior fixation for a number of reasons. The fracture in this patient is displaced, which precludes anterior fixation without prior reduction. As noted earlier, closed reduction of displaced odontoid fractures in the elderly has been demonstrated to be associated with risk of airway compromise,[19] and so any preoperative closed reduction procedure probably carries more inherent risk than it would in a younger patient. Closed reduction in the operating room is possible, but if reduction cannot be achieved, the anterior procedure would need to be aborted. There is a lack of consensus regarding the role of anterior screw fixation in the elderly with respect to the quality of the bone. One large single-center retrospective cohort study reviewed results for 75 acute type II odontoid fractures that were managed surgically and found a statistically significant increase in the rate of airway problems and dysphagia in patients who underwent anterior screw fixation compared with those treated using other techniques.[1] Several reports have suggested that in osteoporotic patients anterior screw fixation may result in suboptimal outcomes due in part to fracture site comminution, as well as the risk of nonunion with subsequent failure of the hardware, and the rate of nonunion is higher in elderly than in younger patients.[22] Anterior screw fixation has not been demonstrated to be superior to posterior C1-C2 instrumentation, and given the conflicting data on the efficacy of the procedure in the elderly, a posterior procedure may provide more consistent results in achieving fusion and stability, which is the ultimate goal of surgical management.

Due to the displacement type of fracture, the patient's age, and the history of osteoporosis, the patient underwent a posterior C1-C2 fusion with lateral mass instrumentation and placement of C2 pars screws, with patellar allograft bone used as the graft source, secured in place with No. 5 fiber wire (modified Gallie technique) (Figure 11-2). The patient was extubated on postoperative day 1 and progressed well enough to be transferred to a skilled nursing facility on postoperative day 5. At the time of 6-month follow-up the patient had returned to living independently with her spouse.

FUNDAMENTAL TECHNIQUE

Surgical planning, positioning of the patient, and use of intraoperative fluoroscopy are procedural variables that are under the control of the surgeon, and proper attention to these details is essential (Tips from the Masters 11-1).

Tips from the Masters 11-1 • Careful preoperative planning using CT reconstructions is essential. The C2 isthmus and foramen must be scrutinized to confirm that the morphology is appropriate for use of a C2 screw, and a thorough understanding of the anatomy is mandatory before surgical intervention is undertaken.

Preoperatively the vertebral artery should be visualized on MRI scan and the foramen identified on CT images of C1 and C2, with careful attention paid to the diameter of the C2 pars. A high-riding foramen in C2 may preclude the safe placement of a pars screw on that side or necessitate use of a shorter screw.

The patient should be positioned prone on chest rolls in Mayfield tongs in reverse Trendelenburg position of sufficient angle to make the cervical spine at least parallel with the floor of the operating room; this will facilitate operative visualization and minimize blood loss. To facilitate fluoroscopy the table may need to be reversed with the patient's head at the opposite end of the table from the anesthesia team, so the anesthesia team should be prepared accordingly for management of the endotracheal tube and intravenous lines.

Surgical dissection should be carried subperiosteally along the posterior elements of C2 and C1. Great care should be taken to maintain the initial midline dissection of the lamina of C1 within 15 mm of midline and along the posterior inferior margin. This will minimize the chance of injury to the vertebral artery as it traverses dorsally along the superior aspect of the posterior arch of C1. The lamina of C2 should be exposed, and the C2 isthmus clearly identified. It is recommended that at this point a Penfield 4 dissector be placed along each side of the C2 isthmus and that lateral fluoroscopic images be obtained. The fluoroscope should be adjusted until the images of the Penfield dissectors are superimposed: this will help to avoid parallax and optimize accurate visualization of the anatomy (Tips from the Masters 11-2).

Tips from the Masters 11-2 • Use two Penfield dissectors to eliminate parallax when orienting for lateral fluoroscopy.

At this point dissection of the soft tissues inferior to the C1 lateral mass, the cavernous sinus, and the C2 greater occipital nerve should be performed, and the C2 greater occipital nerve should be mobilized inferiorly. This can be done with minimal blood loss with the aid of a small thrombin-soaked patty and Penfield dissector, with the patty used to sweep the soft tissues away from the lamina. If the epidural plexus is disturbed, the surgeon should be prepared to encounter brisk venous bleeding; this can be controlled using a thrombin-soaked absorbable gelatin sponge, cottonoid patty, and FloSeal hemostatic matrix (Tips from the Masters 11-3).

Tips from the Masters 11-3 • Careful dissection with a thrombin-soaked patty will minimize epidural bleeding in the C1-2 interval.

After exposure of the C1-C2 articulation, the medial and lateral borders of the inferior articular process of C1 should be palpated with a Penfield 4 dissector, and a 2-mm bur used to score the starting point for drill insertion. Notching of the inferior cortex of the posterior ring of C1 may be necessary to obtain the correct starting point and trajectory. This can be done with either a Kerrison punch or bur, with careful attention to the superior vertebral artery (Figure 11-3). Using real-time fluoroscopy, a drill is then advanced past the starting point to cannulate the lateral mass. It is crucial that the proper sagittal trajectory be maintained. In the sagittal plane the drill should be parallel to the C1 posterior arch, and it should be medially angulated 5 to 10 degrees (Tips from the Masters 11-4). After drilling, a ball-tipped probe is used to confirm that the lateral mass has not been breached. Screws of the appropriate length should be placed. Use of a partially threaded screw is recommended, because the smooth exposed shank will minimize neural irritation.

Tips from the Masters 11-4 • The undersurface of the C1 ring may need to be notched for proper C1 lateral mass instrumentation.

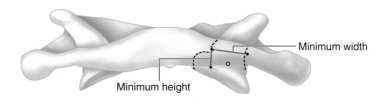

FIGURE 11-3 Starting point for lateral mass screw. Note the posterior overhang of C1, which may need to be notched to facilitate proper screw trajectory.

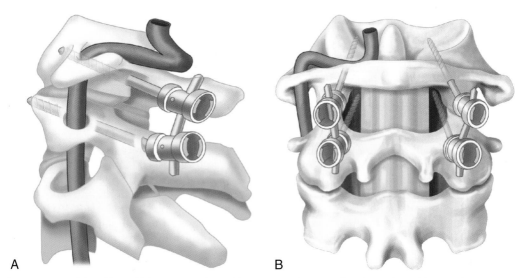

A   B

FIGURE 11-4 AP (**A**) and lateral (**B**) representations of instrumentation. Note the relationship of the vertebral artery. The general starting point for the C2 screw is the intersection of the pars and the midline of the lamina; this must be confirmed with careful palpation of the medial border.

After insertion of the C1 lateral mass screws, the C2 isthmus screws can be placed using palpation of the medial border. Preoperative CT images should be carefully reviewed to confirm that there is adequate space to accommodate a screw. The medial border of the isthmus should be palpated from within the canal, and a 2-mm drill should be used to cannulate the pilot hole. The starting point is proximal to the C2-3 facet and should be confirmed both by palpation of the medial border of the isthmus and by preoperative imaging. A general guide for the starting point is the intersection of the pars interarticularis with a horizontal line through the midline of the lamina of C2; however, there is no universal starting point, and preoperative planning is essential (Figure 11-4). Preferred practice is to bias the starting point superior and medial to the intersection of the pars and midline of the lamina, with careful use of a Penfield 4 dissector to define the medial border of the pars. The starting point should be initiated with a bur, and then a 2-mm drill should be used. The drill should have a medial angulation of 20 to 30 degrees as it is advanced, with the assistant taking care to delineate the medial border of the isthmus with palpation, providing visual confirmation of the trajectory. The pilot hole should be carefully probed, and then the screw placed.

Optimal bone grafting is essential to achieve osseous union. Tricortical iliac crest autograft is the gold standard. However, harvest of tricortical iliac crest is associated with donor site morbidity, and in an elderly patient the quality of the graft may be suboptimal. If the surgeon feels that patient-specific factors preclude autologous iliac crest structural graft harvest, an alternative is allograft. The preference is to use autologous graft whenever possible, but when circumstances require it, good results have been achieved with patellar bone allograft. The graft must be appropriately sized so that it fits securely between the cortical surfaces of the inferior ring of C1 and the C2 lamina; the graft can be notched superiorly to match the contour of C1 and inferiorly to straddle the

C2 spinous process, and then gently wedged into place. With proper dimensions the fit should be tight—compressive force is necessary to promote adequate fusion. The graft can be bolstered in place with suture material looped under the lamina and over the graft in a figure-eight pattern (Tips from the Masters 11-5). Alternatively, the graft may be secured with stainless steel wire or titanium cable using a modified Gallie technique.

Tips from the Masters 11-5 • Graft may be bolstered with suture material to minimize risk of dislodgment.

As with all posterior cervical cases, meticulous hemostasis and wound closure technique are imperative. Preferred practice is to use a cervical orthosis (Philadelphia collar) in the postoperative period and to place a drain deep to the fascia. Patient-specific issues should be considered in determining the length of time the cervical orthosis should be worn. The recommendation is to maintain the orthosis for a minimum of 6 weeks; at that point the relative merits of continued immobilization should be balanced against patient-specific factors such as ease of feeding and activity level. For a minimally active patient who is developing occipital irritation and/or having difficulty eating, it may be reasonable to discontinue use of the orthosis.

DISCUSSION OF BEST EVIDENCE

The current evidence regarding the management of type II odontoid fractures comes primarily from Level III studies as well as from some Level II studies. No Level I evidence is available.

Nonoperative Management

There is a clear consensus that the rate of nonunion is high for displaced type II odontoid fractures treated nonoperatively, particularly in the elderly population.

Level II Studies

Clark and White,[23] in a multicenter study of odontoid fractures, found that displacement greater than 5 mm and angulation greater than 10 degrees correlated with risk of nonunion. Govender and colleagues[24] reported that age older than 40 years, displacement greater than 4 mm, and posterior displacement are risk factors for nonunion. In a study by Stoney and co-workers,[25] more than 3 mm of displacement and more than 30 degrees of angulation were shown to be associated with risk of nonunion. Lennarson and colleagues[26] found that age older than 50 years was associated with poor outcomes with halo vest management.

Level III Studies

Level III evidence consistently demonstrates that nonunion rates are significantly associated with displacement and patient age.[27-32] The use of halo vest immobilization in the elderly has been reported in several Level III studies to be associated with significant morbidity and mortality,[4,33] but good success with halo vest treatment has been reported in others.[34-36]

Surgical Management

There is no Level I evidence comparing surgical options (anterior versus posterior techniques) for the management of type II odontoid fractures.

Level II Studies

No Level II studies have investigated surgical technique. (There is a prospective case series examining use of the anterior odontoid screw technique, but no control group was included.[37]) Bednar and associates,[38] in a **prospective cohort study,** found that surgical management decreased peri-injury mortality compared with nonoperative management in the elderly.

Level III Studies

Numerous Level III studies have demonstrated excellent union rates with anterior odontoid screw fixation.[8,9,12,39] Level III evidence[11,13,22] suggests a higher rate of nonunion and complications in elderly patients, but whether this is due solely to bone quality or age is not clear. Posterior C1-C2 fusion techniques are associated with union rates exceeding 90%.[11,16,40,41] Kuntz and co-workers[30] found that operative management was associated with fewer early failures than nonoperative management, but equivalent overall morbidity and mortality. Peri-injury mortality rates in the octogenarian population were found by Smith and colleagues[3] to be similar for both operative and nonoperative management.

COMMENTARY

The management of type II odontoid fractures is controversial, particularly in the elderly population. There is a lack of Level II follow-up data describing the respective outcomes of surgical and nonsurgical management, and the long-term morbidity of a fibrous nonunion is similarly controversial due in large part to a lack of consensus regarding the relative risk of developing late-onset myelopathy. It is clear that surgical management of these fractures can be safely accomplished in the elderly population via either anterior or posterior approaches. The choice of approach and fixation should be made by the surgeon taking into account fracture geometry, bone quality, and patient-specific considerations. This injury is associated with significant morbidity and mortality in patients undergoing both nonoperative and operative treatment as reported in multiple studies. Optimal management of this injury necessitates careful consideration of the given patient's clinical situation and baseline activity level, so that the patient may make an informed decision regarding operative versus nonoperative management. Long-term follow-up studies of patients treated for this injury are needed to more accurately delineate the outcomes of both surgical and nonsurgical management of odontoid fractures.

REFERENCES

1. Smith HE, Vaccaro AR, Maltenfort M, et al: Trends in surgical management for type II odontoid fracture: 20 years of experience at a regional spinal cord injury center, *Orthopedics* 31:650, 2008.
2. Panjabi MM, Crisco JJ, Vasavada A, et al: Mechanical properties of the human cervical spine as shown by three-dimensional load-displacement curves, *Spine* 26:2692–2700, 2001.
3. Smith HE, Kerr SM, Maltenfort M, et al: Early complications of surgical versus conservative treatment of isolated type II odontoid fractures in octogenarians: a retrospective cohort study, *J Spinal Disord Tech* 21:535–539, 2008. **This study reports on a large cohort of octogenarians with type II odontoid fractures managed either operatively (n = 32) or nonoperatively (n = 40). Significant inpatient morbidity and mortality was noted in both cohorts; patients undergoing surgery experienced significantly more complications, but both groups had similar mortality rates.**
4. Majercik S, Tashjian RZ, Biffl WL, et al: Halo vest immobilization in the elderly: a death sentence? *J Trauma* 59:350–356; discussion, 6–8, 2005. **This study examined data for patients admitted to a trauma center with cervical spine fractures and compared outcomes for younger patients (under 65 years) and older patients (over 65 years). The mortality rate with halo vest management was 40% in older patients, compared with 2% in the younger cohort.**
5. Sasso RC: C2 dens fractures: treatment options, *J Spinal Disord* 14:455–463, 2001.
6. Maak TG, Grauer JN: The contemporary treatment of odontoid injuries, *Spine* 31:S53–S60; discussion, S1, 2006.
7. Crockard HA, Heilman AE, Stevens JM: Progressive myelopathy secondary to odontoid fractures: clinical, radiological, and surgical features, *J Neurosurg* 78:579–586, 1993. **Report on 16 patients with delayed diagnosis of odontoid fracture. A correlation between delayed diagnosis and diminished cord volume was noted, which suggests a causal relationship with late-onset myelopathy. In the majority of cases of nonunion, transposition of the transverse ligament was found.**
8. Bohler J: Anterior stabilization for acute fractures and non-unions of the dens, *J Bone Joint Surg Am* 64:18–27, 1982. **Bohler's initial description of anterior fixation with the use of bone grafting for nonunions.**
9. Apfelbaum RI, Lonser RR, Veres R, et al: Direct anterior screw fixation for recent and remote odontoid fractures, *J Neurosurg* 93:227–236, 2000. **Report on 147 consecutively treated patients who underwent anterior odontoid screw fixation. Excellent fusion rates were noted in fractures treated less than 6 months after injury. There were no differences in outcome related to the number of screws placed. The importance of recognizing anterior-oblique fracture geometry and its correlation with worse outcomes was noted.**
10. Jenkins JD, Coric D, Branch CL Jr: A clinical comparison of one- and two-screw odontoid fixation, *J Neurosurg* 89:366–370, 1998.

11. Andersson S, Rodrigues M, Olerud C: Odontoid fractures: high complication rate associated with anterior screw fixation in the elderly, *Eur Spine J* 9:56–59, 2000.

12. Borm W, Kast E, Richter HP, et al: Anterior screw fixation in type II odontoid fractures: is there a difference in outcome between age groups? *Neurosurgery* 52:1089–1092; discussion, 92–94, 2003.

13. Harrop JS, Przybylski GJ, Vaccaro AR, et al: Efficacy of anterior odontoid screw fixation in elderly patients with type II odontoid fractures, *Neurosurg Focus* 8:E6, 2000.

14. Platzer P, Thalhammer G, Oberleitner G, et al: Surgical treatment of dens fractures in elderly patients, *J Bone Joint Surg Am* 89:1716–1722, 2007. **Retrospective review of outcomes for 56 patients (average age, 71 years) with odontoid fractures managed surgically. This study found that operative management in the elderly can have overall good results, but noted lower union rates and higher frequency of reoperation with anterior screw fixation.**

15. Grob D, Magerl F: Surgical stabilization of C1 and C2 fractures, *Orthopade* 16:46–54, 1987.

16. Harms J, Melcher RP: Posterior C1-C2 fusion with polyaxial screw and rod fixation, *Spine* 26:2467–2471, 2001. **Harms' and Melcher's description that popularized the surgical technique of posterior C1 lateral mass–C2 isthmus fixation.**

17. Wright NM: Posterior C2 fixation using bilateral, crossing C2 laminar screws: case series and technical note, *J Spinal Disord Tech* 17:158–162, 2004.

18. Vender JR, Rekito AJ, Harrison SJ, et al: The evolution of posterior cervical and occipitocervical fusion and instrumentation, *Neurosurg Focus* 16:E9, 2004.

19. Harrop JS, Vaccaro A, Przybylski GJ: Acute respiratory compromise associated with flexed cervical traction after C2 fractures, *Spine* 26:E50–E54, 2001. **A report detailing the high (40%) rate of airway compromise with attempts at closed reduction of posteriorly displaced odontoid fractures. If closed reduction is attempted, one should consider prior nasotracheal intubation.**

20. Muller EJ, Schwinnen I, Fischer K, et al: Non-rigid immobilisation of odontoid fractures, *Eur Spine J* 12:522–525, 2003.

21. Hart R, Saterbak A, Rapp T, et al: Nonoperative management of dens fracture nonunion in elderly patients without myelopathy, *Spine* 25:1339–1343, 2000.

22. Platzer P, Thalhammer G, Ostermann R, et al: Anterior screw fixation of odontoid fractures comparing younger and elderly patients, *Spine* 32:1714–1720, 2007.

23. Clark CR, White AA 3rd: Fractures of the dens. A multicenter study, *J Bone Joint Surg Am* 67:1340–1348, 1985. **Clark's and White's landmark multicenter analysis of odontoid fractures found that displacement of more than 5 mm or angulation of more than 10 degrees correlated with higher risk of nonunion.**

24. Govender S, Maharaj JF, Haffajee MR: Fractures of the odontoid process, *J Bone Joint Surg Br* 82:1143–1147, 2000.

25. Stoney J, O'Brien J, Wilde P: Treatment of type-two odontoid fractures in halothoracic vests, *J Bone Joint Surg Br* 80:452–455, 1998.

26. Lennarson PJ, Mostafavi H, Traynelis VC, et al: Management of type II dens fractures: a case-control study, *Spine* 25:1234–1237, 2000. **An analysis of data for 33 patients with type II odontoid fractures managed with halo vest immobilization. Nonunion cases were compared with union controls, and age older than 50 years was found to be a significant risk factor for nonunion.**

27. Greene KA, Dickman CA, Marciano FF, et al: Acute axis fractures. Analysis of management and outcome in 340 consecutive cases, *Spine* 22:1843–1852, 1997.

28. Hadley MN, Browner C, Sonntag VK: Axis fractures: a comprehensive review of management and treatment in 107 cases, *Neurosurgery* 17:281–290, 1985.

29. Hadley MN: Isolated fractures of the axis in adults, *Neurosurgery* 50:S125–S139, 2002.

30. Kuntz CT, Mirza SK, Jarell AD, et al: Type II odontoid fractures in the elderly: early failure of nonsurgical treatment, *Neurosurg Focus* 8:E7, 2000.

31. Muller EJ, Wick M, Russe O, et al: Management of odontoid fractures in the elderly, *Eur Spine J* 8:360–365, 1999.

32. Maiman DJ, Larson SJ: Management of odontoid fractures, *Neurosurgery* 11:820, 1982.

33. Tashjian RZ, Majercik S, Biffl WL, et al: Halo-vest immobilization increases early morbidity and mortality in elderly odontoid fractures, *J Trauma* 60:199–203, 2006.

34. Bransford RJ, Stevens DW, Uyeji S, et al: Halo vest treatment of cervical spine injuries: a success and survivorship analysis, *Spine* 34:1561–1566, 2009.

35. Koech F, Ackland HM, Varma DK, et al: Nonoperative management of type II odontoid fractures in the elderly, *Spine* 33:2881–2886, 2008.

36. Platzer P, Thalhammer G, Sarahrudi K, et al: Nonoperative management of odontoid fractures using a halothoracic vest, *Neurosurgery* 61:522–529, 2007:discussion, 9-30.

37. ElSaghir H, Bohm H: Anderson type II fracture of the odontoid process: results of anterior screw fixation, *J Spinal Disord* 13:527–530; discussion, 31, 2000.

38. Bednar DA, Parikh J, Hummel J: Management of type II odontoid process fractures in geriatric patients: a prospective study of sequential cohorts with attention to survivorship, *J Spinal Disord* 8:166–169, 1995. **This prospective study of odontoid fractures in geriatric patients found that early operative management resulted in decreased perioperative mortality.**

39. Alfieri A: Single-screw fixation for acute type II odontoid fracture, *J Neurosurg Sci* 45:15–18, 2001.

40. Campanelli M, Kattner KA, Stroink A, et al: Posterior C1-C2 transarticular screw fixation in the treatment of displaced type II odontoid fractures in the geriatric population—review of seven cases, *Surg Neurol* 51:596–600; discussion, 600–601, 1999.

41. Jeanneret B, Magerl F: Primary posterior fusion C1/2 in odontoid fractures: indications, technique, and results of transarticular screw fixation, *J Spinal Disord* 5:464–475, 1992.

Chapter 12 C1-C2 Fusion: Transarticular Screws Versus Harms/Melcher Procedure

Thomas J. Kesman, Bradford L. Currier

The upper cervical spine is a unique portion of the spine that allows great mobility. The distinctive architecture, including the articulation of the dens with the anterior ring of C1, provides much of the rotation of the cervical spine. The atlanto-axial motion segment provides 50% of cervical rotation and additionally provides approximately 10% of cervical flexion-extension.[1,2] This high degree of mobility predisposes the C1-C2 level to instability, particularly in the event of ligamentous or bony pathologic changes.[1]

Congenital malformations, trauma, ligamentous laxity, and inflammatory processes such as rheumatoid arthritis are all potential causes of atlantoaxial instability.[1,3,4] Various techniques have been developed to fuse the C1-C2 segment to avoid the potential consequences of instability, which include pain, deformity, neurologic decline, and even death. Gallie developed a posterior wiring technique in 1939 that used a structural bone graft for support.[4,5] Numerous other techniques have also been developed since that time, including Brooks and Jenkins[6] double-looped wiring method. Both methods are good at reducing flexion, but the Gallie technique reduces axial rotation by only 67%, whereas the Brooks-Jenkins method reduces axial rotation by 91%.[7,8] All of these methods are technically less challenging than some of the more modern techniques, but the results are not as stable. The wiring techniques are also not feasible when the structural integrity of the posterior ring of C1 is compromised.[8] Because of the mobility at these segments, these techniques generally require use of external supplemental immobilization, such as a halo vest.[1]

Cumbersome rigid external immobilization can be avoided with the use of different techniques that provide more rigid internal fixation. This can lead to fewer complications from halo-type immobilization, which is especially critical in the elderly patient. Two of the most prominent modern techniques include posterior C1-C2 transarticular screw fixation, as described by Magerl and Seemann,[9] and posterior C1-C2 fusion with polyaxial screws and rods described by Harms and Melcher.[3] Each of these techniques has advantages and disadvantages, which are the focus of this chapter.

CASE PRESENTATION

An 81-year-old nonsmoking man with a history of chronic lymphocytic leukemia, atrial fibrillation, degenerative joint disease, and dizziness came to the emergency department after falling from a ladder while trimming a tree of unknown height. The patient fell backward directly onto his neck, back, and arm. Upon arrival to the emergency department he complained of neck, back, and right wrist pain. He reported no loss of consciousness.

- PMH: Unremarkable
- PSH: Unremarkable
- Exam: The physical examination revealed a Glasgow Coma Scale score of 15 and normal findings on neurologic assessment. The patient had abrasions on his face and midline tenderness of the entire cervical spine.

FIGURE 12-1 Sagittal CT image showing an odontoid fracture at the time of injury.

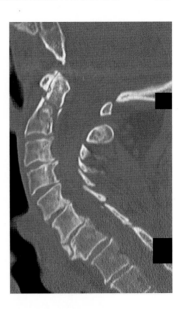

FIGURE 12-2 Axial CT image demonstrating left lateral mass subluxation and fracture.

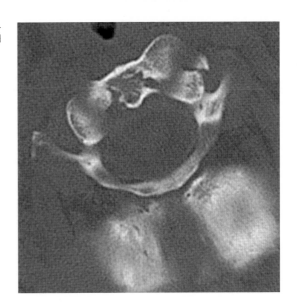

- Imaging: Computed tomography (CT) of the cervical spine with coronal and sagittal reformatted images showed a type II posterior oblique odontoid fracture with 2-mm posterior displacement of the odontoid (Figure 12-1) (Tips from the Masters 12-1). There was posterior subluxation of the left lateral mass of C1 associated with a mildly displaced intraarticular fracture of the lateral mass (Figure 12-2). There were also nondisplaced fractures of the right C7 lamina and extensive degenerative changes with rotatory scoliosis. The patient's other injuries included displaced fractures of the left first and second ribs, a fracture of the left maxillary antrum, and a right distal radius fracture.

Tips from the Masters 12-1 • Anatomic variation is common in the upper cervical spine. Contrast-enhanced CT is advisable in *every* case.

After obtaining appropriate informed consent, the surgeon proceeded with closed reduction and internal fixation of the type II odontoid fracture with a single 4.0 × 38 mm cannulated screw through a right-sided anterior approach. A satisfactory

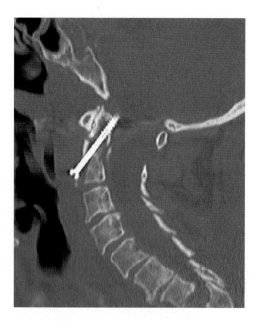

FIGURE 12-3 Sagittal CT image showing post-operative screw fixation of the odontoid fracture.

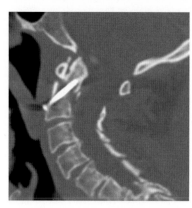

FIGURE 12-4 Sagittal CT image revealing loss of fixation of the odontoid screw.

reduction was obtained at the time of surgery based on intraoperative findings; however, a CT scan done 3 days later showed early signs of loss of solid fixation of the screw (Figure 12-3). The patient's postoperative course was complicated by delirium and swallowing difficulties.

Tips from the Masters 12-2 • All placement of screws in C1 and C2 is a physician-directed (off-label) application and requires disclosure and consent.

The patient's clinical status was monitored carefully, and radiographs taken at 2 weeks postoperatively demonstrated that the odontoid screw continued to lose fixation and the patient developed posterior subluxation of the odontoid fragment (Figure 12-4). At this point, approximately 2 weeks after the index operation, the patient was referred to a cervical spine surgeon.

SURGICAL OPTIONS

Initially, nonoperative care using a collar could have been considered based on the minimal displacement of the fracture.[10,11] The recommendation is to consider that option only in elderly patients with fractures that have minimal displacement and angulation, and that show no change in alignment or fracture gap between radiographs taken in the supine and upright positions. Such radiographs were not made before placement of the odontoid screw, but based on the marked displacement that occurred postoperatively and the fracture of the lateral mass of C1 with posterior displacement of the joint, the spine was obviously unstable, and nonoperative care would also have failed.

Immobilization in a halo is an option for treatment of minimally displaced odontoid fractures in younger age groups. The complication rate associated with halo immobilization is much higher in the elderly, however, so most surgeons have abandoned their use in that population.[12,13] The risk of using a halo would have been exceptionally high in this case considering the patient's rib fractures as well as his age.

C1-C2 fusion with a wiring construct alone also is not a good option in this case, since postoperative immobilization in a halo is often used to achieve an acceptable fusion rate.[3,14]

Although odontoid screw fixation is a reasonable option for type II odontoid fractures (with the appropriate fracture angulation and without comminution), it was not a good choice for the index operation. Studies have shown lower union rates (70% to 88%) and higher complication rates in the elderly with this procedure.[15,16] In addition, the fracture of the lateral mass of C1 and rotatory C1-C2 subluxation in this case are signs of instability and foretold a poor result. Some have recommended using two screws in the odontoid, but adding a second screw provides no significant change in the load to failure[17] and would have been unlikely to prevent the loss of fixation.

Revising the screw as an isolated procedure was not an option at the time of referral for the same reasons that it was not a good choice initially. In addition, the anterior aspect of C2 had then failed, and a screw would not have been able to gain adequate purchase in C2. The screw might need to be removed if it migrates or causes esophageal irritation; otherwise it may be left in place.

There has been a trend in recent years to augment posterior C1-C2 fusions using either transarticular screws as described by Magerl and Seemann[9] or C1 lateral mass screws connected via bilateral rods to C2 pars interarticularis screws (Harms technique).[3] This is true across all age groups and across the full spectrum of pathologic conditions, including odontoid fractures in the elderly.[18] The advantages and disadvantages of these techniques were considered when deciding which procedure to use to salvage this case and are reviewed below.

Transarticular Screw Fixation

The technique of augmenting a C1-C2 fusion with transarticular screws was described by Magerl and Seemann in 1987.[9] It involves placement of bilateral screws, inserted from a posterior approach, through the pars interarticularis of C2 and across the C1-2 joints. The screws achieve excellent fixation because they engage three or four cortices, depending on whether the tip of the screw is bicortical or unicortical in the lateral mass of C1. The increased rigidity conferred by the screws eliminates the need for halo immobilization postoperatively and leads to a higher fusion rate than with wiring constructs.[1,7,9] Furthermore, the screws provide a means for achieving fusion in patients with a deficient posterior arch of the atlas. The traditional wiring techniques are not applicable in that setting, since they rely on the wires encircling the arch to provide stability.

Although the placement of transarticular screws has distinct advantages, the procedure is a technically demanding one that requires substantial preoperative planning to minimize risk to nearby neurovascular structures. Because of variation in patient anatomy, a detailed understanding of the patient's neurovascular and bony anatomy is essential.[19] The course of the vertebral artery through the lateral mass of the axis has been found to be asymmetric in approximately one half of patients.[20] A high-riding transverse foramen is located in the path of a transarticular screw in approximately one fifth of patients.[20-22] In addition, the isthmus of C2 in approximately 10% of patients is less than 5 mm in height and width, which makes fixation with a 3.5-mm screw risky, especially if placed under fluoroscopic guidance alone.[23]

The internal carotid artery (ICA) is also at risk during transarticular screw fixation, especially when bicortical fixation is needed. The center of the lateral mass of C1 is

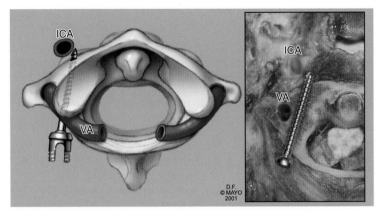

FIGURE 12-5 Diagram (**A**) and axial section from a fresh frozen cadaveric specimen (**B**) showing the risk of C1 screw placement relative to the location of the ICA. *VA*, Vertebral artery. *(From Cyr SJ, Currier BL, Eck JC, et al: Fixation strength of unicortical versus bicortical C1-C2 transarticular screws,* Spine *8(4):661–665, 2008, Figure 2.)*

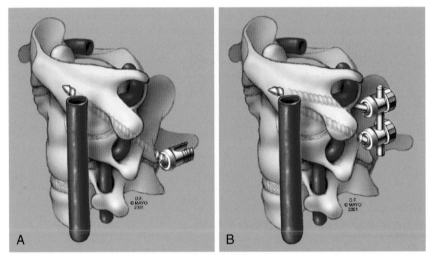

FIGURE 12-6 Diagrams showing the proximity of the ICA and vertebral artery to a C1-C2 transarticular screw (**A**) and a C1 lateral mass screw and a C2 pars interarticularis screw (**B**). *(From Cyr SJ, Currier BL, Eck JC, et al: Fixation strength of unicortical versus bicortical C1-C2 transarticular screws,* Spine *8(4):661–665, 2008, Figure 3.)*

the optimal exit point for transarticular screws. Unfortunately, the ICA may be located within 1 mm of that site[24,25] (Figures 12-5 and 12-6). A transarticular screw with bicortical purchase puts the ICA at moderate risk on at least one side in approximately half of cases and at high risk in 12% of case.[21,25] Therefore, careful planning with contrast-enhanced CT is advised before transarticular screw fixation. If preoperative imaging reveals that the ICA is within 2 mm of the anterior cortex of C1 and medial to the transverse foramen, a unicortical screw or alternative technique should be used.[21] This practice is also supported by biomechanical data, which show no statistically significant difference in pullout strength of unicortical versus bicortical transarticular screws in this setting, if the bone quality is good and the screws are well positioned.[26]

Another limitation of the technique is that spine malalignment must be reduced before the screws are placed. Incomplete C1-C2 reduction may lead to increased risk of vertebral artery injury if C1 is subluxed anteriorly or to failure of fixation in the lateral mass of C1 if the atlas is subluxed posteriorly.[20,22]

Finally, because of the acute angle required for insertion of these screws, it may be difficult or impossible to achieve the correct trajectory in obese patients or patients with increased thoracic kyphosis.

Posterior C1-C2 Fusion with Polyaxial Screw and Rod Fixation

The technique of posterior C1-C2 fusion with polyaxial screw and rod fixation was originally developed in 2001 by Harms and Melcher[3] based on the pioneering work of Goel and Laheri[27] with C1-C2 posterior plates. The technique has many of the advantages of the transarticular screw technique, including its stability and lack of reliance on the arch of the atlas. Biomechanically, transarticular screws and polyaxial screw and rod constructs have been found to be equivalent.[8] The placement of the lateral mass screws in C1 and the pars-pedicle screws in C2 provides solid fixation that spans the entire sagittal dimension of the bones.

The screw and rod construct has several advantages over transarticular screws. The C1 and C2 screws can be placed independently, which allows the spine to be reduced after the screws have been placed. This permits more flexibility in screw positioning, which may make the technique safer and feasible in a larger percentage of cases. It also allows more control over the final alignment of the spine and does not require placing the patient into an awkward position on the operating table. In addition, the C2 pars-pedicle screws of the screw and rod construct are angled more medially than transarticular screws, which provides a greater margin of safety relative to the vertebral arteries. Although the C2 screw is often described as a pedicle screw, the implant is generally placed into the pars interarticularis, because the C2 pedicles may be too small to safely accept a screw[28] and the exaggerated angle required for a pedicle screw is often difficult to achieve. In cases in which neither a pars nor a pedicle screw can be inserted safely, the screw and rod construct may be connected to laminar screws in C2.[29,30] These modular options also give the screw-rod construct the advantage that the screws can be easily connected to fusion levels above and below C1-C2.

Although the screw and rod construct theoretically has a lower risk of injuring the vertebral artery than transarticular screws, the ideal exit points of the screws in the C1 lateral mass are the same and therefore carry a similar risk to the ICA and the hypoglossal nerve. Both techniques require special preoperative imaging and rigorous planning as noted previously (Tips from the Masters 12-3 and 12-4). The primary disadvantages of screw and rod constructs over transarticular screws are the increased cost and complexity of the former.

Tips from the Masters 12-3 • Preoperative planning and proper patient positioning are the keys to success.

Tips from the Masters 12-4 • Rehearse the steps with your operating room team before placing a C1 screw so your eyes can stay focused on the wound.

FUNDAMENTAL TECHNIQUE

Transarticular Screw Technique

Preoperative advanced imaging is required with contrast-enhanced CT to further understand the neurovascular anatomy as well as the bony dimensions of the atlantoaxial complex. In certain cases, especially when a high-riding transverse foramen is present or the ICA is close to the anterior portion of the atlas, transarticular screws with or without bicortical fixation may not be possible.

Once adequate preoperative planning has been completed, the patient is brought to the operating room and intubated. Multimodality neurologic monitoring can be instituted with the patient in the supine position to obtain baseline readings. The patient is then placed prone on a Jackson table with the head held in place with a pinion and Mayfield attachment. Reverse Trendelenburg position can be maximized using the Jackson table by inserting the head of the table in the highest selectable position and the foot of the table in the lowest selectable position. This will help reduce venous pressure and decrease bleeding during the procedure. Fluoroscopy is used to reduce the deformity and place C1 and C2 in the proper orientation for the instrumentation, and to demonstrate that adequate images can be obtained in the chosen position. Rotation of the head should be neutral. A second set of neurologic monitoring tests can be performed once reduction is complete, and a postposition wake-up test can be conducted if deemed necessary.

The posterior scalp and neck are clipped or shaved, and are then prepared and draped in the usual sterile fashion from the occiput proximally to the midthoracic spine distally. Once this has been accomplished, a midline skin incision is made over the C1-C2 level and skin and subcutaneous tissue are retracted to reveal the cervical fascia. The cervical fascia is incised in line with the skin incision. A careful subperiosteal dissection of the C1 arch and C2 lamina are accomplished, and self-retaining retractors are inserted. If possible, the insertion of the semispinalis cervicis should be preserved on C2. If it must be sacrificed, ideally it can be removed with a small piece of bone from the spinous process C2 to provide anchor for repair at the end of the procedure. The arch of the atlas is exposed, with care taken to protect the vertebral artery on its superior surface.[21] The starting point for the screws is located just lateral to the junction of the lamina with the articular mass, close to the lower edge of the caudal articular process of C2 so that the isthmus is crossed close to the posterior surface.[9,31] A caliper and the preoperative CT scan can assist in measuring the distance between the two screws. This should be compared with the medial border of the pars interarticularis so that violation of the canal is avoided. The starting point can be created using a 2-mm high-speed bur to avoid slipping off the axis while using a Kirschner wire (K-wire) or drill bit.[21]

Once the starting point is located, the trajectory needs to be determined. This is done using fluoroscopy in a lateral view or image guidance. Use of the percutaneous technique, described by McGuire and Harkey,[32] makes it unnecessary to expose the entire region from C1 to the entrance point of the screws. Once the trajectory is determined, small vertical stab incisions are made in the upper thoracic spine (around T2) to allow for appropriate placement of the trocar along the correct trajectory. These stab incisions are generally the same width apart as the entrance holes burred in C2, since the trajectories of the transarticular screws are generally parallel to the midsagittal plane. The trocar is then passed through the stab incisions and docked in the entrance holes in C2. On the lateral image, the trocar should be aiming at the anterior tubercle of C1. The ideal target point for the drill, relative to the anterior tubercle, is just below the midpoint in the 20% to 40% region, where 100% represents the cranial border of the arch and 0% the caudal border.[33] A cannula is passed over the trocar and the trocar is removed. A 2.5-mm drill bit is then inserted and under fluoroscopy is passed into the C1 lateral mass. The hole is then tapped, and a 3.5-mm screw is inserted under fluoroscopic guidance. The same process is repeated on the contralateral side. The posterior elements are decorticated and a bone graft with posterior wiring can be placed based on surgeon preference.[21] If the posterior arch of C1 is deficient, then the C1-2 joints are decorticated and packed with bone graft. If a wiring construct can be used, it is not necessary to directly fuse the C1-2 joints.

The semispinalis cervicis is repaired if it was detached during exposure. The wound is irrigated and closed in a layered fashion over a drain. A sterile dressing and collar are applied. The patient's neurologic status is checked postoperatively.

Technique of C1-C2 Fusion Using a Screw and Rod Construct

The setup for C1-C2 fusion using a screw and rod construct technique is the same as for placement of transarticular screws, except that it is not mandatory to reduce the spine before exposure and the head and neck may be placed in physiologic alignment. Refer to the previous section for further details. Once the patient is prepared and draped, an incision is made over the midline of C1 and C2. Dissection is carried down to the C2 spinous process. Again, care should be taken to preserve the attachments of the semispinalis cervicis muscle to the C2 spinous process if possible. The superior aspect of the C2 lamina should be identified and subperiosteally dissected to identify entry points for the C2 pars screws. Dissection of the posterior arch of the atlas is carried out laterally to identify the lateral masses of C1. The vertebral artery should be avoided as described previously. Bleeding often occurs during dissection around the epidural venous plexus near the C1-2 joint. This can be controlled with thrombin-soaked absorbable gelatin sponges and judicious use of bipolar electrocautery (Tips from the Masters 12-5). The C2 pars interarticularis or pedicle screw entry points are identified by locating the medial border of the pars. The entry point is marked with a 2-mm bur. Generally the direction of the bit is approximately 25 degrees medial and cephalad. The entry point should be in the cranial and medial quadrant of the isthmus surface of C2.[3]

Tips from the Masters 12-5 • When the almost inevitable bleeding is encountered during placement of a C1 lateral mass screw, use a hemostatic agent, cottonoid patty, and patience rather than blind or excessive bipolar cautery.

Attention is then turned to the C1 lateral mass screws. The dorsal root ganglion of C2 is retracted caudally to expose the entry point for the C1 lateral mass screw. The analog of the C1 pedicle can be identified with a Penfield 4 dissector to assist in finding the appropriate starting point. The entry point is in the middle of the posterior aspect of the lateral mass of C1 just caudal to the point where the analog of the pedicle becomes confluent with the lateral mass.[3,34] This entry point is marked with a 2-mm bur. A hand drill is then used to drill the screw path. The drill bit should be directed medially 5 to 10 degrees and parallel to the plane of the pedicle analog of C1. Fluoroscopy or image guidance can be used to guide the drill bit; the target point is the same as that described for a transarticular screw (see previous section). The hole is probed, tapped, and probed, and a 3.5-mm polyaxial screw of appropriate length is inserted. Use of a smooth-shanked screw can be useful in reducing potential nerve root irritation from the threads of the screw. These steps are repeated on the contralateral side at C1. An alternative entrance point for the screw is on the inferior one third of the posterior arch to enter the lateral mass through the pedicle analog.[35] Use of this entrance point avoids the troublesome bleeding that is often encountered when dissecting in the region of the lateral mass. Unfortunately, the bone caudal to the groove of the vertebral artery in the arch is often insufficient to allow safe placement of a screw in this location.[34,36-38]

The focus is then shifted back to C2, where the entrance holes are already in place. The hand drill is used to make a pilot hole that is approximately 25 degrees medial and cephalad. This hole is probed, tapped, and probed, and a fully threaded 3.5- to 4.0-mm screw is inserted, depending on preoperative planning. The same steps are repeated on the contralateral side at C2. The location of the vertebral artery in C2 usually necessitates placing the screw cranial and medial in the pars interarticularis, hugging the medial border of the pars. If the bone quality is good, it may be possible to carefully place a shorter screw into the lower pars to avoid the vertebral artery. A prominent or high-riding vertebral artery may preclude placement of a pars screw, in which case a C2 laminar screw may be chosen.[29,30,37]

With four polyaxial screws in place, any further reduction of C1 on C2 can be completed using fluoroscopic guidance. The screws can be used for leverage to assist with the reduction. Once optimal reduction has been achieved, the rods are tightened to maintain this reduction. Decortication of C1 and C2 is followed by placement of bone graft. The recommendation is to use cables to secure a block of iliac crest autograft to the posterior elements of C1 and C2 to provide three-point fixation and optimal biomechanical rigidity, especially when the bone quality is marginal. Others prefer to onlay graft over the decorticated posterior elements without wires or cables.[3] Finally, the wound is irrigated and closed in a layered fashion over a drain. A sterile dressing and collar are applied. The patient's neurologic status is checked postoperatively.

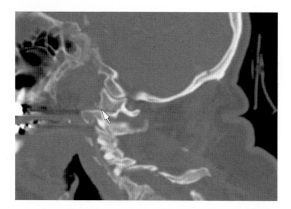

FIGURE 12-7 Sagittal CT image revealing posterior subluxation of the left C1 lateral mass on C2.

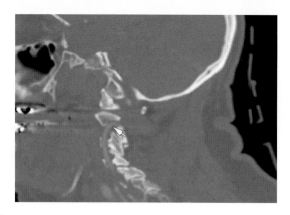

FIGURE 12-8 Sagittal CT image showing a high-riding vertebral artery on the right side.

The patient remains in a cervical collar for 3 months. Weight-lifting restrictions are 10 lb for most patients. The patient is seen at 3 months and flexion and extension cervical spine radiographs are obtained to verify solid fusion of the atlantoaxial complex. After 3 months, the patient is weaned off the collar using isometric neck exercises for strengthening and reconditioning, and the patient is allowed to ease into noncontact activities.[21]

Careful consideration was given to the appropriate type of fixation for this 81-year-old patient in whom closed-reduction internal fixation of a type II odontoid fracture had failed and who was developing subluxation of C1 on C2. Because of the patient's age, extensive medical comorbidities, and rib fractures, it was determined that he would likely do poorly with halo immobilization. Therefore rigid fixation, which would not require halo immobilization, was elected. A screw and rod construct was chosen in this case for several reasons. The patient's thoracic hyperkyphosis and compensatory cervical lordosis would have made the acute angle needed to insert transarticular screws nearly impossible to obtain. In addition, the lateral mass of C1 was posteriorly displaced relative to C2 on the left, and a transarticular screw would not have engaged C1 unless the spine could be reduced before drilling the pilot hole (Figure 12-7). On the right side, a high-riding vertebral artery precluded use of a transarticular screw (Figure 12-8). Since the patient's bone quality was excellent, relatively short screws placed into the lower portion of the pars interarticularis were chosen to avoid injury to vascular structures (Figures 12-9 and 12-10). Had these screws not achieved excellent fixation, an intralaminar C2 screw would have been placed. Using the screw and rod technique, the screws were placed into the ideal locations in C1 and C2 and then the spine was reduced and the construct tightened (Figure 12-11). Anatomic reduction was achieved, and this brought the odontoid screw back into position, which made it unnecessary to remove it (Figures 12-12 and 12-13). In this case, a corticocancellous block of iliac crest bone graft was secured to the posterior elements with a titanium cable to enhance the stability and increase the fusion rate (Figure 12-14).

FIGURE 12-9 Sagittal CT image showing a right vertebral artery path necessitating use of a short screw in the right C2 pars.

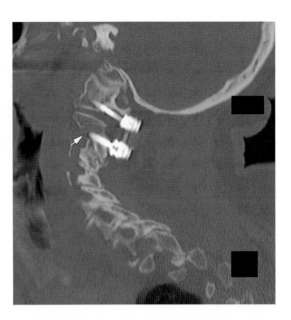

FIGURE 12-10 Sagittal CT image showing a left vertebral artery path necessitating use of a short screw in the left C2 pars.

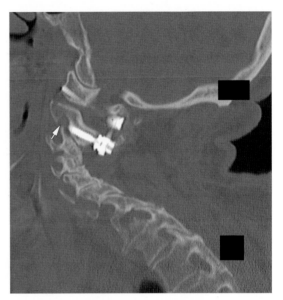

This case illustrates that preoperative planning is paramount to avoid complications in C1-C2 fusions. For the patient in the Case Presentation, the vertebral artery would have been in jeopardy had the surgeon chosen to use transarticular screws instead of a screw and rod construct. Both of these more modern techniques provide greater stability than posterior wiring techniques alone, which eliminates the need for postoperative immobilization with a halo vest. In younger, healthier patients, a cable and graft construct without screws would be a reasonable alternative if augmented with halo immobilization. When it is essential to avoid the use of a halo, the risk and cost of screw augmentation techniques are justified.

DISCUSSION OF BEST EVIDENCE

The current evidence concerning surgical techniques for C1-C2 arthrodesis consists of Level III, IV, and V studies. There is no Level I or Level II evidence from clinical studies to direct treatment. Levels of evidence are generally not assigned to basic science studies, but since the biomechanical and anatomic investigations cited in the

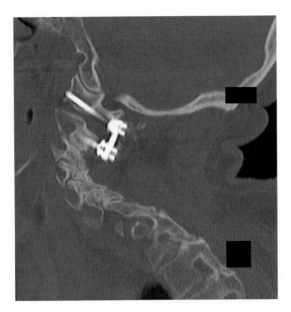

FIGURE 12-11 Sagittal CT image illustrating rod reduction of C1 on C2.

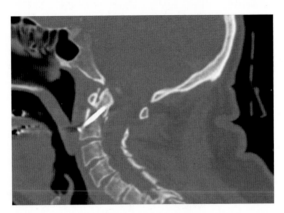

FIGURE 12-12 Preoperative CT lateral view of the odontoid showing malreduction.

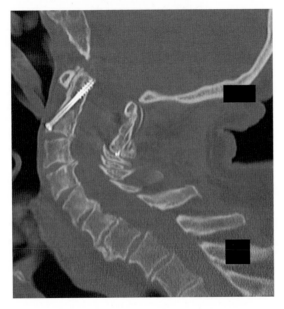

FIGURE 12-13 Postoperative CT lateral view of the odontoid showing re-reduction.

FIGURE 12-14 Postoperative radiograph of the entire construct.

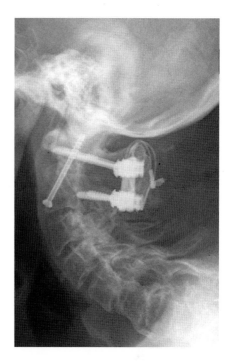

following sections are prospective, well designed, and adequately powered, they will be considered Level I evidence.

Fusion Rate

There is good evidence that the fusion rate is higher when a C1-C2 arthrodesis is augmented with transarticular screws or screw and rod constructs than when posterior wiring alone is used.

Level III Studies

Reilly and colleagues[1] completed a single-center **retrospective study** involving 67 patients who underwent atlantoaxial arthrodesis via posterior wiring or cabling and external rigid immobilization or C1-C2 transarticular screw fixation, mostly with supplemental posterior wiring. The transarticular screw procedure was associated with a significantly higher fusion rate (94% vs. 71%).

Level IV Studies

Several case series have cited high fusion rates with transarticular screws or screw and rod constructs followed by collar immobilization, including Harms and Melcher,[3] Magerl and Seemann,[9] and Grob and associates.[31] The fusion rates are higher than, or equivalent to, the rates in historical control series reporting on patients treated by posterior wiring augmented with halo immobilization.

Biomechanical Stability

The biomechanical stability of transarticular screw and screw-rod constructs is roughly equivalent, and both are superior to posterior wiring constructs. Multiple studies have shown that transarticular screws provide a more stable construct than wiring techniques. Wiring methods such as the Gallie or Brooks-Jenkins technique do a fair job of controlling flexion and extension, but not in lateral bending or rotation.[14,38,39] A combination of transarticular screw fixation and a single posterior cable graft construct was found to create the most stable construct in a study by Naderi and co-workers.[40] A similar biomechanical study compared transarticular screws with posterior wire graft to a posterior screw and rod construct and found

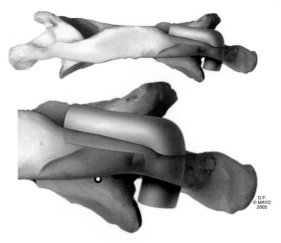

FIGURE 12-15 Posterior view of C1 at the confluence of the posterior ring and the lateral mass. The posterior arch can be seen superimposed over the caudal aspect of the vertebral artery as it passes over the groove. The black-and-white dot denotes the starting point for a screw on the posterior aspect of the lateral mass. *(From Christensen DM, Eastlack RK, Lynch JJ, et al: C1 anatomy and dimensions relative to lateral mass screw placement, Spine 32:844–848, 2007, Figure 1. By permission of Mayo Foundation for Medical Education and Research. All rights reserved.)*

them to be equivalent.[8] One could postulate that adding a posterior bone graft and wire construct to a screw and rod assembly would likely give it better stability than transarticular screw fixation with posterior wire graft.[36]

Level I Studies

Melcher and colleagues[8] completed biomechanical testing on cadaveric spine specimens and found that transarticular screws and screw-rod constructs had equivalent biomechanical properties. These screw constructs had significantly greater stability than posterior wiring constructs. Other studies, including those by Henriques and associates[39] and Naderi and co-workers,[40] showed similar results with slightly different constructs.

Anatomic Characteristics

The anatomy of the atlantoaxial joint is complex and variable. A careful understanding of the C1 and C2 anatomy is critical to the success of any type of screw fixation. Several anatomic studies have described the surgically relevant anatomy of the atlas.

The dimensions of the lateral mass of C1 allow screw fixation in nearly all cases. Christensen and colleagues[34] performed a study of 120 human specimens at the Cleveland Museum of Natural History. The anteroposterior length of the lateral mass averaged 16.93 mm (minimum, 13.13 mm) below the posterior ring of C1. The width of the lateral mass between the vertebral artery foramen and the spinal canal averaged 8.68 mm (minimum, 5.25 mm). The cephalocaudal height from the top of the pedicle analog to the inferior facet averaged 8.99 mm (minimum, 4.73 mm). Others have confirmed these findings.[35,41] Christensen and associates also studied the dimensions of the pedicle analog to see how often it is feasible to insert a screw through the posterior inferior portion of the arch of C1 to avoid dissecting out the lateral mass as described by Resnick and associates.[35] They found that the bone beneath the groove of the vertebral artery in the arch of C1 is less than 4-mm thick in 20% of cases.[34] This would potentially cause a 3.5-mm screw to cut out superiorly, placing the vertebral artery at risk, unless the surgeon intentionally causes the screw to cut out inferiorly[36] (Figures 12-15 and 12-16).

Tan and co-workers[38] published results of a study of 50 dried atlas specimens that identified basic anatomic dimensions, including the posterior arch of the atlas. The thinnest part of the groove as measured by coronal CT scan was 4.72 ± 0.65 mm on the left and 4.72 ± 0.68 mm on the right. Only 8% of the cases in their series had a thickness of less than 4 mm, whereas Lee and co-workers[37] found that the bone in that location was more than 4 mm in only 46% of cases. The preference is to place the screw into that location when the preoperative contrast-enhanced CT scan shows that it can be done safely.

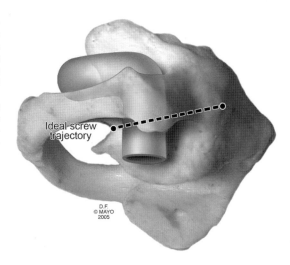

FIGURE 12-16 Lateral view of C1 demonstrating the ideal orientation of screw placement within the sagittal plane (10 to 15 degrees caudad to cephalad). Note the starting position below the posterior ring confluence with the lateral mass. *(From Christensen DM, Eastlack RK, Lynch JJ, et al: C1 anatomy and dimensions relative to lateral mass screw placement, Spine 32:844–848, 2007, Figure 2. By permission of Mayo Foundation for Medical Education and Research. All rights reserved.)*

Level I Studies

Multiple morphometric studies demonstrate the wide anatomic variability of the atlantoaxial complex.[22,23,25,28,34,41] All of these investigations highlight the need to carefully plan the procedure before placing instrumentation in the upper cervical spine.

COMMENTARY

C1-C2 fusions are technically challenging operations, but they are also among the most gratifying procedures spine surgeons do. Nowhere in the spine is the anatomy more exquisite or more important to the success of the operation than in the upper cervical spine. The region is rife with anatomic variations that alter the technique for the informed and lead to complications for the unaware. Preoperative planning is the key to success.

Surgeons should be comfortable with multiple techniques since each one has pros and cons. The primary advantage of using the Harms method or transarticular screw fixation over simple wiring techniques is the added stability conferred by the screws; the enhanced stability allows a comparable or higher fusion rate without halo immobilization. The main advantages of the transarticular screw technique over the Harms technique are lower cost and simplicity. The major advantages of the Harms technique over the transarticular screw technique are broader application (it can be used when transarticular screw fixation is contraindicated by variations in the anatomy) and the ability to place screws before the spine is reduced.

The surgeon should watch an experienced colleague and practice in the cadaver laboratory before attempting these techniques in the operating room. A surgeon who is not yet comfortable with placing C1 and C2 screws should consider referring the patient to a colleague with more experience or using a simple wiring technique, with the following caveats: The use of simple wiring techniques without the added stability of postoperative halo immobilization results in an unacceptably high pseudarthrosis rate. Unfortunately, halo use is associated with a high complication rate in the elderly and should be avoided in that patient group. Nonoperative care may be the best option in the elderly if the spine is stable. Remember that the benefits of an advanced technique outweigh the risks only when the operation is accomplished by a surgeon who is adequately prepared.

REFERENCES

1. Reilly TM, Sasso RC, Hall PV: Atlantoaxial stabilization: clinical comparison of posterior cervical wiring technique with transarticular screw fixation, *J Spinal Disorders Tech* 16(3):248–253, 2003. **Retrospective study involving 67 patients who underwent atlantoaxial arthrodesis using either posterior wiring or cabling and external rigid immobilization, or C1-C2 transarticular screw fixation, mostly with supplemental posterior wiring. Transarticular screw fixation was associated with a significantly higher fusion rate (94% vs. 71%) and significantly lower rate of displacement (0% vs. 16%).**

2. White AA 3rd, Panjabi MM: The clinical biomechanics of the occipitoatlantoaxial complex, *Orthop Clin N Am* 9(4):867–878, 1978.

3. Harms J, Melcher RP: Posterior C1-C2 fusion with polyaxial screw and rod fixation, *Spine* 26(22): 2467–2471, 2001. **Classic article describing posterior screw-rod construct for atlantoaxial fusion. The article provides a retrospective review of results for 37 patients treated with a screw-rod construct along with discussion of prior techniques as well as advantages of using the screw-rod constructs.**

4. Lehman RA, Sasso RC: Current concepts in posterior C1-C2 fixation, *Semin Spine Surg* 19(4):244–249, 2007.

5. Gallie WE: Fractures and dislocations of the cervical spine, *Am J Surg* 46:495–499, 1939.

6. Brooks AL, Jenkins EB: Atlanto-axial arthrodesis by the wedge compression method, *J Bone Joint Surg Am* 60(3):279–284, 1978.

7. Grob D, Crisco JJ 3rd, Panjabi MM, et al: Biomechanical evaluation of four different posterior atlantoaxial fixation techniques, *Spine* 17(5):480–490, 1992.

8. Melcher RP, Puttlitz CM, Kleinstueck FS, et al: Biomechanical testing of posterior atlantoaxial fixation techniques, *Spine* 27(22):2435–2440, 2002. **Study of 10 fresh frozen cadaveric specimens stabilized using a variety of atlantoaxial fusion techniques, including posterior wiring, transarticular screws, and screw-rod constructs. Results demonstrated biomechanical equivalence of transarticular screws and screw-rod constructs, with significantly less stability offered by wiring constructs.**

9. Magerl F, Seemann PS: Stable posterior fusion at the atlas and axis by transarticular screw fixation. In Kehr P, Weiner A, editors: *Cervical spine*, New York, 1987, Springer-Verlag, pp 327–332.

10. Muller EJ: Non-rigid immobilisation of odontoid fractures, *Eur Spine J* 12:522–525, 2004.

11. Smith HE, Kerr SM, Maltenfort M, et al: Early complications of surgical versus conservative treatment of isolated type II odontoid fractures in octogenarians: a retrospective cohort study, *J Spinal Disorders Tech* 21:535–539, 2008.

12. Majercik S, Tashjian RZ, Biffl WL, et al: Halo vest immobilization in the elderly: a death sentence? *J Trauma* 59:350–356: discussion, 356-358; 2005.

13. Taitsman LA, Altman DT, Hecht AC, et al: Complications of cervical halo-vest orthoses in elderly patients, *Orthopedics* 31:446, 2008.

14. Dickman CA, Crawford NR, Paramore CG: Biomechanical characteristics of C1-2 cable fixations, *J Neurosurg* 85(2):316–322, 1996.

15. Harrop JS, Przybylski GJ, Vaccaro AR, et al: Efficacy of anterior odontoid screw fixation in elderly patients with type II odontoid fractures, *Neurosurg Focus* 8:e6, 2000.

16. Platzer P, Thalhammer G, Ostermann R, et al: Anterior screw fixation of odontoid fractures comparing younger and elderly patients, *Spine* 32:1714–1720, 2007.

17. Sasso RC, Doherty BJ, Crawford MJ, et al: Biomechanics of odontoid fracture fixation: comparison of the one and two screw techniques, *Spine* 18:1950–1953, 1993.

18. Smith HE, Vaccaro AR, Maltenfort M, et al: Trends in surgical management for type II odontoid fracture: 20 years of experience at a regional spinal cord injury center, *Orthopedics* 31:650, 2008.

19. Yamazaki M, Koda M, Aramoni MA, et al: Anomalous vertebral artery at the extraosseous and intraosseous regions of the craniovertebral junction: analysis by three-dimensional computer tomography angiography, *Spine* 30:2452–2457, 2005.

20. Madawi AA, Casey AT, Solanki GA, et al: Radiological and anatomical evaluation of the atlantoaxial transarticular screw fixation technique, *J Neurosurg* 86:961–968, 1997. **Study of outcomes for 61 patients who underwent transarticular screw fixation, including a smaller subset evaluated for anatomic variations. Results highlight the need for preoperative planning to avoid neurovascular injury.**

21. Eck JC, Currier BL: Transarticular fixation. In Wang JC, editor: Advanced reconstruction, *Spine*. Rosemont, Ill, 2011, American Academy of Orthopaedic Surgeons, pp C1–C2.

22. Paramore CG, Dickman CA, Sonntag VK: The anatomical suitability of the C1-2 complex for transarticular screw fixation, *J Neurosurg* 85:221–224, 1996.

23. Mandel IM, Kambach BJ, Petersilge CA, et al: Morphologic considerations of C2 isthmus dimensions for the placement of transarticular screws, *Spine* 25(12):1542–1547, 2000.

24. Currier BL, Todd LT, Maus TP, et al: Anatomic relationship of the internal carotid artery to the C1 vertebra: a case report of cervical reconstruction for chordoma and pilot study to assess the risk of screw fixation of the atlas, *Spine* 28:E461–E467, 2003.

25. Currier BL, Maus TP, Eck JC, et al: Relationship of the internal carotid artery to the anterior aspect of the C1 vertebra: implications for C1–C2 transarticular and C1 lateral mass fixation, *Spine* 33:635–639, 2008. **An analysis of 50 random head and neck CT scans to assess the location of the ICA relative to the atlas. The ICA was located 0 to 7 mm (mean, 2.9 mm) from the anterior aspect of the atlas. The ICA was considered to be at moderate risk in 46% of cases and at high risk in 12% (on at least one side) if bicortical transarticular or C1 lateral mass screws were used.**

26. Cyr SJ, Currier BL, Eck JC, et al: Fixation strength of unicortical versus bicortical C1-C2 transarticular screws, *Spine* 8(4):661–665, 2008.

27. Goel A, Laheri V: Plate and screw fixation for atlanto-axial subluxation, *Acta Neurochir (Wien)* 129:47–53, 1994.

28. Ebraheim N, Rollins JR, Xu R, et al: Anatomic consideration of C2 pedicle screw placement, *Spine* 21(6):691–695, 1996.

29. Wright NM: Posterior C2 fixation using bilateral, crossing C2 laminar screws: case series and technical note, *J Spinal Disord Tech* 17:158–162, 2004.

30. Wright NM: Translaminar rigid screw fixation of the axis. Technical note, *J Neurosurg Spine* 3: 409–414, 2005.
31. Grob D, Jeanneret B, Aebi M, et al: Atlanto-axial fusion with transarticular screw fixation, *J Bone Joint Surg* 73B:972–976, 1991.
32. McGuire RA Jr, Harkey HL: Modification of technique and results of atlantoaxial transfacet stabilization, *Orthopedics* 18:1029–1032, 1995.
33. Yeom JS, Buchowski JM, Park KW, et al: Lateral fluoroscopic guide to prevent occipitocervical and atlantoaxial joint violation during C1 lateral mass screw placement, *Spine J* 9:574–579, 2009.
34. Christensen DM, Eastlack RK, Lynch JJ, et al: C1 anatomy and dimensions relative to lateral mass screw placement, *Spine* 32:844–848, 2007. **A total of 240 C1 lateral masses were examined and measurements recorded. The dimensions of the lateral masses were adequate to allow an appropriately placed 3.5-mm screw to be inserted in all cases. The thickness of the posterior arch of C1 beneath the groove of the vertebral artery was less than 4 mm in 20% of cases, which makes screw placement in that location potentially dangerous.**
35. Resnick DK, Lapsiwala S, Trost GR: Anatomic suitability of the C1-C2 complex for pedicle screw fixation, *Spine* 27:1494–1498, 2002.
36. Currier B, Yaszemski M: The use of C1 lateral mass fixation in the cervical spine, *Curr Opin Orthop* 15(3):184–191, 2004.
37. Lee MJ, Cassinelli E, Riew KD: The feasibility of inserting atlas lateral mass screws via the posterior arch, *Spine* 31:2798–2801, 2006. **Over 700 cadaveric atlases were examined and morphometric data compiled. The majority (85%) of specimens had posterolateral arches greater than 3 mm in diameter but a few (14%) had diameters greater than 5 mm. The authors concluded that it is difficult in most patients to insert a screw safely via the posterolateral arch without violating the cortex.**
38. Tan M, Wang H, Wang Y, et al: Morphometric evaluation of screw fixation in atlas via posterior arch and lateral mass, *Spine* 28(9):888–895, 2003.
39. Henriques T, Cunningham BW, Olerud C, et al: Biomechanical comparison of five different atlanto-axial posterior fixation techniques, *Spine* 25(22):2877–2883, 2000.
40. Naderi S, Crawford NR, Song GS, et al: Biomechanical comparison of C1-C2 posterior fixations. Cable, graft, and screw combinations, *Spine* 23:1946–1955, 1998.
41. Dong Y, Hong MX, Jianyi L, et al: Quantitative anatomy of the lateral mass of the atlas, *Spine* 28: 860–863, 2003.

Chapter 13 Multilevel Cervical Corpectomy: Anterior-Only Versus Circumferential Instrumentation

Andrew J. Schoenfeld, Christopher M. Bono

Anterior cervical corpectomy is a well-established procedure that has been used successfully in the treatment of numerous conditions, including infection, deformity, trauma, and cervical spondylotic myelopathy.[1-12] Although posteriorly based procedures were the treatment of choice at the time cervical myelopathy was initially described, over the course of time anterior corpectomy has gained much popularity.[5] Although some meta-analyses have reported equivocal results in comparisons between anterior and posterior decompression for the treatment of myelopathy,[9] several series from single centers demonstrate satisfactory outcomes over long periods of follow-up for anterior cervical corpectomy.[3,5,6,8,10-12] Anterior cervical corpectomy allows a more direct decompression and reduces the number of host-graft interfaces necessary for successful fusion.[1,3,5,6,8] Hilibrand and colleagues[6] demonstrated improved clinical outcomes for anterior cervical corpectomy compared with multilevel diskectomy and fusion, and other studies have documented better neurologic outcomes and less axial neck pain with corpectomy than with posterior procedures.[1,9,11-13]

Potential complications after anterior cervical corpectomy include graft- and hardware-related problems.[3,5,8,14-18] Hardware failure, graft pistoning, graft dislodgment, and pseudarthrosis have all been documented following corpectomy, with the risk of failure increasing with the number of cervical levels involved.[3,5,14,15,18] Vaccaro and colleagues[18] documented a 50% failure rate for corpectomy procedures involving more than two levels.

At present, the question remains regarding the optimal mode of fixation following cervical corpectomy at more than one level. Although anterior-posterior instrumentation is known to enhance stability relative to standalone anterior plate fixation, the added cost, increased operative time, greater blood loss, and less favorable complication profile of posterior instrumentation are not necessarily justified for every multilevel corpectomy. This chapter reviews the existing literature regarding circumferential instrumentation versus standalone anterior fixation after multilevel corpectomy and provides an algorithm based on best available evidence to inform decision making in regard to this issue.

CASE PRESENTATION

A 54-year-old man had a long history of progressive gait instability and upper extremity paresthesias. He had minimal issues with neck pain and had been previously treated with mild conservative measures.

- PMH: Unremarkable
- PSH: Unremarkable
- Exam: The patient had subjectively decreased sensation in the arms and hands bilaterally, and a positive Lhermitte sign. The patient also exhibited the Hoffman sign bilaterally and inverted brachioradialis reflexes. Ambulatory evaluation revealed a frankly ataxic gait.

FIGURE 13-1 Lateral radiograph revealing diffuse spondylosis in the subaxial cervical spine.

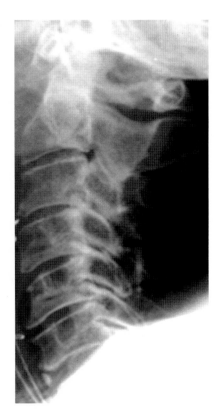

- Imaging: Plain radiographs showed diffuse spondylosis throughout the subaxial cervical spine (Figure 13-1). T2-weighted magnetic resonance imaging (MRI) studies are shown in Figures 13-2 through 13-4. MRI revealed significant cervical stenosis in the setting of degenerative disk disease and broad-based disk bulges from C3 to C7. Cord signal changes were also evident at C3-4 (see Figure 13-3) and C5-6 (see Figure 13-4).

Based on the patient's history, physical examination findings, and radiographic imaging studies the decision was made to proceed with a three-level anterior cervical corpectomy and instrumented fusion.

SURGICAL OPTIONS

For any case in which a multilevel corpectomy is indicated, the operative surgeon can choose to rely on anterior plate fixation alone or apply circumferential instrumentation with an anterior plate and a posterior fixation construct. The use of anterior plate fixation increases stiffness and reduces cervical motion following corpectomy.[15] Such devices have been shown to improve fusion rates and reduce the incidence of strut graft subsidence.[5] The addition of posterior spinal instrumentation further enhances construct stability through a tension-band effect.[19] Posterior lateral mass fixation also improves stability due to the fact that it involves multiple points of segmental fixation, lies further from the axis of motion in the cervical spine, and achieves better fixation in the lateral masses than screws placed within the vertebral bodies.[18] In addition, the presence of multiple points of fixation allows forces to be dissipated across several segments rather than concentrated at the ends of a construct.[18]

For interventions that may warrant corpectomy at three or more levels, the surgeon can also opt to perform a two-level corpectomy in the area of greatest pathologic change combined with an anterior cervical diskectomy and fusion at the remaining level or levels.[17,20,21] This technique, termed *hybrid decompression and fixation* by some,[21] offers the advantage of a single anterior surgery with a theoretically more biomechanically stable anterior construct than multilevel corpectomy with end fixation only.

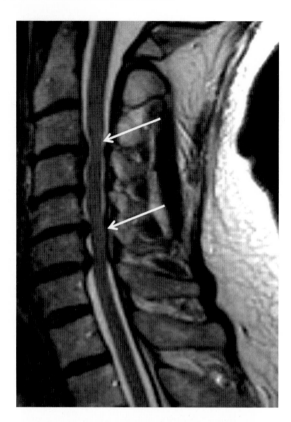

FIGURE 13-2 Sagittal T2-weighted MRI scan showing significant cervical degenerative disk disease with broad-based disk bulging at C3-4, C5-6, and C6-7. Cord signal changes are evident at C3-4 and C5-6 (*arrows*).

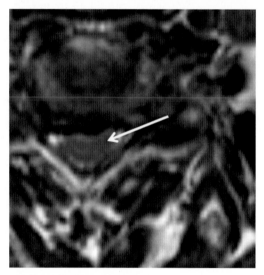

FIGURE 13-3 Axial T2-weighted MRI scan showing significant stenosis at C3-4 with cord signal changes (*arrow*).

FUNDAMENTAL TECHNIQUE

The initial portion of an anterior cervical corpectomy procedure, whether or not hybrid decompression-fixation or circumferential instrumentation will be used, is performed with the patient in a supine position on a radiolucent table. Careful thought should be given preoperatively to whether an awake, fiberoptic-assisted intubation is necessary. Spinal cord monitoring with measurement of somatosensory and motor evoked potentials and electromyography is also recommended during cervical corpectomy procedures.

Once the patient is intubated, an intravenous bag or towels are placed in the interscapular region to hyperextend the cervical spine. The patient's head can be

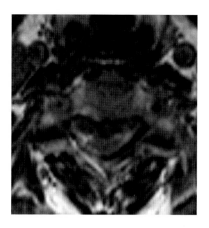

FIGURE 13-4 Axial T2-weighted MRI scan demonstrating significant stenosis at C5-6.

placed in a Mayfield headrest or cushioned head support based on surgeon preference. Importantly, the neck should be maintained in a neutral position within the patient's functional range of motion as assessed before surgery. The arms are padded and secured close to the body by means of tucked sheets or arm sleds attached beneath the operating table. The shoulders may be secured to the end of the bed with tape to facilitate exposure (Tips from the Masters 13-1).

Tips from the Masters 13-1 • Shoulder traction should be performed with extreme caution, especially in cases of severe cervical spondylosis, to avoid neurapraxia of the cervical nerve roots.

The approach for a cervical corpectomy can be performed from the left or right side based on the surgeon's preference. The incision should be plotted using standard anatomic landmarks in the cervical spine and centered over the operative levels. In certain circumstances a two-level corpectomy can be performed using a transverse incision similar to that utilized for an anterior cervical diskectomy. However, in most cases, a longitudinal incision along the anterior border of the sternocleidomastoid is recommended for multilevel corpectomies. The cervical levels to be included are exposed in a fashion identical to that used in the standard anterior exposure of the cervical spine. Exposure should extend to the middle of the vertebral body above and below the fullest extent of the corpectomy. Appropriate surgical levels should be confirmed with intraoperative fluoroscopy.

Once the appropriate surgical levels have been confirmed, Caspar pins can be placed in the middle of the vertebral bodies above and below the corpectomy levels. Pins should be carefully placed so as not to violate the end plates. A Caspar distraction device can then be used to perform gradual distraction across the operative levels, usually after the corpectomy has been completed, to facilitate cage or strut insertion. Care must be taken to avoid overdistraction, because this can lead to neurologic injury. A scalpel with a size 15 blade is then used to perform diskectomies at the disk spaces above, within, and below the corpectomy levels. Disk material is removed with a pituitary rongeur.

Once the diskectomies are complete, a rongeur is used to create an initial trough in the vertebral bodies to be included in the corpectomy. This bone material should be retained for grafting, especially if a titanium mesh or expandable cage is to be used for reconstruction. It is imperative to clearly establish the cervical midline before initiating the corpectomy to minimize the risk of iatrogenic vertebral artery injury during the procedure. Once an adequate trough has been fashioned in the vertebral bodies with the rongeur, a high-speed cutting bur can be used to complete most of the corpectomy, although it is recommended to switch to a diamond-tip bur once the surgeon visualizes posterior cortical bone or nears the posterior longitudinal ligament (PLL). Remaining cortical bone can be elevated from a nonossified PLL using curved curettes. The PLL may then be elevated from its cephalad insertion with a curved curette or nerve hook and removed in piecemeal fashion with Kerrison rongeurs. At this point the dura is exposed and the decompression is completed.

Vertebral end plates at the cephalad and caudal margins of the corpectomy site, and at the adjacent diskectomy site if a hybrid decompression-fixation is performed, should be prepared with curettes and/or a cutting bur. The surgeon's graft of choice (autogenous or allogenic; fibula strut, iliac crest, titanium mesh cage, or expandable cage) is then tailored to span the defect made by the corpectomy (Tips from the Masters 13-2). Unless an expandable cage is being used, the strut is inserted into the superior end plate first, followed by tamp impaction into the end plate at the caudal margin. When nonexpandable cages or struts are used, it is useful to slightly overdistract the corpectomy site before insertion. Once the cage is in an ideal position, the distraction can be relaxed, which will enhance the interference fit at the end plates.

Tips from the Masters 13-2 • Care must be taken to ensure that the graft does not rest too anteriorly on the inferior end plate, because this increases the risk of subsidence and kick-out.

An appropriately sized plate is then placed, spanning the decompression and resting on the vertebral bodies above and below the corpectomy. The plate is provisionally secured while screw holes are drilled and locking screws are placed. In a standard corpectomy four screws are placed to secure the plate. With hybrid decompression-fixation, six screws can be placed: two above and below the corpectomy site and two in the vertebral body adjacent to the site where the standard diskectomy was performed (Tips from the Masters 13-3).[16,20,21]

Tips from the Masters 13-3 • In situations in which a two- or three-level corpectomy is warranted, a more rigid standalone anterior construct can be fashioned by performing hybrid decompression-fixation.

If circumferential fixation is necessary, the anterior incision is closed in standard fashion and the patient is then transferred to the prone position on a Jackson table. The patient's head may be placed in a standard headrest or Mayfield tongs. A midline approach to the posterior cervical spine is then performed, extending from one level above to one level below the corpectomy levels. Lateral mass screws are placed using one of the techniques described in the literature. If the corpectomy includes C7 or ends at the C6-7 disk space, it may be advantageous to extend the posterior instrumentation to the level of T2.[22]

If this is done, lateral mass screws do not need to be inserted at C7, because they provide little additional biomechanical stability to cervicothoracic constructs (Tips from the Masters 13-4).[22] Appropriately sized rods are contoured and secured in place with locknuts. The lateral masses, spinous processes, and laminae can be decorticated, and bone graft, including cancellous bone retained from the corpectomy sites, should be placed to potentiate fusion.

Tips from the Masters 13-4 • If the multilevel corpectomy extends to C7 or T1, consideration should be given to extending the posterior instrumentation to the level of T2.

DISCUSSION OF BEST EVIDENCE

The neurologic benefits of a corpectomy procedure are achieved via the extent and quality of decompression performed. Although numerous studies have documented successful outcomes following these procedures,[1-12,23] high failure rates have been reported, particularly in multilevel corpectomies with standalone strut grafting or anterior plate fixation.[3,5,14,18,24] Pseudarthrosis after corpectomy has been shown to correlate with unsatisfactory outcomes and an increased risk of axial neck pain.[5] Catastrophic construct failures can result in graft subsidence or kick-out that can lead to esophageal perforation, neurologic injury, and/or life-threatening airway compromise.[3-5]

In a **retrospective review** of data for patients treated with multilevel corpectomy, Vaccaro and colleagues reported a 9% early failure rate for two-level corpectomies reconstructed with strut graft and anterior plate fixation, as opposed to a 50% failure rate for three-level corpectomies treated in the same manner.[18] Similar findings were reported by Kristof and colleagues[13] and Sasso and co-workers.[14] In a **retrospective review** published by Sasso and co-workers, failure rates were reported for 40 patients undergoing multilevel anterior cervical corpectomy with iliac crest autograft and locked plate fixation. A 6% failure rate was documented in the two-level corpectomy group, whereas 71% of patients undergoing three-level corpectomies in this series experienced catastrophic failure, including subsidence and anterior dislodgment.[14]

In a **prospective study** conducted by ElSaghir and Bohm,[24] anterior corpectomy with titanium cage reconstruction and anterior plate fixation was found to be associated with a 23% incidence of screw breakage and implant subsidence. In this investigation, the authors reported a significantly higher risk of hardware failure after this anterior procedure than after posteriorly based reconstruction. Findings in these clinical reports are substantiated by numerous **biomechanical investigations.**[15-17,22,25,26] DiAngelo and associates[15] reported that anterior plating following multilevel corpectomy resulted in a reversal of loading patterns in the cervical spine. Under flexion, the strut graft is shielded from loading, but excessive forces are applied to the graft during extension. DiAngelo and colleagues[15] proposed that this biomechanical phenomenon could be responsible for inferior end-plate cavitation and anterior strut extrusion.

Investigators have hypothesized that longer corpectomies, reconstructed with strut grafts and anterior plate fixation, have concomitantly increased rates of failure owing to longer lever arms and cantilever forces acting on the construct.[5,16,17,27,28] In a **cadaveric biomechanical study,** Isomi and colleagues found a significantly increased range of motion, and consequent failure risk, in three-level corpectomies reconstructed with anterior plates compared with single-level corpectomies.[27] Similar biomechanical findings were also reported by Singh and co-workers.[17]

Many surgeons maintained that the risk of failure following multilevel anterior corpectomy could be mitigated by the application of posterior instrumentation. The use of posterior fixation, particularly lateral mass screw-rod constructs, would create a posterior tension band in the cervical spine, limiting the forces felt to be responsible for graft failures.[4,5,16,19,26] Schmidt and co-workers[26] compared anterior plate fixation with circumferential instrumentation in a C4 to C6 corpectomy model. A statistically significant reduction in range of motion was found for circumferential instrumentation compared with anterior plate fixation, which led these authors to conclude that circumferential procedures were preferential to standalone anterior plating.[26]

In a biomechanical model simulating corpectomy following cervical flexion-extension injury, Do Koh and associates[25] reported a structural advantage for circumferential fusion over anterior fixation in terms of limiting flexion, extension, rotation, and lateral bending across involved motion segments. Ames and colleagues[22] reported like findings in a similar model representing severe flexion-compression injury at C7. In this **biomechanical investigation,** circumferential instrumentation was found to significantly limit cervical flexion, extension, lateral bending, and rotation compared with anterior fixation alone. These authors also recommended that, when the C7 vertebral body is compromised by trauma or involved in a corpectomy, consideration be given to extending the posterior fusion to T2.[22]

Adams and colleagues[28]. characterized limitations in range of motion for anterior cervical plating and circumferential instrumentation in a C5 corpectomy model. The addition of anterior plate fixation produced significant range of motion limitations compared with a normal spine, but only in flexion and extension. Circumferential instrumentation led to a significant reduction in range of motion compared with a normal spine in flexion, extension, rotation, and lateral bending. Compared with anterior plate fixation, circumferential instrumentation was associated with a significant reduction in range of motion for all tested parameters except axial rotation.

Adams and co-workers[28] maintained that circumferential fixation was not indicated for every patient undergoing multilevel corpectomy, but recommended that strong consideration be given to this procedure in individuals with osteoporosis, those with significant deformity, and those requiring early mobilization after surgery.

Singh and co-workers[16] examined the biomechanical performance of anterior cervical locking plates with circumferential instrumentation in a two-level (C4 and C5) corpectomy model. Results of this study indicated that anterior plate fixation was significantly less rigid than circumferential instrumentation in flexion, extension, lateral bending, and axial rotation. These findings led the authors to conclude that circumferential instrumentation was justified in instances in which patient factors might compromise the integrity of a standalone anterior plate construct.[16]

Porter and co-workers[20] compared the rigidity of three-level corpectomy (C5 through C7) with anterior plate fixation, and two-level corpectomy (C5 and C6) plus anterior cervical diskectomy (C7 through T1) with anterior plate fixation (hybrid decompression-fixation). The hybrid decompression-fixation construct provided more rigidity in flexion, extension, and lateral bending, although only limitations in flexion-extension were considered significant. Singh and associates[17] have also shown that a hybrid decompression-fixation construct performs better under biomechanical testing than a two-level corpectomy and anterior plate fixation. The rationale for hybrid decompression-fixation includes the fact that additional fixation can dissipate forces that otherwise would be borne by the inferior end plate in a multilevel corpectomy.[17,20,21] In a cohort of 25 patients treated with hybrid decompression-fixation, Ashkenazi and co-workers[21] reported a 96% fusion rate and no instances of construct failure.

Although no comparative studies presently exist investigating outcomes in patients with multilevel corpectomies treated with anterior plate fixation or circumferential instrumentation, several **case series** report improved outcomes in patients undergoing stabilization with anterior-posterior fixation after multilevel corpectomies.[1,2,8,10] In a **prospective study** by McAfee and colleagues[8] investigating outcomes after anterior decompression and circumferential instrumentation for myelopathy, 15 of 100 patients underwent multilevel corpectomies. In this subset of patients, no instances of construct failure or graft dislodgment were reported.

In a series of 26 myelopathic patients treated with multilevel anterior cervical decompression, Sevki and co-workers[10] included 12 cases in which circumferential instrumentation was used for stabilization. Eight patients treated with anterior-posterior fixation in this study had undergone three-level corpectomies, whereas the remaining four had undergone two-level corpectomies. No instances of hardware failure, graft migration, or nonunion were reported for this cohort.[10] These authors advocated routine circumferential instrumentation for all corpectomies involving three or more levels.

Acosta and co-workers[1] published one of the few reports to document outcomes solely for individuals undergoing multilevel corpectomies and circumferential instrumentation. This **retrospective review** included 20 patients who underwent corpectomy at three or more levels with a mean follow-up of 33 months. Neurologic improvement was documented in all patients, and there were no instances of hardware or graft failure. The fusion rate for individuals in this series was 100%.[1] Acosta and colleagues echoed the sentiments of Sevki and associates in recommending that anterior-posterior fixation be utilized on a routine basis for stabilization following anterior cervical corpectomy exceeding two levels.[1,10]

At present, the threat of anterior construct failure after multilevel cervical corpectomy must be weighed against the added surgical risks and morbidity of circumferential instrumentation. Unfortunately, no prospective or comparative studies are available to contrast the performance of these reconstructive options, and guidance must be derived from biomechanical investigations and small case series. Nonetheless, based on the best available evidence it is possible to make a strong recommendation for circumferential fixation in multilevel corpectomies involving three or more levels.[1,10,16,18,26,28] If anterior-posterior instrumentation is not desirable, it may be prudent to perform hybrid decompression-fixation with a two-level corpectomy and adjacent-level diskectomy.[17,20,21]

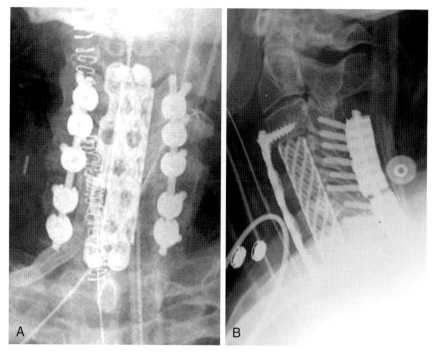

FIGURE 13-5 Postoperative anteroposterior (**A**) and lateral (**B**) plain radiographs. The patient was treated with a C4 through C6 anterior corpectomy and reconstruction with circumferential instrumentation. Lateral mass screws were placed posteriorly from C3 to C7. Because the patient did not have osseoligamentous abnormalities or preoperative deformity, the posterior construct was not extended across the cervicothoracic junction.

For multilevel corpectomies involving two vertebral bodies it could be possible to reconstruct the spine with a strut graft and anterior plate fixation. However, in patients with significant kyphosis, osteoporosis, or compromised posterior osseoligamentous structures the optimal construct may still be a circumferential instrumentation.[1,10,16,28]

Based on the evidence reviewed in this chapter, the patient was treated with an anterior cervical corpectomy of C4 through C6 and circumferential instrumentation (Figure 13-5). Lateral mass screws were placed posteriorly at C3 through C7. Because good lateral mass fixation was achieved at C7 intraoperatively, the construct was not extended across the cervicothoracic junction.

COMMENTARY

A successful outcome after multilevel anterior corpectomy depends on an adequate decompression and stable reconstruction. Pseudarthrosis, hardware failure, and graft subsidence lead to unacceptable failure rates following surgery. Based on the best available evidence in the literature, it is clear that circumferential instrumentation provides more significant rigidity to the cervical spine than standalone anterior plate fixation, even following one-level corpectomy. The questions of how much rigidity is necessary to facilitate fusion and when the critical threshold of risk-benefit is reached for additional posterior fixation cannot be definitively answered based on the current research data.

Nonetheless, it would appear that in light of the significant risk of failure for corpectomies involving three or more levels reconstructed using standalone anterior plate fixation,[3,5,14,18,24] routine circumferential instrumentation for these cases can be justified. Another alternative would be to perform a hybrid decompression-fixation with anterior plate fixation, a procedure that has been found to perform well in both clinical and biomechanical investigations.[17,20,21] In cases that warrant only two-level corpectomy, standalone anterior plate fixation may be appropriate, although patients with compromised bone or ligaments, or significant preoperative deformity may still benefit from anterior-posterior fixation.

REFERENCES

1. Acosta FL Jr, Aryan HE, Chou D, et al: Long-term biomechanical stability and clinical improvement after extended multilevel corpectomy and circumferential reconstruction of the cervical spine using titanium mesh cages, *J Spinal Disord Tech* 21(3):165–174, 2008. **Retrospective review of results for 20 patients treated with multilevel corpectomy and anterior-posterior fixation. All patients showed improvement following surgery and there were no instances of failure. This represents the largest clinical series to address the biomechanical stability of multilevel corpectomy constructs.**
2. Acosta FL Jr, Aryan HE, Ames CP: Successful outcome of six-level cervicothoracic corpectomy and circumferential reconstruction. Case report and review of literature on multilevel cervicothoracic corpectomy, *Eur Spine J* 15(Suppl 5):S670–S674, 2006.
3. Emery SE, Bohlman HH, Bolesta MJ, et al: Anterior cervical decompression and arthrodesis for the treatment of cervical spondylotic myelopathy. Two- to seventeen-year follow-up, *J Bone Joint Surg Am* 80(7):941–951, 1998.
4. Epstein NE: Anterior approaches to cervical spondylosis and ossification of the posterior longitudinal ligament: review of operative technique and assessment of 65 multilevel circumferential procedures, *Surg Neurol* 55:313–324, 2001.
5. Geck MJ, Eismont FJ: Surgical options for the treatment of cervical spondylotic myelopathy, *Orthop Clin North Am* 33:329–348, 2002.
6. Hilibrand AS, Fye MA, Emery SE, et al: Increased rate of arthrodesis with strut grafting after multilevel anterior cervical decompression, *Spine* 27(2):146–151, 2002.
7. Matz PG, Holly LT, Mummaneni PV, et al: Joint Section on Disorders of the Spine and Peripheral Nerves of the American Association of Neurological Surgeons and Congress of Neurological Surgeons. Anterior cervical surgery for the treatment of cervical degenerative myelopathy, *J Neurosurg Spine* 11(2):170–173, 2009.
8. McAfee PC, Bohlman HH, Ducker TB, et al: One-stage anterior cervical decompression and posterior stabilization. A study of one hundred patients with a minimum of two years of follow-up, *J Bone Joint Surg Am* 77(12):1791–1800, 1995. **Of the 100 patients in this prospective study who underwent anterior decompression and circumferential instrumentation for myelopathy, 15 had undergone multilevel corpectomies; no construct failure or graft dislodgment was noted in this patient subgroup.**
9. Mummaneni PV, Kaiser MG, Matz PG, et al: Joint Section on Disorders of the Spine and Peripheral Nerves of the American Association of Neurological Surgeons and Congress of Neurological Surgeons. Cervical surgical techniques for the treatment of cervical spondylotic myelopathy, *J Neurosurg Spine* 11(2):130–141, 2009.
10. Sevki K, Mehmet T, Ufuk T, et al: Results of surgical treatment for degenerative cervical myelopathy: anterior cervical corpectomy and stabilization, *Spine* 29(22):2493–2500, 2004. **Retrospective series of 26 patients undergoing anterior cervical corpectomy and stabilization for myelopathy. A 100% success rate was reported for the 12 patients in this series who received circumferential instrumentation.**
11. Wada E, Suzuki S, Kanazawa A, et al: Subtotal corpectomy versus laminoplasty for multilevel cervical spondylotic myelopathy: a long-term follow-up study over 10 years, *Spine* 26(13):1443–1447, 2001.
12. Yonenobu K, Hosono N, Iwasaki M, et al: Laminoplasty versus subtotal corpectomy. A comparative study of results in multisegmental cervical spondylotic myelopathy, *Spine* 17(11):1281–1284, 1992.
13. Kristof RA, Kiefer T, Thudium M, et al: Comparison of ventral corpectomy and plate-screw–instrumented fusion with dorsal laminectomy and rod-screw–instrumented fusion for treatment of at least two vertebral-level spondylotic cervical myelopathy, *Eur Spine J* 18:1951–1956, 2009.
14. Sasso RC, Ruggiero RA, Reilly TM, et al: Elderly reconstruction failures after multilevel cervical corpectomy, *Spine* 28(2):140–142, 2003. **Retrospective review of failure rates for two- and three-level corpectomies reconstructed with anterior plate fixation. Seventy-one percent of patients in the three-level corpectomy group experienced construct failure within 2 months of surgery.**
15. DiAngelo DJ, Foley KT, Vossel KA, et al: Anterior cervical plating reverses load transfer through multilevel strut-grafts, *Spine* 25(7):783–795, 2000. **Biomechanical investigation that demonstrated reversal of loading patterns for long anterior strut grafts instrumented with stand-alone anterior plates.**
16. Singh K, Vaccaro AR, Kim J, et al: Biomechanical comparison of cervical spine reconstructive techniques after a multilevel corpectomy of the cervical spine, *Spine* 28(20):2352–2358, 2003. **Biomechanical investigation comparing rigidity of anterior plates with that of circumferential instrumentation in a two-level corpectomy model. Anterior plate fixation was found to be significantly less rigid than circumferential instrumentation in flexion, extension, lateral bending, and axial rotation.**
17. Singh K, Vaccaro AR, Kim J, et al: Enhancement of stability following anterior cervical corpectomy: a biomechanical study, *Spine* 29(8):845–849, 2004.
18. Vaccaro AR, Falatyn SP, Scuderi GJ, et al: Early failure of long segment anterior cervical plate fixation, *J Spinal Disord* 11(5):410–415, 1998. **Retrospective review of failure rates in patients undergoing two- or three-level corpectomies and anterior plate fixation. The failure rate in the two-level corpectomy group was 9% compared with a 50% failure rate in the three-level corpectomy group.**
19. Kirkpatrick JS, Levy JA, Carillo J, et al: Reconstruction after multilevel corpectomy in the cervical spine. A sagittal plane biomechanical study, *Spine* 24(12):1186–1190, 1999.

20. Porter RW, Crawford NR, Chamberlain RH, et al: Biomechanical analysis of multilevel cervical corpectomy and plate constructs, *J Neurosurg* 99(Suppl 1):98–103, 2003. **Biomechanical study that showed hybrid decompression-fixation to provide better stability than three-level corpectomy and anterior plate fixation.**

21. Ashkenazi E, Smorgick Y, Rand N, et al: Anterior decompression combined with corpectomies and discectomies in the management of multilevel cervical myelopathy: a hybrid decompression and fixation technique, *J Neurosurg Spine* 3(3):205–209, 2005. **Clinical case series documenting satisfactory outcomes in 25 patients treated with hybrid decompression-fixation. Ninety-six percent of patients showed clinical improvement following surgery, and the fusion rate in this series was also 96%.**

22. Ames CP, Bozkus MH, Chamberlain RH, et al: Biomechanics of stabilization after cervicothoracic compression-flexion injury, *Spine* 30(13):1505–1512, 2005. **Biomechanical study that compared the performance of circumferential instrumentation and anterior plate fixation in a model simulating corpectomy following traumatic three-column injury. Anterior-posterior fixation performed better than anterior plate fixation, and the authors also found that, in the event of C7 corpectomy, extension of the posterior construct to T2 provided increased stability.**

23. Ikenaga M, Shikata J, Tanaka C: Long-term results over 10 years of anterior corpectomy and fusion for multilevel cervical myelopathy, *Spine* 31(14):1568–1574, 2006.

24. ElSaghir H, Bohm H: Anterior versus posterior plating in cervical corpectomy, *Arch Orthop Trauma Surg* 120(10):549–554, 2000. **In a prospective study, anterior corpectomy with titanium cage reconstruction and anterior plate fixation were found to be associated with a 23% incidence of screw breakage and implant subsidence.**

25. Do Koh Y, Lim TH, Won You J, et al: A biomechanical comparison of modern anterior and posterior plate fixation of the cervical spine, *Spine* 26(1):15–21, 2001.

26. Schmidt R, Wilke HJ, Claes L, et al: Pedicle screws enhance primary stability in multilevel cervical corpectomies: biomechanical in vitro comparison of different implants including constrained and nonconstrained posterior instrumentations, *Spine* 28(16):1821–1828, 2003. **Biomechanical study examining the rigidity of seven different constructs in a three-level corpectomy model. Circumferential instrumentation was associated with statistically significant reductions in cervical range of motion compared with all other constructs, including stand-alone anterior plate fixation.**

27. Isomi T, Panjabi MM, Wang JL, et al: Stabilizing potential of anterior cervical plates in multilevel corpectomies, *Spine* 24(21):2219–2223, 1999.

28. Adams MS, Crawford NR, Chamberlain RH, et al: Biomechanical comparison of anterior cervical plating and combined anterior/lateral mass plating, *Spine J* 1:166–170, 2001.

Chapter 14 Cervical Jumped Facets and Incomplete Neurologic Deficit: Closed Reduction Versus Urgent Surgery

Michael A. Finn, Paul A. Anderson

Cervical facet dislocations, also known as *jumped facets,* are the result of a hyperflexion or flexion distraction injury, often associated with a component of rotation. In cases of unilateral dislocation, patients most often escape neurologic injury, whereas bilateral facet dislocations are frequently associated with significant neurologic deficit.[1] Neurologic deficits in the setting of cervical dislocation with jumped facets are attributable to both the primary injury, or the initial trauma and disruption of neural tissue, and to the secondary injury, or injury attributable to the ongoing compression of neural elements. Although the primary neurologic injury is irreversible, the secondary injury represents a treatable source of neurologic dysfunction and is thought to occur in proportion to the length of time and the magnitude of physical compression.[2-6] One cause of this secondary injury is spinal cord ischemia due to compression of the anterior spinal artery and radicular feeders. Simple spinal realignment may at a minimum reestablish blood flow to partially damaged tissue, thereby reducing the severity of secondary injury. Timely decompression of neural elements has been shown to be critical in minimizing secondary neurologic injury and maximizing the chances of neurologic recovery in animal studies, although proof of this in humans is lacking except in anecdotal case reports.[7-9]

Patients with either unilateral or bilateral jumped facets and incomplete neurologic injury present a situation in which the primary neurologic injury is subtotal; thus the goal of initial treatment is to minimize secondary injury, that is, to lessen the chances of neurologic decline from further spinal cord necrosis and to maximize the chances of recovery. Neurologic decompression should be carried out in an expeditious fashion to meet this goal. Closed reduction of the cervical fracture dislocations via traction provides the most rapid means of reducing the traumatic deformity and decompressing the neural elements, and its safe use has been well reported.[10-14] Despite its well-documented efficacy, however, the closed reduction of cervical fracture dislocations has been the focus of much debate in the literature because of the fear of precipitating a neurologic decline through the displacement of extruded disk material.[15-18] Although this risk may be real, it is relatively small and should not delay the prompt closed reduction of a traumatic deformity in the awake, examinable patient.

CASE PRESENTATIONS

Case 1

A 35-year-old woman came for treatment after a high-velocity fall over the handlebars in a mountain biking accident. She experienced a brief loss of consciousness and was transported for medical evaluation using full spinal precautions. She complained of numbness in bilateral C7 distributions.

- PMH: Unremarkable
- PSH: Unremarkable

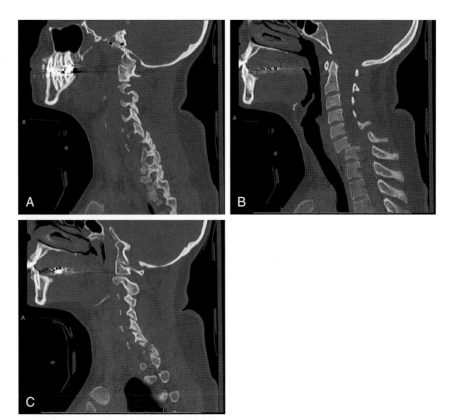

FIGURE 14-1 Sagittal CT reconstructions demonstrating C6-7 fracture dislocation with C5-6 and C6-7 dislocated facets on the left (**A**) and a fractured C7 facet on the right (**C**). Approximately 50% anterolisthesis of C6 on C7 can be seen (**B**).

- Exam: Strength in the triceps was 4/5 bilaterally with full strength in all other muscle groups and decreased sensation to light touch from C7 down. Rectal tone was normal, and reflexes were symmetric and nonpathologic.
- Imaging: Computed tomography (CT) revealed a fracture dislocation at C6-7 with 50% anterolisthesis of C6 on C7, a dislocated facet on the left, a fractured dislocated facet on the right, and a complex fracture of C5 with fracture through the pedicle and posterior elements resulting in a floating lateral mass (Figure 14-1).

The patient was placed in Garner-Wells tongs and 10 lb of traction was applied. Traction was increased in 10-lb increments, with radiography and a thorough physical examination performed at each interval increase in weight, until 30 lb was reached, at which point there was some concern for overdistraction at the C6-7 interspace (Figure 14-2). CT with the patient in traction demonstrated a 25% reduction in dislocation, but persisting facet dislocation of C6-7 (Figure 14-3).

The patient was then taken to the operating room for a C6 corpectomy with C5-C7 anterior fusion followed by posterior fixation from C5 to C7 on the right (Figure 14-4). Reduction was obtained with distraction using distraction posts during the anterior portion of the procedure. Left-sided posterior instrumentation was precluded by the fracture pattern. The patient's sensory and motor deficits had resolved completely by 1-month follow-up.

Case 2

A 16-year-old gymnast fell from parallel bars onto a hyperflexed neck. She was immediately quadriplegic and was brought to the emergency department within 45 minutes of injury.

FIGURE 14-2 Lateral radiograph taken with the patient in 30 lb of traction. Note widening of the C6-7 interspace.

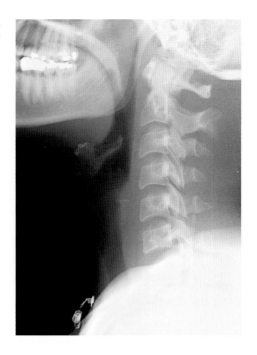

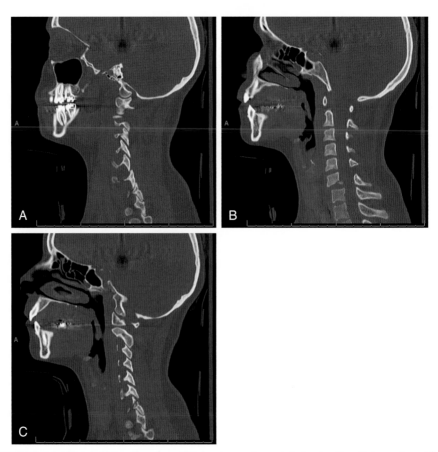

FIGURE 14-3 Sagittal reconstructions from CT scanning performed during traction. Note continued facet dislocation on left (**A**).

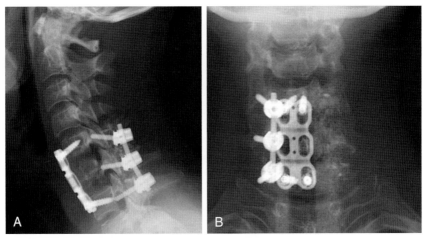

FIGURE 14-4 Radiographs obtained after anterior and posterior fixation via C6 corpectomy, anterior plating, and posterior lateral mass instrumentation.

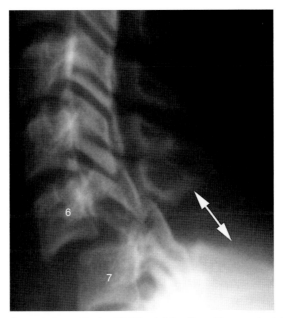

FIGURE 14-5 Lateral radiograph demonstrating C6-7 facet dislocation with approximately 50% anterolisthesis.

- PMH: Unremarkable
- PSH: Unremarkable
- Exam: Neurologic examination revealed a complete C6 cord-level injury except for patchy sensation on her chest. The bulbocavernosus reflex was absent.
- Imaging: A lateral radiograph revealed bilateral facet dislocations at C6-7 (Figure 14-5).

   Cranial tong traction was immediately applied, and reduction was achieved at 40 lb of traction weight within 20 minutes after the patient entered the emergency

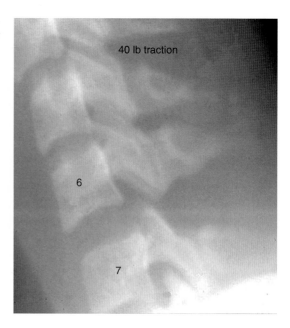

FIGURE 14-6 Lateral radiograph demonstrating reduction of dislocation in 40 lb of traction.

department (Figure 14-6). She noted an instantaneous return of sensation to her arms and legs when reduction occurred. Within 6 hours she began to regain motor function, and by the next day had normal motor strength but residual spasticity. Five days later she underwent a posterior C6-7 fusion and maintained normal motor and sensory function.

TREATMENT OPTIONS

Reduction of facet dislocations may be accomplished using cranial tong traction, and surgically using either an anterior or posterior approach.

Closed Reduction

The closed cranial tong traction technique is faster and is preferred in patients with severe neurologic injury. Disadvantages include a failure rate of between 5% and 25% and a small risk of neurologic deterioration.

Surgical Reduction

Surgical reduction via a posterior approach was traditionally used, which allowed open reduction by manual means or with removal of small amounts of the facet to allow unlocking and then fusion. More recently with the development of rigid anterior cervical plates the anterior approach has been advocated and safely performed. This allows diskectomy and theoretically prevents neurologic deterioration from retained disk fragments that may compress the cord after reduction. It also allows reduction using anterior distraction pins and manual leverage. Disadvantages are lack of familiarity with techniques of open anterior reduction and failure of the construct in the presence of vertebral body fractures, which occur frequently.

FUNDAMENTAL TECHNIQUE

Reduction with Tong Traction

Before traction is initiated, images of the cervical spine should be scrutinized closely for the presence of injuries cephalad to the dislocated level, with specific attention directed to the occipitocervical junction (Tips from the Masters 14-1). The presence of skull fractures underlying the site of application of the tongs should also be ruled out if clinically suspected (Tips from the Masters 14-2). Finally, the presence of an ankylosed cervical spine, as in the case of ankylosing spondylitis, is a relative contraindication to the use of traction. In these cases, attempts at reduction should be performed using fluoroscopy and a slow escalation of traction weights.

Tips from the Masters 14-1 • Carefully assess the cervical spine for rostral injuries. Odontoid and hangman fractures and atlantooccipital dislocation are contraindications to closed reduction.

Tips from the Masters 14-2 • Patients who are neurologically intact should, if possible, undergo magnetic resonance imaging (MRI) before reduction to evaluate the location of the intervertebral disk. If there is a herniated disk behind the body of the dislocated vertebrae, an anterior diskectomy should be performed before reduction.

The patient is positioned supine on a hospital bed that accepts a traction apparatus. The skin overlying the pin insertion site is prepared in the normal fashion. Hair shaving is not necessary. Local anesthesia is injected into the skin and down to the periosteum in awake patients. For Gardner-Wells or similar tongs, the standard site of pin placement is approximately 1 cm superior to the pinna and 1 cm anterior to the external auditory canal, a location which places the tongs below the equator of the skull and thereby reduces the risk of pullout. More anterior placement can lead to penetration of the superficial temporal artery. Of note, stainless steel tongs are less susceptible to deformation and should be used if high traction weights (more than 50 lb) are anticipated rather than graphite and titanium MRI-compatible tongs.[19] Alternatively, a standard halo ring can be used with traction if halo immobilization is likely to be required after reduction. When Gardner-Wells tongs are used, the pins are tightened until the spring indicator protrudes 1 mm. Care should be taken to ensure that pins are placed symmetrically.

Before traction is initiated, a thorough neurologic examination is performed (Tips from the Masters 14-3). Traction is typically started at 10 lb and increased in 5- to 10-lb increments until reduction is achieved. A neurologic examination is performed and a lateral cervical radiograph is scrutinized after each increase in weight. Fluoroscopy can also be useful to obtain real-time evaluation of traction maneuvers. Specific attention should again be paid to more cephalad levels to ensure that there is no distraction, defined as widening of the disk space to more than 1.5 times that of the adjacent levels, or an occult injury. Although many authors report using weight of approximately 10 lb per level of injury in addition to the initial 10 lb (e.g., 60 lb total for a C5-6 injury), weights of up to 140 lb have been reported to be used safely and successfully.[10,14,20] Placing the bed in reverse Trendelenburg position is useful with the application of higher weights to counteract the tendency to pull the patient cephalad in the bed. For bilateral facet dislocations it can also be helpful to place the Gardner-Wells pins slightly posterior to the angle of the vector of traction and allow for the creation of a greater flexion moment.

Tips from the Masters 14-3 • Before and after each addition of traction weight a careful neurologic examination is performed. Increasing paresthesias or decreased sensation are warning signs of potential neurologic deterioration and should result in discontinuation of the reduction attempt. Further lateral radiographs taken after each addition of weight are scrutinized for signs of overreduction such as diastasis of the facets or distraction across the intervertebral disk.

In the event of failure of traction, manual maneuvers may prove helpful. Manual maneuvers should be undertaken with traction weight removed to reduce the possibility of overdistraction. Administration of a small amount of a muscle relaxant (e.g., diazepam [Valium]) may be helpful in difficult cases. In patients with bilateral jumped facets, manual pressure may be applied behind the neck at a level beneath the injury. In combination with traction and a flexion moment, anteriorly directed pressure in this location may aid in reduction. Alternatively, the head can be turned approximately 30 degrees in each direction in an attempt to sequentially relocate facets. In the case of unilateral dislocation, manual traction can be applied with rotation in the direction of the jumped facet. Closed reduction under general anesthesia is a final nonoperative means of obtaining reduction. The advantage of this technique is that complete muscle relaxation can be obtained.[21] This technique is controversial, however, because the patient is not examinable and neurologic decline may be unrecognized (Tips from the Masters 14-4). Reduction under general anesthesia should be undertaken after fiberoptic intubation and under fluoroscopic guidance. In either case, once reduction is obtained the patient is placed in extension and the traction weight can be reduced to 15 to 25 lb with a final radiograph taken to confirm alignment.

Tips from the Masters 14-4 • Once reduction is obtained, the patient is brought to the operating room in traction. An anterior approach for stabilization is preferred, because it eliminates the risk associated with rotating the patient prone and allows removal of any potentially herniated disk material.

Open Reduction

Failure of reduction with the aforementioned nonoperative maneuvers requires surgical reduction. Although a posterior approach has traditionally been advocated,[22] anterior approaches are effective and may even be preferred, because any herniated disk fragments can be removed.[20,23] Intraoperative reduction can be obtained anteriorly with the use of distraction, applied either through distraction posts or with a laminar spreader (Tips from the Masters 14-5).[20,24] This procedure is monitored by fluoroscopy and by measurement of spinal evoked potentials to decrease the risk of neurologic deterioration.

Tips from the Masters 14-5 • Expandable cages can be used to help provide further distraction to release locked facets.

Once reduction has been obtained, complete decompression and interbody fusion is performed. Fixation is achieved using an anterior cervical plate. In most cases this is sufficient, and combined anterior-posterior techniques are not needed.

Open reduction through a posterior approach can usually be achieved by manual manipulation of the spinous processes, with flexion moments applied initially to unlock the joints and then compression to fully reduce kyphosis. A curette or elevator can be placed into the joint to act as a lever to elevate and reduce the dislocated vertebra. Difficult cases may require the removal of a small amount of the overriding facet with a bur to aid in reduction. After reduction a posterior fusion using lateral mass screws is performed. In some patients with extensive lateral mass comminution that precludes secure screw placement across the involved segments, additional levels may need to be incorporated into the fusion.

DISCUSSION OF BEST EVIDENCE

The goal of treatment of any incomplete spinal cord injury is the prevention of further injury and the optimization of the chances for neurologic recovery (Figure 14-7). Rapid decompression of neural elements is paramount in accomplishing these goals and is supported not only by empiricism, but also by animal and Level III clinical studies. Several animal studies have demonstrated that the severity and permanence of spinal cord injury is directly related to the duration and magnitude of compression.[2,3,6,25] Carlson and colleagues[4] demonstrated in an **animal model** that a critical time period of 1 to 3 hours may exist beyond which neurologic recovery may not be possible in the setting of ongoing compression. These results are consistent with those of Delamarter and associates, who showed recoverability of function when neurologic

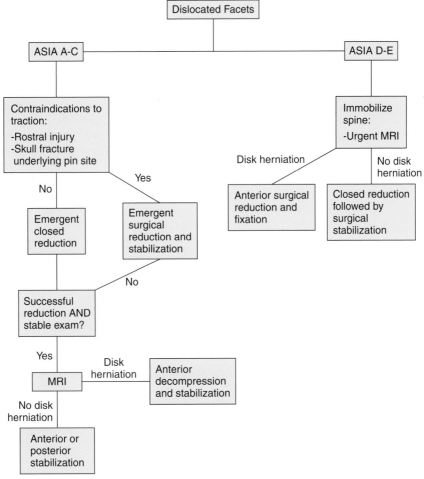

FIGURE 14-7 Treatment algorithm for dislocated facets. *ASIA,* American Spinal Injury Association Impairment Scale.

compression was relieved within 1 hour and no recoverability after 6 or more hours of compression.[5]

Clinical evidence supporting early cord decompression is composed of case reports and series. Several large **retrospective studies** have reported on the safe and effective use of closed reduction in cervical facet fracture dislocations. Hadley and co-workers[12] reported on the treatment of 68 patients with facet fracture dislocation, with closed reduction attempted on 66. Although reduction was successful in only 58% of patients, neurologic improvement was seen in 78%, and it appeared that the timing of the reduction, whether by open or closed means, was the most important factor influencing recovery. Grant and associates[11] reported a 97.6% success rate in reduction in their series of 82 patients with cervical subluxations secondary to facet dislocations or other fractures. Postreduction MRI revealed disk herniation in 22% of patients and disk space disruption in 24%, although these findings had no effect on outcome. Lee and colleagues reported on a series of 210 patients, of whom 91 were treated by manipulation under anesthesia and 119 were treated by rapid traction.[13] They reported a greater success rate with rapid traction (88% vs. 73%) as well as greater safety, with six patients experiencing declining neurologic function with reduction under anesthesia versus one with rapid traction. Several other series have corroborated the safety and efficacy of closed reduction.[26-28]

Closed reduction of cervical facet dislocations with traction is not without risk. The most feared complication is neurologic deterioration, thought to be most often secondary to disk herniation. Two **case reports** have described neurologic deterioration from herniation and have caused physicians much pause in instituting traction, with some arguing for prereduction MRI in all patients.[16,17] This well-publicized risk has led to several investigations of disk herniations and traction. In a **prospective study,** Vaccaro and colleagues[18] obtained prereduction and postreduction MRI scans for 11 patients with cervical dislocations. Among the nine patients undergoing success reductions, disk herniations were found in two before reduction and in five after reduction. No patient, however, experienced a neurologic worsening. Darsaut and associates reported on the use of MRI guidance in the reduction of cervical dislocations and observed an increase in spinal canal diameter in 11 of 17 patients undergoing traction, with herniated disk material being pulled back toward the disk space.[15]

The usefulness of MRI before traction in patients with incomplete neurologic deficit is thus debatable. In patients with incomplete neurologic injuries, a delay in treatment while MRI is performed can theoretically lead to an exacerbation of injury or the conversion of a reversible injury into an irreversible one, because the duration of neurologic compression is inversely related to the probability of recovery in animal models, as discussed earlier. Furthermore, exactly what findings on an MRI scan would preclude the application of traction is unclear, because traction has certainly been applied without adverse effect in the setting of disk disruption and herniation.

MRI remains an option in patients with incomplete neurologic injury if it is readily available and will not substantially delay reduction. MRI can be more strongly considered in patients who are unexaminable due to a head injury, intoxication, or other causes, because in such cases a neurologic decline will not be detectable if it should occur during the application of traction. If a herniated disk fragment is detected, thought should be given to operative decompression and reduction at the earliest possible time.

The application of traction can also cause neurologic decline through overdistraction, which can occur with the use of too much weight or the failure to recognize a more rostral lesion.[22,29-33] A missed atlantooccipital dislocation is a well-reported and serious cause of deterioration when traction is used, and the patient must be carefully screened for such a dislocation before application of traction.[22,34] In total, the risk of permanent neurologic deterioration from closed reduction appears to be less than 1.0%[16,26,27,35,36]; transient neurologic deficits occur with a slightly higher frequency (2% to 4%) and are mostly reversible with reduction of traction.[26,37] Moreover, no permanent neurologic injury has been described in an awake and examinable patient undergoing closed reduction of a cervical facet dislocation. This underscores the importance of the examination of the patient when traction is used, and for this reason reduction in the awake, examinable patient may actually be safer than reduction under general anesthesia at the time of operation.

Surgical reduction of cervical jumped facets is performed when traction is unsuccessful and can be accomplished using either an anterior or posterior approach.[38] Advantages of a posterior approach include the ability to obtain reduction of jumped facets directly and the greater biomechanical strength of posterior stabilization constructs compared with anterior constructs.[39] Anterior approaches, on the other hand, enable the direct removal of herniated disk material and allow the dislocation to be stabilized with the fusion of only the involved levels, whereas the posterior approach may necessitate instrumentation of additional levels, especially if significant amounts of facet are removed to accomplish reduction. Although anterior constructs are not as robust biomechanically as posterior constructs, fusion rates of more than 90% are reported, and outcomes for the two techniques are similar.[38,40,41] Combined anterior and posterior approaches may be preferred by some, but circumferential stabilization is usually not necessary.

In summary, the best animal and clinical human evidence indicates that there is an advantage to early decompression of the spinal cord in cases of spinal cord injury. In the case of jumped cervical facets decompression can be accomplished most rapidly in a closed fashion, with the use of cranial tongs and traction. In an awake, examinable patient, such reduction should be carried out as soon as possible. In cases in which closed reduction is not possible, early open reduction from an anterior or posterior approach is indicated.

COMMENTARY

Closed traction of facet dislocations in patients with neurologic injuries is the most expeditious means to improve local spinal cord flow and reduce secondary effects of spinal cord injury and compression. Anecdotal case reports have shown that rapid reduction within 1 to 2 hours may reverse quadriplegia. Delaying reduction to perform imaging such as MRI or to prepare for surgery may increase the duration of neural compression, exceeding the small window of opportunity to obtain the benefits of immediate reduction.

Closed reduction with tong traction is safe and effective in realigning the spine in the majority of patients. Contraindications include skull fractures and unstable injuries rostral to the cervical dislocation, including atlantooccipital dislocations, odontoid fractures, and hangman's fractures. Ankylosing spondylitis represents a relative contraindication to traction. Large retrospective case series of closed reduction via cranial tongs in awake patients have shown that neurologic worsening occurs in 1% to 2% of cases. This is usually transient and is secondary to overdistraction. Reduction of all fracture types is achieved in 75% to 95% of cases, although large traction weights may be required. Once reduction is achieved, traction weights can generally be reduced and definitive treatment performed.

REFERENCES

1. Sonntag VK: Management of bilateral locked facets of the cervical spine, *Neurosurgery* 8(2):150–152, 1981.
2. Tarlov IM, Klinger H: Spinal cord compression studies. II. Time limits for recovery after acute compression in dogs, *AMA Arch Neurol Psychiatry* 71(3):271–290, 1954.
3. Dolan EJ, Tator CH, Endrenyi L: The value of decompression for acute experimental spinal cord compression injury, *J Neurosurg* 53(6):749–755, 1980.
4. Carlson GD, Minato Y, Okada A, et al: Early time-dependent decompression for spinal cord injury: vascular mechanisms of recovery, *J Neurotrauma* 14(12):951–962, 1997.
5. Delamarter RB, Sherman J, Carr JB: Pathophysiology of spinal cord injury. Recovery after immediate and delayed decompression, *J Bone Joint Surg Am* 77(7):1042–1049, 1995. **Delamarter and colleagues demonstrate the critical correlation between time of neurologic compression and histologic neurologic damage, and electrophysiologic and clinical recovery. Their results are consistent with those of other animal and human studies indicating that prolonged neurologic compression leads to greater injury. Conversely, timely decompression allows improved recovery.**
6. Tarlov IM: Spinal cord compression studies. III. Time limits for recovery after gradual compression in dogs, *AMA Arch Neurol Psychiatry* 71(5):588–597, 1954.
7. Cowan JA Jr, McGillicuddy JE: Images in clinical medicine. Reversal of traumatic quadriplegia after closed reduction, *N Engl J Med* 359(20):2154, 2008.
8. Brunette DD, Rockswold GL: Neurologic recovery following rapid spinal realignment for complete cervical spinal cord injury, *J Trauma* 27(4):445–447, 1987.
9. Wolf A, Levi L, Mirvis S, et al: Operative management of bilateral facet dislocation, *J Neurosurg* 75(6):883–890, 1991.
10. Cotler JM, Herbison GJ, Nasuti JF, et al: Closed reduction of traumatic cervical spine dislocation using traction weights up to 140 pounds, *Spine* 18(3):386–390, 1993.
11. Grant GA, Mirza SK, Chapman JR, et al: Risk of early closed reduction in cervical spine subluxation injuries, *J Neurosurg* 90(Suppl 1):13–18, 1999. **Grant and colleagues report on a large retrospective study of the utility of closed reduction in treatment of cervical spine injuries. Ninety-seven percent of 82 patients underwent successful reduction using closed methods. Although 22% of patients had postreduction disk herniation evident on MRI scans, this was not found be clinically significant.**
12. Hadley MN, Fitzpatrick BC, Sonntag VK, et al: Facet fracture-dislocation injuries of the cervical spine, *Neurosurgery* 30(5):661–666, 1992. **Hadley and colleagues reported on the use of closed and open reduction techniques in a series of 68 patients with cervical facet fracture-dislocation injuries. Although closed techniques were successful only 58% of the time in this study, the timing of reduction by any method was the strongest variable correlating with neurologic outcome.**
13. Lee AS, MacLean JC, Newton DA: Rapid traction for reduction of cervical spine dislocations, *J Bone Joint Surg Br* 76(3):352–356, 1994.
14. Rizzolo SJ, Vaccaro AR, Cotler JM: Cervical spine trauma, *Spine* 19(20):2288–2298, 1994.
15. Darsaut TE, Ashforth R, Bhargava R, et al: A pilot study of magnetic resonance imaging–guided closed reduction of cervical spine fractures, *Spine* 31(18):2085–2090, 2006.
16. Farmer J, Vaccaro A, Albert TJ, et al: Neurologic deterioration after cervical spinal cord injury, *J Spinal Disord* 11(3):192–196, 1998.

17. Maiman DJ, Barolat G, Larson SJ: Management of bilateral locked facets of the cervical spine, *Neurosurgery* 18(5):542–547, 1986.

18. Vaccaro AR, Falatyn SP, Flanders AE, et al: Magnetic resonance evaluation of the intervertebral disc, spinal ligaments, and spinal cord before and after closed traction reduction of cervical spine dislocations, *Spine* 24(12):1210–1217, 1999. **Vaccaro and colleagues obtained prereduction and postreduction MRI scans for 11 patients with cervical spine dislocations and noted an increase in the incidence of disk herniations after reduction. No neurologic deficits were attributed to this finding. These results should alert clinicians to disk herniation as a potential cause of neurologic decline after closed reduction, and this possibility should be examined.**

19. Blumberg KD, Catalano JB, Cotler JM, et al: The pullout strength of titanium alloy MRI-compatible and stainless steel MRI-incompatible Gardner-Wells tongs, *Spine* 18(13):1895–1896, 1993.

20. Vital JM, Gille O, Sénégas J, et al: Reduction technique for uni- and biarticular dislocations of the lower cervical spine, *Spine* 23(8):949–954; discussion, 955, 1998.

21. Lu K, Lee TC, Chen HJ: Closed reduction of bilateral locked facets of the cervical spine under general anaesthesia, *Acta Neurochir (Wien)* 140(10):1055–1061, 1998.

22. Bohlman HH: Acute fractures and dislocations of the cervical spine. An analysis of three hundred hospitalized patients and review of the literature, *J Bone Joint Surg Am* 61(8):1119–1142, 1979.

23. de Oliveira JC: Anterior reduction of interlocking facets in the lower cervical spine, *Spine* 4(3):195–202, 1979.

24. Fazl M, Pirouzmand F: Intraoperative reduction of locked facets in the cervical spine by use of a modified interlaminar spreader: technical note, *Neurosurgery* 48(2):444–445; discussion, 445-446, 2001.

25. Jelsma RK, Rice JF, Jelsma LF, et al: The demonstration and significance of neural compression after spinal injury, *Surg Neurol* 18(2):79–92, 1982.

26. Initial closed reduction of cervical spine fracture-dislocation injuries, *Neurosurgery* 50(Suppl 3):S44–S50, 2002.

27. Mahale YJ, Silver JR, Henderson NJ: Neurological complications of the reduction of cervical spine dislocations, *J Bone Joint Surg Br* 75(3):403–409, 1993.

28. Star AM, Jones AA, Cotler JM, et al: Immediate closed reduction of cervical spine dislocations using traction, *Spine* 15(10):1068–1072, 1990.

29. Scher AT: Overdistraction of cervical spinal injuries? *S Afr Med J* 59(18):639–641, 1981.

30. Gruenberg MF, Rechtine GR, Chrin AM, et al: Overdistraction of cervical spine injuries with the use of skull traction: a report of two cases, *J Trauma* 42(6):1152–1156, 1997.

31. Key A: Cervical spine dislocations with unilateral facet interlocking, *Paraplegia* 13(3):208–215, 1975.

32. Schaefer DM, Flanders A, Northrup BE, et al: Magnetic resonance imaging of acute cervical spine trauma. Correlation with severity of neurologic injury, *Spine* 14(10):1090–1095, 1989.

33. Fried LC: Cervical spinal cord injury during skeletal traction, *JAMA* 229(2):181–183, 1974.

34. Guigui P, Milaire M, Morvan G, et al: Traumatic atlantooccipital dislocation with survival: case report and review of the literature, *Eur Spine J* 4(4):242–247, 1995.

35. Fehlings MG, Tator CH: An evidence-based review of decompressive surgery in acute spinal cord injury: rationale, indications, and timing based on experimental and clinical studies, *J Neurosurg* 91 (Suppl 1):1–11, 1999.

36. Mahale YJ, Silver JR: Progressive paralysis after bilateral facet dislocation of the cervical spine, *J Bone Joint Surg Br* 74(2):219–223, 1992.

37. Wimberley DW, Vaccaro AR, Goyal N, et al: Acute quadriplegia following closed traction reduction of a cervical facet dislocation in the setting of ossification of the posterior longitudinal ligament: case report, *Spine* 30(15):E433–E438, 2005.

38. Brodke DS, Anderson PA, Newell DW, et al: Comparison of anterior and posterior approaches in cervical spinal cord injuries, *J Spinal Disord Tech* 16(3):229–235, 2003.

39. Coe JD, Warden KE, Sutterlin CE 3rd, et al: Biomechanical evaluation of cervical spinal stabilization methods in a human cadaveric model, *Spine* 14(10):1122–1131, 1989.

40. Garvey TA, Eismont FJ, Roberti LJ: Anterior decompression, structural bone grafting, and Caspar plate stabilization for unstable cervical spine fractures and/or dislocations, *Spine* 17(Suppl 10):S431–S435, 1992.

41. Johnson MG, Fisher CG, Boyd M, et al: The radiographic failure of single segment anterior cervical plate fixation in traumatic cervical flexion distraction injuries, *Spine* 29(24):2815–2820, 2004.

Chapter 15 Laminectomy Across the Cervicothoracic Junction: Fusion Versus Nonfusion

Timothy E. Link, Rahul Jandial, Volker K.H. Sonntag

Surgery involving the cervicothoracic junction (CTJ) is universally accompanied by questions about postoperative stability. This junction must be crossed in treating many pathologic conditions: tumors, trauma, infections, and inflammatory, degenerative, and congenital disorders. Anterior access to this region is complex and associated with morbidity, requiring significant surgical skill. Posterior approaches provide a simpler alternative, but the complex biomechanics requires thoughtful preoperative planning. Laminoplasty is acceptable when preoperative cervical lordosis is present and facet disruption is minimized. However, even when lordotic alignment is normal, the ability of laminoplasty to maintain cervical range of motion (ROM) remains questionable, and doing so is even considered counterproductive by some authors.[1,2] Furthermore, the more accepted forms of laminoplasty (i.e., open-door and double-door) have a narrow range of indications. Standalone cervical laminectomy in the setting of kyphosis (i.e., "reverse lordosis"), sigmoid deformity (i.e., "swan neck"), straightening of the normal cervical lordosis, or crossing of the CTJ remains controversial and recently has largely been abandoned. Laminectomy involving segments rostral to or including C7, in which there is disruption of the C7-T1 interspinous ligament, is particularly controversial. Many cases of postlaminectomy instability, characterized by progressive kyphotic deformity or, more severely, by cervical stenosis with accompanying neurologic deficits from kyphosis or listhesis, have been reported after this procedure. With improved understanding of the complex biomechanics of the CTJ, particularly the inherent stresses in this region of transition from the mobile cervical spine to the relatively immobile thoracic spine, ways to minimize postoperative structural failure become clearer. The stresses here are only compounded with partial disruption of the posterior elements (interspinous ligaments and ligamentum flavum) as required for effective laminectomy.

Alternatives to formal laminectomy (e.g., arcocristectomy, myoarchitectonic spinolaminoplasty) may provide a solution for those limited cases involving only stenosis, but the long-term benefits have not been confirmed by formal longitudinal study.[3,4] An improved understanding helps to reinforce surgeons' comfort with stabilization of this region. Those well versed in spinal neurosurgery now accept that destabilization of the cervicothoracic spine (including posterior element disruption only) typically should be followed with a subsequent procedure to provide adequate stabilization.

CASE PRESENTATION

A 54-year-old man with a history of cerebral palsy came for treatment of progressive neck pain and right upper extremity radicular pain.

- PMH: Unremarkable
- PSH: Unremarkable
- Exam: His neurologic examination revealed bilateral deltoid weakness, spasticity in all four extremities, and pathologic reflexes.

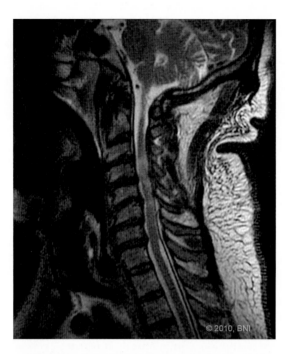

FIGURE 15-1 Sagittal T2-weighted MRI scan of the cervical spine showing straightening of the spine with circumferential stenosis secondary to spondylosis. *(Courtesy Barrow Neurological Institute.)*

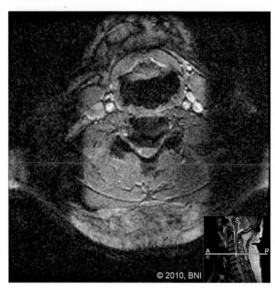

FIGURE 15-2 Axial T2-weighted MRI scan showing a representative axial view of the circumferential stenosis and spinal cord impingement and deformity. *(Courtesy Barrow Neurological Institute.)*

- Imaging: Magnetic resonance imaging (MRI) of the cervical spine (Figures 15-1 and 15-2) revealed diffuse central stenosis from the second to the seventh cervical segments secondary to marked spondylosis with both anterior and posterior compression. The patient's MRI scans also showed loss of the normal lordotic curvature with straightening. Flexion and extension radiographs revealed no hypermobility or instability.

SURGICAL OPTIONS

Surgical options include the following: anterior decompression via multilevel diskectomies or corpectomies, laminoplasty, laminectomy without posterior fusion, or laminectomy with posterior fusion (and/or posterior-anterior fusions if there is significant athetoid motion).

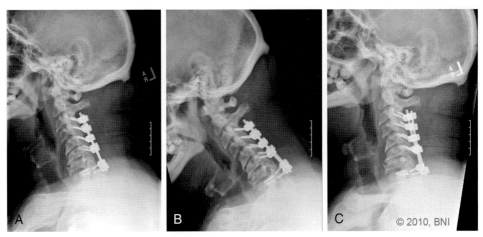

FIGURE 15-3 Lateral cervical spine radiographs in neutral position (**A**), flexion (**B**), and extension (**C**) showing the fractured T1 screws bilaterally. Note the persistent motion as evidenced by angulation and displacement of the screw fragments on the flexion and extension views. *(Courtesy Barrow Neurological Institute.)*

Given the patient's loss of lordosis and circumferential compression, a multilevel cervical laminectomy with lateral mass fusion was recommended. Intraoperatively, his habitus prevented optimal intraoperative imaging. He ultimately underwent a decompressive laminectomy from C3 through C7. Given the disruption of his C7-T1 interspinous ligament, it was deemed that fusion would need to include T1. C7 was skipped to facilitate instrumentation.

Postoperatively, the patient's myelopathic findings did not progress and his deltoid weakness improved modestly. He did well for several months until he fell from standing height. He noted immediate neck pain. Examination revealed no significant change in his baseline neurologic status. Radiographs (Figure 15-3) revealed bilateral fracture of the T1 screws at the interface between the pedicle and pars interarticularis. Flexion and extension radiographs showed persistent motion (see Figure 15-3) despite salvage attempts with a rigid cervical orthosis and strict adherence to treatments with an external bone growth stimulator. Ultimately, his fusion had to be extended to more caudal thoracic segments without anterior supplementation.

This case raises several questions that will be addressed using published evidence:

- Would standalone laminectomy have been appropriate in this patient?
- Was there a place for laminoplasty in this case?
- Should the initial fusion have been longer? If so, how far caudally should it have been extended? What type of instrumentation would have been optimal in this case?
- Would anterior stabilization have helped?
- Would intraoperative navigation (use of three-dimensional [3D] systems rather than two-dimensional [2D] fluoroscopy) have been helpful in this case?

FUNDAMENTAL TECHNIQUE

Laminectomy is performed using established techniques. Subsequent lateral mass fusion is facilitated by wide exposure of facets. An appropriate starting point can be determined by creating an imaginary **X** over the lateral mass (Figure 15-4). Superior and inferior boundaries are the facet joints, and medial and lateral boundaries of the lateral mass serve as the other boundaries. The ideal starting point is 1 mm medial to the middle of the imaginary **X**. A "matchstick" bur is used to penetrate the cortex and create a starting point (Figure 15-5). An up-and-out technique is used for the hand drill trajectory (Figure 15-6). A medial to lateral trajectory at 30 degrees avoids injury to the vertebral artery, and a cephalad to caudal trajectory at 20 degrees avoids injury to the nerve root. Before placement of screws, the facet joints of the segments

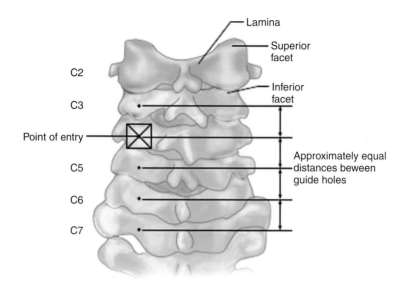

FIGURE 15-4 An appropriate starting point can be determined by creating an imaginary X over the lateral mass. Superior and inferior boundaries are the facet joints, and medial and lateral boundaries of the lateral mass serve as the other boundaries. The ideal starting point is 1 mm medial to the middle of the imaginary X. *(From Chen MY, Duenas MJ, Jandial R: Procedure 62: Lateral mass fixation. In Jandial R, McCormick P, Black P, editors:* Core techniques in operative neurosurgery, *Philadelphia, 2011, Saunders, pp 440-444, Figure 62-3.)*

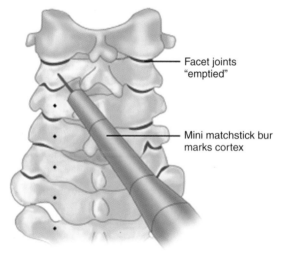

FIGURE 15-5 "Matchstick" bur is used to penetrate the cortex and create a starting point. *(From Chen MY, Duenas MJ, Jandial R: Procedure 62: Lateral mass fixation. In Jandial R, McCormick P, Black P, editors:* Core techniques in operative neurosurgery, *Philadelphia, 2011, Saunders, pp 440-444, Figure 62-4.)*

included in the fusion are decorticated (Figure 15-7). The dorsal cortical surfaces are decorticated for onlay arthrodesis as well. Polyaxial screws are placed and can be measured before placement during the hand drill and feeler steps. A medial trajectory risks injury to the vertebral artery (Figure 15-8). Failing to aim cephalad places the nerve root at risk. Starting too far laterally risks fracture of the lateral mass. When extension to the upper thoracic region is necessary, upper thoracic pedicle screws are placed using anatomic landmarks, because visualization with fluoroscopy at these levels can be difficult in the sagittal plane. T1 pedicle screw trajectory is described in Figure 15-9; a large lateral mass screw can be used to avoid the need for a transitional rod in the construct.

Tips from the Masters 15-1 • The caudal trajectory for thoracic pedicle screws decreases from 20 degrees to 5 degrees from T1 to T12.

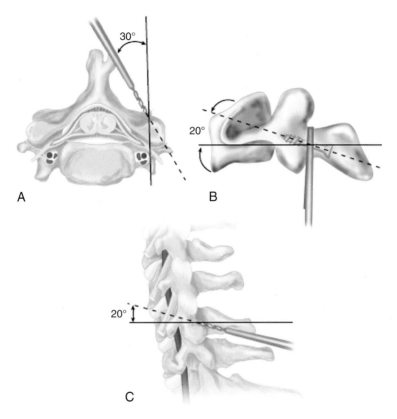

FIGURE 15-6 Up-and-out technique is used for hand drill trajectory. A medial to lateral trajectory at 30 degrees avoids injury to the vertebral artery, and a cephalad to caudal trajectory at 20 degrees avoids injury to the nerve root. *(From Chen MY, Duenas MJ, Jandial R: Procedure 62: Lateral mass fixation. In Jandial R, McCormick P, Black P, editors:* Core techniques in operative neurosurgery, *Philadelphia, 2011, Saunders, pp 440-444, Figure 62-5.)*

FIGURE 15-7 Before placement of screws, the facet joints of the segments included in the fusion are decorticated. Dorsal cortical surfaces are decorticated for onlay arthrodesis as well. *(From Chen MY, Duenas MJ, Jandial R: Procedure 62: Lateral mass fixation. In Jandial R, McCormick P, Black P, editors:* Core techniques in operative neurosurgery, *Philadelphia, 2011, Saunders, pp 440-444, Figure 62-6.)*

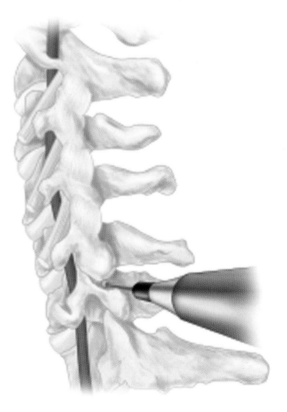

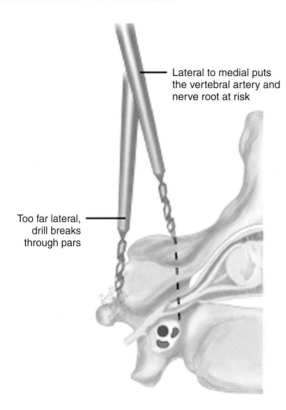

Lateral to medial puts
the vertebral artery and
nerve root at risk

Too far lateral,
drill breaks
through pars

FIGURE 15-8 Medial trajectory risks injury to the vertebral artery. Failing to aim cephalad places the nerve root at risk. Starting too far laterally risks fracture of the lateral mass. *(From Chen MY, Duenas MJ, Jandial R: Procedure 62: Lateral mass fixation. In Jandial R, McCormick P, Black P, editors: Core techniques in operative neurosurgery, Philadelphia, 2011, Saunders, pp 440-444, Figure 62-8.)*

DISCUSSION OF BEST EVIDENCE

Would Standalone Laminectomy Have Been Appropriate?

When used appropriately in the cervical spine, laminectomy is an effective procedure. Laminectomy that spans multiple segments, is performed in an unstable spine, crosses the CTJ, or is undertaken in a patient who has lost the normal cervical lordotic curvature can be problematic. Postlaminectomy kyphotic deformity is a well-known entity.[5-10] Lonstein[8] first brought attention to this undesirable complication. He noted an incidence rate of 100% in children undergoing cervical, cervicothoracic, and thoracic laminectomies for the treatment of intradural or extradural spinal mass lesions. He surmised that the pediatric population is at high risk for this complication given the immaturity of the spinal elements. Yasuoka and colleagues[10] also implicated the immaturity of the pediatric spine. They suggested that deformity developed owing to the wedging of cartilaginous portions of the vertebral bodies allowed by the increased viscoelasticity of the posterior ligamentous complexes in children.

Such deformity is also common in adults, however. The reported incidence of spinal deformity after laminectomy ranges from 33% to 100% in children and is about 20% in adults.[5,6,11,12] Removal of the lamina and spinous process with the accompanying ligamentous complexes completely disrupts the posterior tension band. Saito and associates[13] used finite-element analysis to simulate these disruptions. They found that removal of one or more spinous processes and/or posterior ligaments (i.e., ligamenta flava, supraspinous, and interspinous ligaments) transferred the tensile stresses to the facets, which ultimately leads to stress imbalance and deformity. Therefore, the ultimate development of postlaminectomy kyphosis or spinal deformity depends on the number of involved segments and on the degree of facet disruption.

Certain regions of the spine, namely the CTJ, are particularly dependent on the posterior elements to maintain biomechanical integrity. The CTJ is less well studied

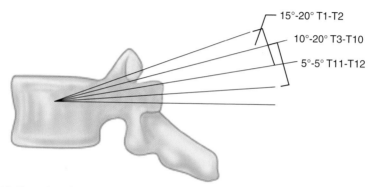

15°-20° T1-T2
10°-20° T3-T10
5°-5° T11-T12

FIGURE 15-9 Thoracic pedicle screws are placed by using established landmarks and trajectories. The caudal trajectory decreases from T1 to T12. *(From Link T, Jandial R, Sonntag V: Procedure 63: Posterior cervicothoracic osteotomy. In Jandial R, McCormick P, Black P, editors:* Core techniques in operative neurosurgery, *Philadelphia, 2011, Saunders, pp 440-444, Figure 63-5.)*

than some other regions, and the risks factors associated with surgical failure have not been adequately defined. Nonetheless, laminectomy alone can create instability and ultimately postlaminectomy spinal deformity with subsequent neurologic deterioration. Steinmetz and co-workers[12] illustrated this point by **retrospectively** reviewing outcomes in patients who underwent various procedures on the CTJ for treatment of different pathologic conditions. Of their 14 treatment failures, 3 involved uninstrumented laminectomy. These patients developed postoperative junctional kyphosis and myelopathy although there was no preoperative loss of lordosis. Interestingly, only 11 of 593 patients underwent uninstrumented laminectomy across the CTJ. Of these, more than 25% developed a spinal deformity requiring further correction and stabilization. Based on these results, Steinmetz and colleagues[12] concluded that treatment failure was significantly associated with laminectomy.

Uninstrumented laminectomy of the CTJ is usually inadequate because of the unique biomechanical forces present in this area. As mentioned, this junction is a zone of transition from a mobile lordotic cervical spine to a rigid kyphotic thoracic spine. There are substantial stresses in the static and dynamic states, particularly during flexion and translation.[11,12] This vulnerability is only magnified after uninstrumented dorsal surgery. However, it is important to remember that laminectomy alone may be the only option in elderly patients with poor bone quality in whom fusion would not be plausible or safe. Typically, postlaminectomy stability can be improved with instrumentation and fusion. This perspective is supported by the following quotes from the few authors who have studied laminectomy of the CTJ:

- "If laminectomy is required, fusion and stabilization should also be performed because of inherent instability after laminectomy of the cervicothoracic spine."[11]
- "Findings of the present study provide further evidence that uninstrumented laminectomy involving the CTJ should not be performed."[12]
- "Almost any posterior procedures involving the CTJ should be followed by fusion of the CTJ."[14]

Was There a Place for Laminoplasty in This Case?

There are many variations of laminoplasty, such as en bloc, open-door, and double-door (also know as French door). The indication for each varies. En bloc laminoplasty is typically used when intradural or extradural access is required, because it allows temporary removal of the lamina–spinous process complex. However, disconnection of the cranial and caudal ends obviates its utility for maintaining the posterior tension band, despite reconstruction efforts with interlaminar wires or sutures. Thus, its biomechanical utility is questionable. Open-door or double-door laminoplasties are useful when the spinal cord needs to be decompressed from the posterior bony-ligamentous complex or ossification of the posterior longitudinal ligament (OPLL). Typically, this procedure is indicated only when cervical lordosis is present. Straightened, sigmoid, or kyphotic cervical alignments are contraindications for laminoplasty.[15] Even in the lordotic cervical spine, kyphosis is a known complication of laminoplasty.[15-18] In addition, laminoplasty offers minimal immediate stability.

Laminoplasty spanning the CTJ specifically has not been well studied. Few reports strictly address this issue. Recently, Komagata and colleagues[19] retrospectively reviewed data for 13 patients who underwent open-door laminoplasty for OPLL that spanned the CTJ. Results were favorable, showing neither restenosis nor progression to spinal deformity at an average follow-up of 75 months. Longer follow-up and larger patient series are required to answer this question adequately. One perceived advantage of laminoplasty over laminectomy with fusion is maintenance of ROM. However, ROM is significantly reduced after laminoplasty compared with intact cervical spines.[2] Disruption of the posterior tension band with denervation and atrophy of the cervical musculature has deleterious effects, such as postoperative axial pain, loss of ROM, or need for further surgery to correct deformity. Several authors offer some modifications (e.g., myoarchitectonic spinolaminoplasty) that avoid disruption of these elements, but the long-term results involving the CTJ have not been scrutinized.[4]

Should the Instrumentation Have Been Longer Initially? If So, How Far Caudally? What Type of Instrumention Should Have Been Used?

The treatment of choice when laminectomy is required to decompress or access the sublaminar space across the CTJ involves stabilization and fusion. Stabilization techniques have evolved immensely even over the past decade. Early constructs involving sublaminar wires or hooks were semirigid and associated with a higher rate of pseudarthrosis than more rigid, contemporary lateral mass systems. Furthermore, after laminectomy sublaminar constructs lose their utility unless levels are included above and below laminectomized levels. This characteristic can significantly increase the length of the fused segment and reduce the proportion of fixation points to fused levels. Sublaminar hooks can also further reduce the spinal canal diameter by as much as 27%.[14] Presently, sublaminar hooks or wires are unnecessary unless the quality of the bony pedicle/lateral mass or the anatomy in which these constructs can act as an anchor at the caudal and cranial ends of the construct is suboptimal.

The lateral mass/pedicle screw and rod system is currently the favorite choice among contemporary spinal surgeons. However, important iterations in the evolution of this current configuration need to be revisited. This evolution is a result of the transitional anatomy in this region. A **morphometric study** by Stanescu and associates reviewed the changes in the posterior elements in this transitional zone.[20] This group showed that from C5 to C7 the lateral mass decreased from 11 to 8.7 mm, but the width of the pedicle increased from 5.2 to 6.5 mm. From C7 to T2, the pedicle width/height averaged as follows: 6.5/6.7 mm, 7.8/8.8 mm, and 6.5/10.5 mm, respectively. Interestingly, on average, the pedicle at T1 was wider than that at T2. From C5 to T1 the angles of the pedicles changed from 50 to 34 degrees, an average of 5 degrees per level. These are important anatomic changes to consider when instrumenting the CTJ.

Tips from the Masters 15-2 • If a three-column injury exists at the CVJ, consider a 360-degree fusion.

As surgeons' understanding of and comfort with instrumenting this transitional anatomy improved, posterior lateral mass plates gained acceptance over laminar hooks or wire constructs. Plates proved to be more robust and practical in patients undergoing laminectomy. In a cadaveric study of the destabilized CTJ by Bueff and co-workers,[21] the stiffness of the construct consisting of lateral mass plate with cervical lateral mass screws and thoracic pedicle screws was superior to that of anterior constructs and posterior fixation with hooks when subjected to 3D and rotational displacements. The posterior constructs were significantly stiffer than anterior constructs, but there was no significant difference between posterior constructs. Chapman and colleagues further confirmed the viability of this system in 23 patients with CTJ instability in whom they used a posterior plate fixed to cervical lateral mass screws and thoracic pedicle screws.[22] All of their patients achieved solid arthrodesis. As illustrated by these studies, the posterior cervical plate was found to be equivalent if not superior to the previously used hook and wire constructs. This point is particularly important with regard to postlaminectomy patients for whom sublaminar constructs are not possible. More importantly, as Houten and Cooper showed, fusion with lateral mass plating prevented the development of spinal deformity associated with laminoplasty or noninstrumented laminectomy of the CTJ.[16]

Rod-screw systems were then developed to circumvent the constraints inherent in the use of plates with fixed hole intervals. Kreshak and co-workers showed that these systems can restore almost 100% of the strength in a two-column but not in a three-column injury pattern and are equivalent to screw-plate constructs.[23] Placantonakis and colleagues showed the superiority of newer rod-screw configurations compared with older systems.[24] They **retrospectively** reviewed outcomes for 90 patients who underwent laminectomy for primary or metastatic tumors crossing the CTJ supplemented with posterior instrumentation over a 10-year period. During this period, their use of constructs shifted from rod–sublaminar hook and lateral mass/plate systems to rod-screw (lateral mass/pedicle) constructs. The rate of fixation failure decreased from 29% to 0% with the transition to a rod-screw system from a lateral mass/plate-screw system and decreased from 15% to 2% with the switch from rod–laminar hook to rod-screw configurations.

Except in the case of a three-column injury, posterior rod-screw systems provide adequate stabilization. As Kreshak and co-workers suggested,[23] a three-column injury involving C7, C7-T1, or T1, as in the case of trauma or tumor, requires further stabilization. Ames and colleagues investigated this issue in a cadaveric study of three-column injury by comparing the following conditions: intact, destabilized, posterior instrumentation from C6 to T1 or T2, and corpectomy with plate with or without posterior supplementation.[25] Combined instrumentation outperformed anterior or posterior constructs alone when subjected to pure moments of flexion, extension, lateral bending, and axial rotation. The length of the construct also affected stability, with stability greater when T2 was included than when instrumentation stopped at T1. Interestingly, exclusion of C7 did not affect stability significantly.

Tips from the Masters 15-3 • Recommend posterior fusion at the CTJ to extend to at least T2.

Prybis and associates agreed with this assessment.[26] They found that anterior supplementation is necessary with three-column disruption and that inclusion of C5 and T3 significantly increases the stiffness of the construct. They concluded that posterior instrumentation alone is "inadequate" in three-column injury involving the CTJ.

How long constructs should be has not been well studied nor specific recommendations supported. There are few biomechanical data to guide decisions about fusion length. Reviewing the literature, Lapsiwala and Benzel also found a paucity of evidence.[27] Although they could find no significant data to support particular recommendations, they suggested the following fundamental guidelines:

- A long fusion should not end at an apical vertebra or at the CTJ.
- Long cervical fusions should be extended to traverse the CTJ to a neutral vertebra.

As discussed, inclusion of T2 or T3 can increase stability, although there is no consensus on the optimal length. When the bulk of the laminectomy is thoracic and involves only the C7-T1 interspace and hence C7 must be included in the fixation, the use of pedicle screws is adequate.

If pedicle screws are not an option and C7 lateral mass screws are used, they should be supplemented with C6 lateral mass screws.[28] Typically, fusion should involve laminectomized levels at a minimum and should traverse the CTJ if it is involved.

Tips from the Masters 15-4 • C7 pedicle fixation is biomechanically superior to lateral mass.

During discussions of instrumentation, one dilemma that often surfaces is the type of rod construct to use: tapered rod, dual-diameter rods connected with a domino or axial connector, or a single-diameter rod. In a **biomechanical study,** Tatsumi and colleagues found dual-diameter rods (3.5 mm to 5.5 mm), whether tapered or connected via a domino connector, to be superior in stiffness and ultimate yield force compared with 3.5-mm single-diameter rods.[29] Dual-diameter rods typically fail at the transition point or point of connection. When possible, the preferred practice is to use the largest-diameter rods if larger-head screws can be used on the cephalad aspects of the construct (e.g., 4-mm pedicle screws at C7). Further comparisons of large-diameter rods versus dual-diameter rods are needed.

In regard to the patient in the Case Presentation, perhaps the length of the fusion above the CTJ should have been matched below as well. The fusion from C3 to C7 created a large moment arm, which placed enormous stress on the T1 pedicle screws. This stress may have been better shared over several caudal levels, particularly given the magnitude of the moment arm. The moment arm in this case takes into account the weight of the patient's head and neck, which is already in positive balance over the T1 vertebral body. This is a point reiterated by Lapsiwala and Benzel in their review.[27]

Would Intraoperative Navigation (3D Systems Rather Than 2D Fluoroscopy) Have Been Helpful in This Case?

Overall, the use of posterior instrumentation is safe. The anatomy of the CTJ changes in a predictable manner, despite facet asymmetry.[30] Pedicle breaches are relatively uncommon. When they occur, they tend to be lateral (44%) and potentially damaging to important neurovascular structures. Intraoperative navigation tends to reduce their incidence.[31] Richter showed that the incidence of pedicle breach, as documented by postoperative computed tomography, could be reduced from 9% to 3% by the use of navigation.[32] In a retrospective study of results for 60 patients with a total of 86 cervicothoracic pedicle screws, Lee and co-workers showed that reduction could be accomplished as well with 2D (fluoroscopy) or 3D navigation as with open evaluation of pedicle anatomy (laminotomy or partial facetectomy).[31] Although in the patient in the Case Presentation screws were placed without breaching the pedicle, operative time potentially could have been reduced if 3D navigation had been used.

COMMENTARY

One of the controversies in spinal surgery is whether to fuse across transitional areas—such as the CTJ, craniocervical junction, or thoracolumbar junction—when they are violated either iatrogenically or by a pathologic process. This chapter addresses this issue with respect to the CTJ. As this chapter emphasizes, this area, where normal cervical lordosis meets thoracic kyphosis, is unique. Consequently, if possible, it is recommended that fusion proceed across the junction if C7-T1 instability is present. The preference for fusion is especially strong in the presence of a two-column injury, and fusion is definitely needed if a three-column injury is observed. In the latter scenario, both posterior and anterior instrumentation should be considered. The anatomy of the region is also unique, and the small size of the C7 lateral mass precludes its use. Therefore, the options are to implement C7 pedicle fixation (preferred) or to skip C7. As this chapter demonstrates, once the decision is made to fuse the CTJ, the construct should extend caudally to at least T2. When fusion proceeds across the CTJ, the preference is to use a rod and screw construct rather than hooks and rods or laminoplasty, which is associated with lower rates of successful fusion.

If C7 must be included, an alternative to fusion is to proceed with a laminectomy to C7 while maintaining the ligamentous continuity between C7 and T1. This strategy might prevent postoperative instability at the CTJ. Obviously, the findings of diagnostic imaging studies, such as the presence of lordosis versus no lordosis and the presence of instability versus no instability, as well as the patient's symptoms, such as the presence of severe neck pain, must be analyzed before surgery to determine the need for fusion across the CTJ.

REFERENCES

1. Chiba K, Ogawa Y, Ishii K, et al: Long-term results of expansive open-door laminoplasty for cervical myelopathy—average 14-year follow-up study, *Spine* 31:2998–3005, 2006.
2. Kang SH, Rhim SC, Roh SW, et al: Postlaminoplasty cervical range of motion: early results, *J Neurosurg Spine* 6:386–390, 2007.
3. Amaral SH, Silva MN, Giraldi M, et al: Multiple cervical arcocristectomies for the treatment of cervical spondylotic myelopathy: surgical technique and results, *J Neurosurg Spine* 7:503–508, 2007.
4. Kim P, Murata H, Kurokawa R, et al: Myoarchitectonic spinolaminoplasty: efficacy in reconstituting the cervical musculature and preserving biomechanical function, *J Neurosurg Spine* 7:293–304, 2007.
5. Amhaz HH, Fox BD, Johnson KK, et al: Postlaminoplasty kyphotic deformity in the thoracic spine: case report and review of the literature, *Pediatr Neurosurg* 45:151–154, 2009.
6. Deutsch H, Haid RW, Rodts GE, et al: Postlaminectomy cervical deformity, *Neurosurg Focus* 15:E5, 2003.
7. Herkowitz HN: A comparison of anterior cervical fusion, cervical laminectomy, and cervical laminoplasty for the surgical management of multiple level spondylotic radiculopathy, *Spine* 13:774–780, 1988. **This study compared the results and complications of 45 patients with at least a 2-year follow-up who had undergone anterior fusion, cervical laminectomy, or cervical laminoplasty for the surgical management of multiple level cervical radiculopathy due to cervical spondylosis. Of the 45 patients, 18 (58 levels) underwent anterior fusion, 12 (38 levels) had a cervical laminectomy, and 15 (57 levels) underwent a cervical laminoplasty. Roentgenograms indicated spinal stenosis (sagittal diameter <12 mm) at 28 levels (15 patients) for the anterior fusion group, 14 levels (nine patients) in the laminectomy group, and 24 levels (13 patients) in the laminoplasty group. Subluxation (2 mm or less) was present at 14 levels (13 patients) in the anterior fusion group, nine levels (nine patients) in the laminectomy group, and 15 levels (eight patients) in the laminoplasty group. Loss of lordosis was present in nine patients undergoing anterior fusion, six undergoing laminectomy, and six who had a laminoplasty.**
8. Lonstein JE: Post-laminectomy kyphosis, *Clin Orthop Relat Res* 128:93–100, 1977.
9. McGirt MJ, Chaichana KL, Atiba A, et al: Incidence of spinal deformity after resection of intramedullary spinal cord tumors in children who underwent laminectomy compared with laminoplasty, *J Neurosurg Pediatr* 1:57–62, 2008.
10. Yasuoka S, Peterson HA, Laws ER Jr, et al: Pathogenesis and prophylaxis of postlaminectomy deformity of the spine after multiple level laminectomy: difference between children and adults, *Neurosurgery* 9:145–152, 1981.
11. An HS, Vaccaro A, Cotler JM, et al: Spinal disorders at the cervicothoracic junction, *Spine* 19:2557–2564, 1994.
12. Steinmetz MP, Miller J, Warbel A, et al: Regional instability following cervicothoracic junction surgery, *J Neurosurg Spine* 4:278–284, 2006.
13. Saito T, Yamamuro T, Shikata J, et al: Analysis and prevention of spinal column deformity following cervical laminectomy. I. Pathogenetic analysis of postlaminectomy deformities, *Spine* 16:494–502, 1991.
14. Wang VY, Chou D: The cervicothoracic junction, *Neurosurg Clin N Am* 18:365–371, 2007.
15. Uchida K, Nakajima H, Sato R, et al: Cervical spondylotic myelopathy associated with kyphosis or sagittal sigmoid alignment: outcome after anterior or posterior decompression, *J Neurosurg Spine* 11:521–528, 2009.
16. Houten JK, Cooper PR: Laminectomy and posterior cervical plating for multilevel cervical spondylotic myelopathy and ossification of the posterior longitudinal ligament: effects on cervical alignment, spinal cord compression, and neurological outcome, *Neurosurgery* 52:1081–1087, 2003.
17. Raab P, Juergen K, Gloger H, et al: Spinal deformity after multilevel osteoplastic laminotomy, *Int Orthop* 32:355–359, 2008.
18. Saruhashi Y, Hukuda S, Katsuura A, et al: A long-term follow-up study of cervical spondylotic myelopathy treated by "French window" laminoplasty, *J Spinal Disord* 12:99–101, 1999.
19. Komagata M, Inahata Y, Nishiyama M, et al: Treatment of myelopathy due to cervicothoracic OPLL via open door laminoplasty, *J Spinal Disord Tech* 20:342–346, 2007.
20. Stanescu S, Ebraheim NA, Yeasting R, et al: Morphometric evaluation of the cervico-thoracic junction. Practical considerations for posterior fixation of the spine, *Spine* 19:2082–2088, 1994.
21. Bueff HU, Lotz JC, Colliou OK, et al: Instrumentation of the cervicothoracic junction after destabilization, *Spine* 20:1789–1792, 1995. **To find an efficient way in restoring stability of the cervicothoracic junction in cases with and without laminectomy, six human spines were tested nondestructively in**

axial torsion, flexion, and extension with the C6-T2 motion segments left unconstrained. The 3D displacements and rotations between C7 and T1 vertebrae were measured using a sonic digitizer. After intact testing, a distractive-flexion Stage 3 cervical spinal injury was simulated surgically between C7 and T1. Posterior stabilization techniques had statistically more stiffness than anterior plates.

22. Chapman JR, Anderson PA, Pepin C, et al: Posterior instrumentation of the unstable cervicothoracic spine, *J Neurosurg* 84:552–558, 1996.

23. Kreshak JL, Kim DH, Lindsey DP, et al: Posterior stabilization at the cervicothoracic junction: a biomechanical study, *Spine* 27:2763–2770, 2002. Twenty-one human cadaveric spines (C3-T3) were loaded in flexion, extension, lateral bending, and axial torsion. A posterior two-column injury was created at C7-T1. One of three posterior fixation systems was applied (two rod-screw systems, one plate-screw system, all with screws at C5, C6 and T1, T2). The spines were tested again. A three-column injury was created by transecting the remaining anterior structures; the spines were tested a final time. In flexion-extension, there were no significant differences in stiffness between intact and instrumented two-column injury specimens for all systems; the instrumented three-column injury was significantly ($P < 0.05$) less stiff than intact specimens in extension. Ranges of motion and neutral zones decreased from intact to instrumented two-column injuries and increased from intact to three-column constructs. In lateral bending and axial rotation, all systems were stiffer than intact spines for both injuries; ranges of motion and neutral zones were reduced for both injuries compared with intact specimens. All three systems stabilized the cervicothoracic junction with a posterior two-column injury in flexion-extension, lateral bending, and axial rotation; none was adequate for a three-column injury, particularly in extension. A three-column injury at this level would warrant supplemental anterior fixation.

24. Placantonakis DG, Laufer I, Wang JC, et al: Posterior stabilization strategies following resection of cervicothoracic junction tumors: review of 90 consecutive cases, *J Neurosurg Spine* 9:111–119, 2008.

25. Ames CP, Bozkus MH, Chamberlain RH, et al: Biomechanics of stabilization after cervicothoracic compression-flexion injury, *Spine* 30:1505–1512, 2005.

26. Prybis BG, Tortolani PJ, Hu N, et al: A comparative biomechanical analysis of spinal instability and instrumentation of the cervicothoracic junction: an in vitro human cadaveric model, *J Spinal Disord Tech* 20:233–238, 2007.

27. Lapsiwala S, Benzel E: Surgical management of cervical myelopathy dealing with the cervical-thoracic junction, *Spine J* 6:268S–273S, 2006.

28. Rhee JM, Kraiwattanapong C, Hutton WC: A comparison of pedicle and lateral mass screw construct stiffnesses at the cervicothoracic junction: a biomechanical study, *Spine* 30:E636–E640, 2005. To determine whether augmenting C7 lateral mass screws with spinous process wires or additional fixation in the C6 lateral mass can create constructs of similar normalized stiffness to that of C7 pedicle screws, 12 cadaveric cervicothoracic specimens (C5-T2) were randomly assigned to one of three experiments: Experiment A (Part 1 and Part 2), Experiment B, and Experiment C (Part 1 and Part 2) ($n = 4$ for each experiment). First, the intact specimens were biomechanically tested according to a seven-part loading protocol. The specimens were destabilized, and then restabilized with the following constructs in conjunction with bilateral T1 pedicle screws and biomechanically tested again using the same seven-part biomechanical protocol as was applied to the intact specimens. Experiment A, Part 1: lateral mass screw fixation at C7 (C7LM); then Part 2: retested after augmentation with triple wiring (C7LM+W). Experiment B: pedicle screw fixation at C7 (C7PS). Experiment C, Part 1: C6 and C7 lateral mass screws (C6C7LM); then Part 2: retested after augmentation with triple wiring (C6C7LM+W). Thus five different constructs were biomechanically compared in these three experiments. Results indicate C7 pedicle screw fixation provides the construct with the highest normalized stiffness for stabilizing the cervicothoracic junction. If C7 pedicle fixation is not possible, then performing two-level lateral mass fixation at C6 and C7 will achieve a construct with similar normalized stiffness except in axial compression. The addition of triple wiring to the spinous processes does not significantly increase lateral mass construct normalized stiffness.

29. Tatsumi RL, Yoo JU, Liu Q, et al: Mechanical comparison of posterior instrumentation constructs for spinal fixation across the cervicothoracic junction, *Spine* 32:1072–1076, 2007.

30. Bailey AS, Stanescu S, Yeasting RA, et al: Anatomic relationships of the cervicothoracic junction, *Spine* 20:1431–1439, 1995.

31. Lee GY, Massicotte EM, Rampersaud YR: Clinical accuracy of cervicothoracic pedicle screw placement: a comparison of the "open" lamino-foraminotomy and computer-assisted techniques, *J Spinal Disord Tech* 20:25–32, 2007.

32. Richter M: Posterior instrumentation of the cervical spine using the neon occipito-cervical system. Part 2: Cervical and cervicothoracic instrumentation, *Oper Orthop Traumatol* 17:579–600, 2005.

Chapter 16

Vertebral Metastases: Ventral and Dorsal Approach Versus Lateral Extracavitary Transpedicular Approach

John H. Shin, Edward C. Benzel

The surgical management of vertebral metastases has evolved in recent decades with the refinement of surgical techniques and advancements in spinal instrumentation. Despite these advances, debate exists regarding the best surgical approach for the treatment of thoracolumbar metastases. Improvements in adjuvant treatment strategies have enhanced local and regional tumor control, increasing the survival of patients and redefining the role of surgery. As a result, patients with metastatic disease are living longer, and disease control plays a significant role in their overall prognosis and quality of life. Early diagnosis and management of these lesions become more important not only in improving survival but in controlling pain.

For surgeons treating these lesions, operative management is critical, since surgery may help improve quality of life, preserve existing neurologic function, and reduce pain. With the development of advanced surgical techniques and a greater understanding of tumor biology, the approaches and instruments available to surgeons now offer better alternatives to laminectomy.

Early studies comparing outcomes for laminectomy and radiation therapy found virtually equivalent results for the two modalities. Because morbidity rates were higher in patients treated operatively, surgery fell out of favor, and radiotherapy became the primary treatment modality for vertebral metastasis.[1,2] Now that the biomechanics of metastatic vertebral disease are better understood, surgery has increasingly been shown to benefit selected patients.[3] In a **randomized, multicenter, nonblinded trial** comparing external beam radiation with decompressive surgery and instrumentation followed by external beam radiation in symptomatic patients with spinal cord compression, Patchell and colleagues[4] concluded that aggressive resection of spinal metastases in highly selected patients accompanied by postoperative radiotherapy is superior to radiotherapy alone. Patients treated with surgery retained ambulatory and sphincter function significantly longer than patients in the radiation-only group. In addition, 56% of nonambulatory patients in the surgical group regained the ability to walk, compared with 19% in the radiation-only group. As surgical techniques have evolved, several approaches, including the ventral transthoracic and various dorsal forms, have shown surgical outcomes superior to those of radiation treatment in historical controls when used alone or in combination.[3,5-8]

The optimal surgical treatment for solitary and multiple metastases is controversial and continues to be argued. Both en bloc and palliative strategies have been discussed. Indications for these interventions continue to change with the advent of stereotactic radiosurgery and cement augmentation. When surgery is indicated, surgical technique is largely defined by several factors, including tumor histologic features, tumor location, number of levels involved, the patient's neurologic condition, and the presence of deformity. Medical comorbidities, extent of systemic disease, and anticipated life expectancy also factor into the decision-making process. Since their introduction, the Tokuhashi and Tomita algorithms have been used by surgeons to help determine the potential benefit of surgery for selected patients.[9-12] Surgical intervention has traditionally been recommended in cases of progressive neurologic deficit, mechanical instability, an enlarging radioresistant tumor, and intractable pain unrelieved by nonsurgical treatment.

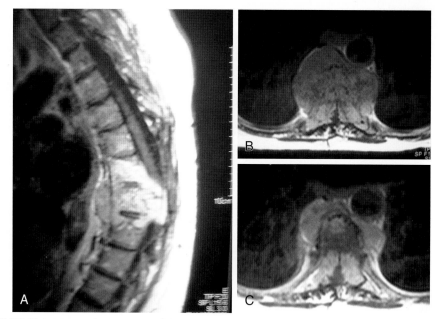

FIGURE 16-1 Preoperative MRI scans of the thoracic spine demonstrating diffuse metastases involving T7, T8, and T9. There is marked compression and encasement of the spinal cord by tumor.

Debate continues over the approach that best minimizes overall morbidity in patients who have limited survival. Given the heterogeneous nature of these tumors, the surgical treatment for patients with metastatic spinal tumors remains highly individualized, with tumor histologic characteristics being the main determinant of survival. Each patient requires a thorough diagnostic and medical assessment, and the decision to operate must consider the risks of surgical morbidity and death along with the potential for gains in both the duration and quality of survival.

Using the best available evidence, this chapter compares the combined ventral and dorsal approach with the lateral extracavitary approach. Through a case illustration, the advantages of the lateral extracavitary approach are highlighted.

CASE PRESENTATION

A 50-year-old woman had recurrent breast metastases to the thoracic spine following previous laminectomy, decompression, and radiotherapy for epidural metastases. At initial presentation she had high-grade paraparesis that improved with surgery and radiation. No other systemic metastases were identified either initially or upon recurrence.

- PMH: Estrogen receptor–positive invasive ductal carcinoma of the breast treated with resection and hormonal therapy; mitral valve prolapse
- PSH: Laminectomy and decompression at T8 followed by radiotherapy at 30 Gy in 10 fractions to the thoracic spine
- Exam: At the time of recurrence, she had worsening gait instability, numbness, and weakness in her lower extremities.
- Imaging: Magnetic resonance imaging (MRI) of the thoracic spine demonstrated bulky, infiltrating metastases from T7 to T9 with paraspinal and epidural extension. Circumferential encasement of the spinal cord was evident, with marked compression and cord edema (Figure 16-1). A preoperative angiogram was obtained that demonstrated arterial supply to the tumor by the right T7 and bilateral T8 radicular arteries. Successful embolization was performed with no tumor blush evident after embolization (Figure 16-2).

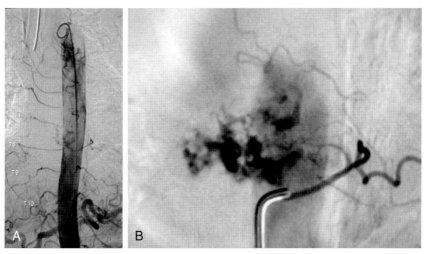

FIGURE 16-2 Preoperative spinal angiogram demonstrating vascular blush of the tumor.

SURGICAL OPTIONS

Combined Ventral and Dorsal Approaches

In the treatment of thoracolumbar metastasis, several surgical options exist for resection, decompression, and stabilization. Thoracic corpectomies have traditionally been performed from a ventral approach via sternotomy or thoracotomy. These approaches allow for direct decompression of the spinal cord, correction of kyphosis, reconstruction of the spinal column, and stabilization.

In general, the ventral approach provides excellent exposure for the resection of epidural extension of vertebral metastases ventral to the spinal canal. These can be visualized directly and decompressed with complete resection of the involved body. For resection of lesions at T1 to T3, a sternotomy or manubrial window can be used if needed. This is performed from the patient's left side, because the recurrent laryngeal nerve has a deeper course on the right side and there is less chance of injury. However, the thoracic duct is at risk for injury with the left-sided approach. The great vessels may be retracted to allow visualization of T1 to T3, and the brachiocephalic vein may need to be ligated and incised for better visualization. Following corpectomy, structural grafts are positioned and a plate may be applied. Due to variances in anatomy and thoracic kyphosis, this may preclude placement of ventral instrumentation, which then necessitates dorsal fixation.

For lesions below T3, a thoracotomy provides access at multiple levels. The side of operation often depends on the location of the lesion. The right side is preferable when approaching T3 and T4 because the aortic arch limits visualization of the left side. For lesions located at T5 through T10, the left side is often chosen because the aorta is easier to mobilize and repair than the inferior vena cava if injured.

Combined ventral and dorsal approaches allow circumferential tumor decompression and spinal stabilization. However, this method is associated with greater morbidity, because it requires a staged approach and two separate incisions. Despite the advantages of ventral approaches, the morbidity of thoracotomy and the risk of complications such as pneumothorax, hemothorax, and vascular injury often prohibit their use. Chest tubes are required postoperatively, and patients may require prolonged ventilatory support.

Lateral Extracavitary Transpedicular Approach

Dorsal approaches, including the transpedicular corpectomy, costotransversectomy, lateral extracavitary approach, and modifications thereof, have been used to access the ventral thoracic spine from a dorsal approach.[13,14] The lateral extracavitary

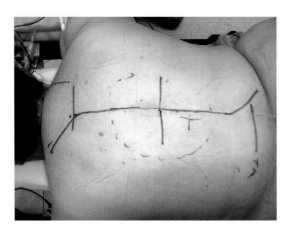

FIGURE 16-3 Planned skin incision for the bilateral lateral extracavitary approach.

approach was first introduced by Capener in 1954 and subsequently modified and popularized by Larson.[14] Initially described for the treatment of tuberculous spondylitis, this approach has been used for various pathologic conditions, including metastatic vertebral disease. It provides lateral exposure to the thoracic and lumbar vertebrae without entering the pleural or abdominal cavity, which allows better visualization of the ventral dural surface than with other dorsal approaches. In addition to permitting ventral spinal cord decompression, this approach allows the placement of dorsal instrumentation without a second incision. It is usually performed from one side, but can be done bilaterally to facilitate complete spondylectomy, including complete removal of the dorsal elements. Often, it can be combined with a less extensive contralateral transpedicular decompression or costotransversectomy.

Advantages of this approach include the ability to complete the surgery in a single stage, avoidance of a thoracotomy, and a potentially faster recovery period. Rigid dorsal instrumentation is readily accomplished through the same incision and eliminates the need for an additional operation. The ability to remain extrapleural in the thoracic spine eliminates the need for chest tubes and division of the diaphragm.

Despite these advantages, corpectomies from a dorsal approach present specific challenges. Sufficient ventral access, adequate decompression, and risk of pleural and vascular injuries are factors that must be taken into consideration. Resnick and Benzel[15] reported on complications associated with this technique in 33 trauma patients. Eighteen patients experienced complications, with the most common being hemothorax or pleural effusion requiring the use of a chest tube. Other complications included pneumonia, wound infections, cerebrospinal fluid leaks, and incisional hernias.[15]

With this approach, preoperative angiography is sometimes useful in identifying the artery of Adamkiewicz for lesions between T7 and L2, because this artery is located at the level of the lesion in approximately 20% of cases and may provide critical blood supply to the spinal cord.[16] It is also valuable in characterizing the vascular supply to tumors in this region. Endovascular embolization of arterial feeders to these lesions is a useful surgical adjunct that lessens the morbidity of excessive blood loss during surgery.

In this patient a bilateral lateral extracavitary approach was performed with complete spondylectomies and tumor resection at T7, T8, and T9. A curved hockey stick incision was used to obtain adequate dorsal and lateral exposure (Figure 16-3). This allowed pedicle screws to be placed at multiple levels above and below the pathologic levels and provided ventral access to the tumor through a single incision. Pedicle screws were placed bilaterally at T4, T5, T6, T10, T11, and T12. The ventral vertebral column was reconstructed with an expandable titanium cage packed with morselized rib graft (Figure 16-4). The patient was discharged after 10 days and experienced no complications. Her symptoms and neurologic findings continued to improve postoperatively, and at 5-year follow-up there was no evidence of recurrence or instrumentation failure.

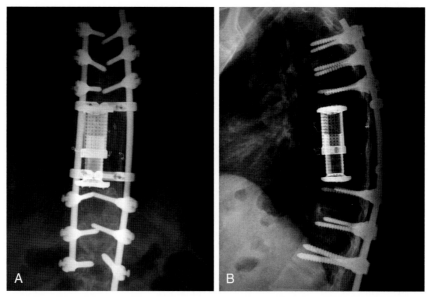

FIGURE 16-4 AP (**A**) and lateral (**B**) radiographs following tumor resection; complete spondylectomy at T7, T8, and T9; reconstruction with an expandable titanium cage; and placement of pedicle screws.

FUNDAMENTAL TECHNIQUE

After induction of general anesthesia, the patient is positioned prone on a Jackson table and a preoperative radiograph is taken to localize the appropriate level. Several types of incisions can be made, and this is left to the discretion of the surgeon. Variations include straight midline, curved hockey stick, and S- and L-shaped incisions. Regardless of the incision used, sufficient exposure for placement of dorsal instrumentation above and below the pathologic level is planned (Tips from the Masters 16-1).

Tips from the Masters 16-1 • An exposure that is medial to the erector spinae muscle may provide the desired exposure—without the associated obligatory injury to the erector spinae muscle.

After skin incision, the subcutaneous tissue, thoracolumbar fascia, and paraspinal muscles are stripped from the spinous processes, laminae, facet joints, and transverse processes bilaterally by subperiosteal dissection (Tips from the Masters 16-2). This standard exposure allows for dorsal decompression and placement of pedicle screws. The thoracolumbar fascia is then elevated from the underlying erector spinae muscle and is retracted laterally with the skin and subcutaneous tissue. A plane is developed using blunt dissection under the lateral aspect of the erector spinae muscle.[14] These muscles are then retracted medially off of the underlying ribs. A self-retaining retractor is used to hold the erector spinae muscle medially and the skin flap laterally. At this point, the initial subperiosteal dissection from the midline structures is continuous with the lateral dissection beneath the erector spinae muscle. This allows for simultaneous exposure of the midline dorsal elements and the lateral elements removed subsequently for a lateral approach to the lateral and ventral vertebral body.[13]

Tips from the Masters 16-2 • A bilateral exposure can provide an enhanced ventral exposure while minimizing blood loss, which often originates from the contralateral ventral epidural space when a unilateral exposure is employed.

The lateral dissection of the erector spinae muscle allows exposure of 8 to 10 cm of rib.[14] This is dissected free from the surrounding soft tissues, including the neurovascular bundle, using a Doyne instrument. The rib head is then disarticulated at the costovertebral joint with a periosteal elevator. Meticulous dissection is performed to avoid tearing the underlying pleura. A rib cutter is used to cut the ribs laterally and the bone is saved for potential graft material. Care is taken to prevent injury to the intercostal nerves and the pleura. This dissection, including rib removal, allows access to the lateral aspect of the vertebral body and pedicle. Three to four vertebral levels can be reached by removing two ribs. The periosteum of the involved vertebrae is bluntly dissected away to identify the disk spaces rostral and caudal to the lesion, and the pleura is retracted to allow proper visualization. Developing this exposure allows an unobstructed view of the lateral aspect of the spine. Similar exposure can be done simultaneously on the contralateral side.

The nerve roots are identified, followed medially to their respective foramina, tied, and incised proximal to the dorsal root ganglia to avoid neuroma formation.[13] The pedicle of the pathologic vertebral body is then removed with a rongeur or drill following dissection of the nerve roots to the medial aspect of the pedicle (Tips from the Masters 16-3). Pedicle removal exposes the lateral aspect of the thecal sac. Compression of the thecal sac by the vertebral tumor is then visualized. The tumor and vertebral body are removed piecemeal and drilled as needed. Downwardly angled curettes are used to push epidural contents into the resection cavity. After the corpectomy is completed, an expandable cage packed with autograft can be placed. Thoracic pedicle screws are then inserted into the levels above and below the pathologic levels.

Tips from the Masters 16-3 • The surgeon can, in fact, go back and forth between the ventral and dorsal components of the operation to fine-tune and tailor the surgical procedure to the needs of the patient.

DISCUSSION OF BEST EVIDENCE

There is debate regarding the best surgical approach for vertebral metastases, and the methodology for selecting the optimal approach has been the subject of recent study.[17,18] As mentioned earlier, both combined ventral-dorsal and lateral extracavitary approaches have been used to treat these lesions effectively. Many factors should be considered when planning an operative strategy, and the patient needs to be involved in the decision-making process, because each approach is associated with morbidity that may affect the quality of the patient's remaining life.

In a recent review of the literature supported by the Spine Oncology Study Group, Polly and colleagues[18] sought to determine the impact of different surgical approaches on local recurrence, adverse effects, pain alleviation, and neurologic recovery. After selecting studies based on certain inclusion criteria, they reviewed a total of 32 articles and found no Level I studies, 1 Level II study, 5 Level III studies, and 26 Level IV studies. They concluded that the existing literature provides only low-quality evidence supporting the superiority of one approach over another.

Although a number of prospective and retrospective studies have detailed the advantages, disadvantages, and complications of these techniques, almost all have evaluated one technique in isolation without comparing it with the others. Because of this limitation, comparisons between techniques have been made by contrasting data from different institutions and often from different generations. This leads to a lack of control within the reported evidence, because institutional biases, surgeon preference, variations in technique, and patient demographics may have an untoward effect on rates of treatment success and failure. Similarly, variations in the types of tumors treated differ in reported series, which makes it difficult to draw conclusions from these reports regarding the superiority of one technique over the other when tumor histologic features are considered. This is critical, because tumor histologic type is known to have the greatest prognostic significance and influence on overall outcomes.

This section discusses the evidence available for each of the named approaches and makes an argument for the lateral extracavitary approach, as illustrated in the case described earlier. The morbidity and complications associated with each are emphasized, because these have the greatest impact on the remaining quality of life in these patients and are factors that must be considered when planning surgery.

Combined Ventral and Dorsal Approaches

Ventral surgery is appealing because it provides the most direct route for decompression and tumor resection. In addition, with current instrumentation techniques, this approach allows for adequate reconstruction of the ventral vertebral column, permitting correction of the loss of height and kyphotic deformity often present with metastatic involvement of the vertebrae.[19] Theoretically, this approach also reduces surgery-related blood loss, because epidural venous pressures are lower in patients in the lateral decubitus position than in the prone position. Another advantage is that segmental vessels feeding a tumor may be identified and ligated before resection.

Despite these advantages, numerous potential complications have been reported with the ventral approaches, including respiratory insufficiency, pneumothorax, pneumonia, hematoma, gastrointestinal bleeding, cerebrospinal fluid leak, renal failure, pulmonary embolism, infection, pleural effusion, surgical defects within the diaphragm leading to visceral herniation, vascular injury, neural injury, and instrumentation failure. Overall complication rates range from 10% to 50%.

To date, many studies have reported results of ventral approaches for the treatment of spinal metastases and have demonstrated high rates of neurologic improvement and pain control.[6,7,20,21] These studies have consistently demonstrated higher rates of neurologic improvement compared to laminectomy with or without fusion. Overall, motor function has been found to improve in 70% to 100% of patients, and pain has also been found to improve in 85% to 97%.[6,8,21-25] In these series, rates of instrumentation failure range from 0% to 11%, and mortality ranges from 0% to 8%.[6,8,21,22,25,26] In contrast to postirradiation laminectomy, which has been associated with wound-related complication rates of around 28%, rates of wound-related complications for ventral approaches are approximately 0% to 16%.[8]

Sundaresan and associates[24] reported a **prospective series** of 54 patients who underwent surgery before radiation or chemotherapy. Patients whose life expectancy was less than 3 months were excluded. Eighty-three percent of the patients underwent decompressive surgery via thoracotomy. Reconstruction following corpectomy consisted of stabilization with Steinman pins augmented with methyl methacrylate. Forty-four percent of patients were nonambulatory before surgery. Most were unable to walk because of weakness, and the second most common reason for inability to ambulate was pain. After surgery, all patients were ambulatory. Pain improved in 90%. Forty-six percent of patients were alive after 2 years, the majority of whom remained ambulatory. Additional dorsal stabilization was required in five patients. The overall complication rate was 20%, and complications included hematoma, respiratory insufficiency requiring prolonged ventilation, pneumonia, deep vein thrombosis, and deep wound infection.

In a **retrospective study** Harrington[7] reported on 77 patients with spinal instability caused by metastatic pathologic fractures of one or more vertebrae. Treatment consisted of ventral decompression and stabilization with methyl methacrylate augmented by Knodt distraction rods positioned ventrally. The follow-up period ranged from 31 to 146 months. Of the 63 patients with major preoperative neurologic impairment, 26 experienced complete neurologic recovery, 16 showed significant improvement, the condition of 20 remained unchanged, and 1 patient experienced deterioration. Relief of pain was obtained in 72 patients. Five patients experienced instrumentation failure and required dorsal stabilization. There was one case of wound infection among the 83 ventral stabilization procedures. Other complications included pulmonary emboli, myocardial infarction, aspiration pneumonia, and cerebrospinal fluid hydrothorax. The overall complication rate was 23%.

Cooper and co-workers[22] studied 28 patients who underwent ventral decompression for spinal metastasis. Surgery was performed in those with spinal cord compression, spinal instability, rapidly progressive neurologic deficit, and failure of radiation therapy. Seventy-five percent of patients were ambulatory preoperatively and 88% postoperatively. Pain improved in 97% of patients. Motor function remained the same or improved in 94% of patients. The mean survival time was 10 months, and the overall complication rate was 22%. Complications included pneumonia, respiratory failure, cerebrospinal fluid leak, pulmonary embolus, gastrointestinal bleeding, and septicemia.

Gokaslan and colleagues[6] published a **retrospective report** on 72 patients with thoracic spine metastatic tumors. Indications for surgery included symptomatic spinal cord compression or intractable axial spinal pain resulting from spinal instability. Life expectancy exceeded 3 months. Treatment consisted of ventral decompression and stabilization with methyl methacrylate injected into a 36F chest tube placed within the corpectomy defect. Preoperatively, 13 patients were nonambulatory. Postoperatively 10 were able to ambulate. Pain improved in 92% of patients. Thirty-five (76%) of 46 patients who had neurologic impairment at presentation experienced significant improvement following surgery. The overall complication rate was 28%, and the 1-year survival rate was 62%. The median chest tube requirement was 4 days (range, 1 to 26 days), and complications included epidural hematoma, pneumonia, gastrointestinal bleeding, cerebrospinal fluid leak, renal failure, cecal perforation, pulmonary embolism, and respiratory failure.

Although a ventral approach alone may suffice in some patients, radiographic studies frequently demonstrate three-column involvement or marked instability of the spine. In such patients, a strictly ventral approach does not provide sufficient access for tumor resection or correction of deformity and instability. This view is consistent with previously published reports of series of patients who underwent ventral surgeries but subsequently required dorsal stabilization for worsening pain or kyphosis following the index procedure. For these reasons, a combined ventral-dorsal approach is often necessary for the treatment of patients with spinal metastases.

Few studies have reported results for a combined approach. Most of these are retrospective reviews of single-institution experiences at large specialty centers. To date, there have been no prospective multicenter studies evaluating indications, clinical results, and outcomes. The available evidence therefore is lacking in quality, and data specific to combined approaches are usually found within larger studies reviewing ventral approaches. Subgroup analyses of combined approaches assessing complications and outcomes are missing from these studies, which typically report data for the group as a whole.

The indications for and results of the combined approach for treatment of spine tumors were reported by Sundaresan and associates[25] for the largest published series of such patients. This was a **retrospective analysis** of the data for patients at a single institution who underwent combined ventral-dorsal surgery. Indications included radiographic demonstration of three-column involvement, significant vertebral instability, marked kyphosis, involvement of more than one vertebral body, junctional site involvement, and previous laminectomy. Fifty-three patients underwent surgery via a combined approach. The majority of procedures were performed in two stages done 1 week apart. Reconstruction was performed using methyl methacrylate, autografts, or tibial allografts. Of 48 patients who were nonambulatory before surgery, 32 became ambulatory after surgery. Fifty-two percent of patients with severe paraparesis showed improvement postoperatively. The overall median survival was 16 months, with 46% surviving 2 years.

The complication rate was 62%, with wound breakdown and infection being most common. However, two intraoperative deaths, deep infections, cerebrospinal fluid leak, respiratory failure, and intraoperative vascular and visceral injury also occurred. Complications were statistically correlated with age older than 65, prior radiotherapy or chemotherapy, and the presence of paraparesis. The authors suggest that despite the high morbidity associated with this combined approach, the high rate of wound breakdown was reflective of previous chemotherapy, radiotherapy, and laminectomy in their referral population.

Fourney and co-workers[27] also reported on results for a single-stage combined approach to the thoracic spine for resection of tumors, both primary and metastatic.

In their **retrospective review** they found this procedure to be both safe and effective in cases of tumors involving both the ventral and dorsal columns of the spine. In this series, 15 patients underwent combined ventral-dorsal surgery for metastatic disease. There was no significant change in Frankel grade postoperatively because all patients with metastatic disease were ambulatory before surgery. Pain assessed at 1 month after surgery was reduced in all but one patient.

The overall complication rate was 53%, with three wound complications. Other complications included cerebrospinal fluid leak, meningitis, deep wound infection, gastrointestinal hemorrhage, and pneumonia. The median chest tube requirement was 5 days (range, 2 to 16 days). Four patients died within 6 months of surgery, and mean survival was 22.5 months.

As illustrated by the results of these representative studies, the combined ventral-dorsal approach has provided alternative techniques to address metastatic tumors that had previously been treated by laminectomy alone. Despite data reflecting improvements in pain and survival, use of this approach is limited by its high complication rate.

Lateral Extracavitary Transpedicular Approach

Although the lateral extracavitary approach has been used to treat spinal metastases for years and the technique for doing so is well described, few have reported clinical outcomes for this specific approach. Most reports concern trauma patients. Unlike for the ventral or combined approaches, there are limited data regarding this technique. Most of the reported series that examine dorsal approaches describe a transpedicular approach with or without costotransversectomy. Within these studies, there are few cases in which a lateral extracavitary approach was used, and specific details regarding these outcomes are rarely provided. In their series of patients who underwent a variety of dorsal procedures for spinal metastasis at the M.D. Anderson Cancer Center, Akeyson and McCutcheon[5] used lateral extracavitary approaches with dorsal instrumentation in a total of 11 patients. These patients, however, were not included in their analysis. In recent years, case reports have been published and modifications of this technique have been described.[28-30] Variations in technique and loose definitions of these approaches cloud the interpretation of such series and make meaningful comparisons difficult.

In a multicenter consecutive case series of **prospectively** followed patients, Shen and colleagues[31] used a lateral extracavitary approach to treat metastatic tumors. A total of 21 patients underwent corpectomy and stabilization with expandable cages and pedicle screw fixation through the same dorsal exposure. Average estimated blood loss was 1360 mL and average length of surgery was 5.3 hours. No chest tubes or postoperative bracing was required. Twenty patients were ambulatory preoperatively and remained ambulatory after surgery. One patient was not ambulatory preoperatively and had not shown improvement by the time he died 1 month after surgery. Nine patients had improvement of at least one partial motor grade. All complications were associated with the implanted cages. One cage required repositioning on the second postoperative day and one cage demonstrated radiographic evidence of subsidence but did not require surgical intervention. The average postoperative stay was 4.7 days. There were no occurrences of deep vein thrombosis, pulmonary embolism, pneumothorax, or hemothorax, and the complication rate for the series was 14.3%.

In the only reported series that compared outcomes for patients who underwent surgery for thoracic metastases via a combined approach or a strictly dorsal approach, Xu and associates[32] found comparable rates of complications for the two procedures.

A **retrospective review** of cases treated at a single institution examined data for 24 patients who underwent a combined ventral-dorsal procedure and 45 who underwent a dorsal procedure alone. The combined approach was defined as a two-stage procedure, with the stages often done 2 weeks apart, or done on the same day. The dorsal approach was defined as transpedicular corpectomies, accompanied by either costotransversectomies or lateral extracavitary techniques. Ventral spinal column reconstruction was achieved with both distractible and nondistractible cages as well as the chest tube and methyl methacrylate technique. Preoperative morbidity, neurologic scores on both on the Nurick and American Spinal Injury Association (ASIA) Impairment scales, as well as ambulatory status were not significantly different between the two groups.

Postoperatively, the cohort under going the combined procedure demonstrated the best ambulatory improvement, with a 25% change compared with a 4.4% change in the cohort undergoing the dorsal procedure. Preoperatively, 71.1% and 75.5% were ambulatory in the dorsal procedure and combined procedure groups, respectively. There was also statistically significant improvement in the Nurick scale score in the combined group.

Overall, the complication rate was 46% for the combined approach and 36% for the dorsal approach. In patients undergoing the combined procedure, the most frequent complications were pulmonary, with 55% experiencing pleural effusions, 14% developing pneumonia, and 18% requiring new chest tube placement. The total number of complications, as judged from the need for reoperation, amount of blood loss, days of chest tube drainage, and occurrence of durotomy, pleural effusion, and pneumothorax, was highest for the combined approach. The dorsal approach was associated with a higher incidence of wound infections and deep vein thromboses. Overall, as in other retrospective series, pulmonary complications were associated with significantly worse postoperative neurologic outcomes.

Vertebrectomy Reconstruction Options

Regardless of surgical approach, corpectomy (or vertebrectomy) with subsequent vertebral body reconstruction is the foundation for restoration of the ventral spinal column during surgery for metastatic tumors. This operative strategy facilitates correction of deformity and immediate stabilization. An ideal vertebral body graft resists axial loading, maintains stability, restores height and sagittal alignment, and has a large bone-interbody interface to prevent graft migration.

Although obtaining a fusion is ideal, specific aspects of the medical management of metastatic spine tumors, including radiation therapy, chemotherapy, and corticosteroid use, create a biologically unfavorable environment for fusion. The nutritional status of patients undergoing this surgery is often poor, so the biologic substrate required for adequate soft tissue and bony healing is limited. These factors should be considered when planning the timing of surgery. The effect of radiotherapy on fusion, whether administered before or after surgery, has not been studied prospectively. Due to the known effect of radiation on wound healing, radiation treatment is usually withheld for several weeks following surgery. Similarly, the timing of chemotherapy and its effect on fusion and soft tissue healing has not been studied prospectively. Many patients undergo cycles of chemotherapy that either precede or are concurrent with surgery. Due to these considerations, as well as the limited life expectancy of patients with metastatic disease, surgical reconstruction constructs need to provide rigid stabilization in anticipation of death before bony fusion.

A number of interbody graft types can be used to reconstruct the ventral spinal column after vertebrectomy. These include bone, cement, metal, and synthetic materials. Bone-interbody grafts include autologous or allogeneic tricortical bone of varying origin. Cement products are often composed of polymethylmethacrylate (PMMA), used in combination with either metal cages, Steinman pins, or chest tubes. Theoretical and practical disadvantages of cement include thermal injury, dislodgment, and extravasation. A large variety of metallic and synthetic materials now exist, including metal alloy, carbon fiber, synthetic materials (e.g., polyetheretherketone), and ceramics. These spacers can be trimmed, stacked, or expanded as needed.

Although case reports have described the use of specific interbody graft types following tumor resection and vertebrectomy in the spine, no study to date has prospectively compared the use of different interbody graft types after vertebrectomy in patients with metastatic tumors. Without a direct comparison of grafts, conclusions regarding graft failure rates and the ability to maintain correction of deformity cannot be made at this time. Therefore, determining which interbody graft to use is a matter of clinical judgment, with consideration given to factors such as patient anatomy, surgical approach, and surgeon preference.

The successful placement of a graft can be greatly influenced by the surgical exposure used. For example, when the dorsal approach is used, expandable cages are advantageous, because the adjustable nature of these devices allows the surgeon to pass the implant safely into the intervertebral space without retraction of the spinal cord. After the device is placed within the vertebrectomy defect, it is expanded to the desired length, with the ends contacting each adjacent end plate. Use of such expandable devices has facilitated reconstruction of the vertebral body from the dorsal approach, because this method is far less cumbersome than attempting to accurately size a structural autograft or allograft that is less flexible.

Placement of either an autologous or allogenic bone graft is also a viable interbody grafting option. However, obtaining a good fit can be more challenging depending on the approach, the type of graft used, and the quality of the bone. These grafts are fixed and nonadjustable, which makes placement through a dorsal approach difficult. Because of the rigid nature of these grafts, they can be placed crooked, which leads to eventual construct failure. These grafts are easier to place via ventral approaches in which the spinal cord is not subjected to manipulation during placement of the graft. Given the number of options available, surgeons must carefully consider the needs of the individual patient when selecting an intervertebral graft.

COMMENTARY

The combined ventral and dorsal approach offers many advantages and historically provided surgeons with better tools to treat metastatic spinal tumors. However, the high risk of complications has made this strategy less attractive to surgeons and patients. The lateral extracavitary approach offers the advantage of circumferential tumor decompression, reconstruction, and stabilization through a single incision and is associated with fewer complications overall. The clinical data reviewed in this chapter illustrate the low quality of evidence currently available. A recent review by the Spine Oncology Study Group[18] failed to make any evidence-based recommendation with regard to the superiority of one technique over the other.

Clearly, surgeon experience, surgeon preference, and institutional practices affect the reported results in the retrospective series reviewed. As illustrated by the case presented in this chapter, when applied appropriately, the lateral extracavitary approach can achieve the goals of combined ventral and dorsal surgery while minimizing overall morbidity. The retrospective nature of the available data must be kept in mind, and consideration must be given to the appropriate surgical approach in patients with limited life expectancy and reserve for recovery.

The choice of operative approaches for the complex surgical endeavors discussed in this chapter is indeed a difficult task. Surgeon comfort with any given surgical strategy, as alluded to here, is paramount. If a surgeon has success with a particular surgical approach, it is difficult to argue with the continued use of that approach. This is so even if the surgeon is in the minority, with respect to his or her colleagues, in determining a surgical strategy. A chemistry exists that cannot be studied. Surgical decision making cannot be totally dictated by the results of randomized clinical trials. Allowing "wiggle room" for surgeon preference in strategy determination is imperative. We, as a profession, must not lose sight of the fact that the preservation of individuality is critical to our success as a profession.

So, which surgical approach is best? Each case must be carefully scrutinized, based on its own particular features. Each surgeon must weigh the pros and cons of each surgical strategy. Each surgeon must also consider his or her own comfort zone and honestly appraise his or her ability to truly help the patient via surgical intervention (honest self-reflection). Finally, the patient must be brought into the decision-making process. This converts an "informed consent" situation into one of "informed decision making."

REFERENCES

1. Findlay GF: Adverse effects of the management of malignant spinal cord compression, *J Neurol Neurosurg Psychiatry* 47:761–768, 1984.
2. Gilbert RW, Kim JH, Posner JB: Epidural spinal cord compression from metastatic tumor: diagnosis and treatment, *Ann Neurol* 3:40–51, 1978.
3. Klimo P Jr, Thompson CJ, Kestle JR, et al: A meta-analysis of surgery versus conventional radiotherapy for the treatment of metastatic spinal epidural disease, *Neurol Oncol* 7:64–76, 2005.
4. Patchell RA, Tibbs PA, Regine WF, et al: Direct decompressive surgical resection in the treatment of spinal cord compression caused by metastatic cancer: a randomised trial, *Lancet* 366:643–648, 2005. **This often-cited article reports results from a randomized multicenter trial demonstrating that surgery using current instrumentation techniques is superior to radiation therapy alone in select patients with metastatic spine disease. These findings refute those of previous reports which suggested that laminectomy is equivalent to radiation therapy.**
5. Akeyson EW, McCutcheon IE: Single-stage posterior vertebrectomy and replacement combined with posterior instrumentation for spinal metastasis, *J Neurosurg* 85:211–220, 1996.
6. Gokaslan ZL, York JE, Walsh GL, et al: Transthoracic vertebrectomy for metastatic spinal tumors, *J Neurosurg* 89:599–609, 1998.
7. Harrington KD: Anterior decompression and stabilization of the spine as a treatment for vertebral collapse and spinal cord compression from metastatic malignancy, *Clin Orthop Relat Res* 233:177–197, 1988.
8. Siegal T: Surgical decompression of anterior and posterior malignant epidural tumors compressing the spinal cord: a prospective study, *Neurosurgery* 17:424–432, 1985.
9. Tokuhashi Y, Ajiro Y, Oshima M: Algorithms and planning in metastatic spine tumors, *Orthop Clin North Am* 40:37–46, v-vi, 2009.
10. Tokuhashi Y, Matsuzaki H, Oda H, et al: A revised scoring system for preoperative evaluation of metastatic spine tumor prognosis, *Spine* 30:2186–2191, 2005.
11. Tokuhashi Y, Matsuzaki H, Toriyama S, et al: Scoring system for the preoperative evaluation of metastatic spine tumor prognosis, *Spine* 15:1110–1113, 1990.
12. Tomita K, Kawahara N, Kobayashi T, et al: Surgical strategy for spinal metastases, *Spine* 26:298–306, 2001.
13. Benzel EC: The lateral extracavitary approach to the spine using the three-quarter prone position, *J Neurosurg* 71:837–841, 1989.
14. Larson SJ, Holst RA, Hemmy DC, et al: Lateral extracavitary approach to traumatic lesions of the thoracic and lumbar spine, *J Neurosurg* 45:628–637, 1976. **This is the description of the lateral extracavitary approach to the thoracic and thoracolumbar spine as modified by Larson. Although originally described for treatment of traumatic lesions, this method has been applied to metastatic spinal tumors as well.**
15. Resnick DK, Benzel EC: Lateral extracavitary approach for thoracic and thoracolumbar spine trauma: operative complications, *Neurosurgery* 43:796–802, 1998: discussion, 802-803. **This article details the operative complications associated with the lateral extracavitary approach. This is the largest series for which results have been published.**
16. Champlin AM, Rael J, Benzel EC, et al: Preoperative spinal angiography for lateral extracavitary approach to thoracic and lumbar spine, *AJNR Am J Neuroradiol* 15:73–77, 1994. **This article describes the usefulness of preoperative angiography when planning a lateral extracavitary approach to the thoracic and lumbar spine. The vascular anatomy of the spine and the variability of the artery of Adamkiewicz are discussed in relation to this surgical approach.**
17. Fourney DR, Gokaslan ZL: Use of "MAPs" for determining the optimal surgical approach to metastatic disease of the thoracolumbar spine: anterior, posterior, or combined. Invited submission from the Joint Section Meeting on Disorders of the Spine and Peripheral Nerves, *J Neurosurg Spine* 2:40–49, 2005. **An algorithm for presurgical planning for metastatic disease to the spine is outlined. Emphasis is given to (1) method of resection, that is, en bloc, piecemeal, or palliative; (2) anatomy of spinal disease; (3) patient's level of fitness; and (4) need for and method of stabilization.**
18. Polly DW Jr, Chou D, Sembrano JN, et al: An analysis of decision making and treatment in thoracolumbar metastases, *Spine* 34:S118–S127, 2009. **This is a recent review of the best available evidence regarding various surgical treatment options for thoracolumbar metastases. Supported by the Spine Oncology Study Group, this review highlights the lack of high-quality evidence for selecting any surgical option, whether it be anterior, posterior, or combined.**
19. Krishnaney AA, Steinmetz MP, Benzel EC: Biomechanics of metastatic spine cancer, *Neurosurg Clin N Am* 15:375–380, 2004.
20. Chen LH, Chen WJ, Niu CC, et al: Anterior reconstructive spinal surgery with Zielke instrumentation for metastatic malignancies of the spine, *Arch Orthop Trauma Surg* 120:27–31, 2000.
21. Hosono N, Yonenobu K, Fuji T, et al: Vertebral body replacement with a ceramic prosthesis for metastatic spinal tumors, *Spine* 20:2454–2462, 1995.
22. Cooper PR, Errico TJ, Martin R, et al: A systematic approach to spinal reconstruction after anterior decompression for neoplastic disease of the thoracic and lumbar spine, *Neurosurgery* 32:1–8, 1993.
23. Perrin RG, McBroom RJ: Anterior versus posterior decompression for symptomatic spinal metastasis, *Can J Neurol Sci* 14:75–80, 1987.
24. Sundaresan N, Digiacinto GV, Hughes JE, et al: Treatment of neoplastic spinal cord compression: results of a prospective study, *Neurosurgery* 29:645–650, 1991.

25. Sundaresan N, Steinberger AA, Moore F, et al: Indications and results of combined anterior-posterior approaches for spine tumor surgery, *J Neurosurg* 85:438–446, 1996.
26. Sundaresan N, Galicich JH, Lane JM, et al: Treatment of neoplastic epidural cord compression by vertebral body resection and stabilization, *J Neurosurg* 63:676–684, 1985.
27. Fourney DR, Abi-Said D, Rhines LD, et al: Simultaneous anterior-posterior approach to the thoracic and lumbar spine for the radical resection of tumors followed by reconstruction and stabilization, *J Neurosurg* 94:232–244, 2001.
28. Chou D, Eltgroth M, Yang I, et al: Rib head disarticulation for multilevel transpedicular thoracic corpectomies and expandable cage reconstruction, *Neurol India* 57:469–474, 2009.
29. Chou D, Wang VY: Trap-door rib-head osteotomies for posterior placement of expandable cages after transpedicular corpectomy: an alternative to lateral extracavitary and costotransversectomy approaches, *J Neurosurg Spine* 10:40–45, 2009.
30. Keshavarzi S, Aryan HE: Multilevel lateral extra-cavitary corpectomy and reconstruction for non-contiguous metastatic lesions to the spine: case report and literature review, *J Surg Oncol* 99:314–317, 2009.
31. Shen FH, Marks I, Shaffrey C, et al: The use of an expandable cage for corpectomy reconstruction of vertebral body tumors through a posterior extracavitary approach: a multicenter consecutive case series of prospectively followed patients, *Spine J* 8:329–339, 2008.
32. Xu R, Garces-Ambrossi GL, McGirt MJ, et al: Thoracic vertebrectomy and spinal reconstruction via anterior, posterior, or combined approaches: clinical outcomes in 91 consecutive patients with metastatic spinal tumors, *J Neurosurg Spine* 11:272–284, 2009. **This is a retrospective single-institution study that compares clinical outcomes in patients who underwent surgery for thoracolumbar metastases using either an anterior, posterior, or combined approach. The complications associated with each approach are discussed.**

Chapter 17 Degenerative Scoliosis: Anterior and Posterior Fusion Versus Posterior Fusion

Krishna Gumidyala, Sigurd Berven

Degenerative lumbar scoliosis is a common spinal disorder with variable presentation and treatment options. Degenerative scoliosis has important differences from adult idiopathic scoliosis, including a new onset of deformity, a lumbar predominance in the curve pattern, degenerative changes within the deformity, and a steady progression of deformity with age.[1-3] Degenerative scoliosis is an important spinal disorder affecting the aging spine, and an evidence-based approach to the nonoperative and operative care of the disorder has not been well established. This chapter discusses the evidence related to the relative merits of a combined anterior and posterior approach to treatment of degenerative scoliosis compared with a posterior approach to deformity correction.

CASE PRESENTATION

A 57-year-old woman had progressive spinal deformity with imbalance in the sagittal and coronal plane. She reported that the onset of her spinal deformity was in adulthood and that she had had back pain for over 30 years. Over the past 5 years she had noted progression of leg pain, with the left leg more affected than the right. She reported that her left leg frequently gave way with walking and that she had a walking tolerance of less than two blocks. She had undergone several treatments with epidural injections and selective nerve blocks with only temporary and partial improvement of her pain. In the past year she was bothered most by her ribs' abutting the pelvis on her right side. She also noted mild subjective weakness as well as numbness and tingling distally in her lower extremities, with pain and paresthesia symptoms worse in the left lower extremity. Other nonoperative care included physical therapy, yoga, and chiropractic care, which led to no significant improvement in her pain or disability. Her medications included extended-release oxycodone (OxyContin) and hydrocodone/acetaminophen (Vicodin) for pain.

- PMH: Medication-controlled hypertension

- PSH: Unremarkable

- Exam: The patient had an obvious deformity with a right rib hump. While standing she had a significant sagittal plane deformity with significant kyphosis as well as left lumbar level prominence. She had abutment of her right ilium into the anterior aspect of her right costal margin. On supine examination she was noted to have significantly less kyphosis. Her thoracolumbar spine area was nontender. Findings of motor, sensory, and reflex examinations were normal. No gait abnormalities were noted.

- Imaging: Radiographs obtained included full-length images of the spine showing marked scoliosis, with lumbar scoliosis measuring 68 degrees with the left-sided apex at L2 (Figure 17-1). The images demonstrated the sagittal deformity with plumb line 8 cm to the right and a positive sagittal imbalance of 17 cm. For preoperative planning traction radiographs and lateral radiographs with the patient over a bolster were also obtained, which revealed some reduction of her kyphosis (Figure 17-2).

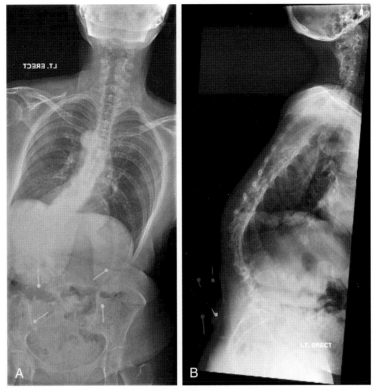

FIGURE 17-1 Preoperative AP (**A**) and lateral (**B**) radiographs showing degenerative scoliosis.

CLINICAL PRESENTATION

The patient with symptomatic degenerative scoliosis characteristically has symptoms of back and leg pain, and progression of deformity, including sagittal and coronal plane imbalance. Consistent findings in a review of data for 200 patients by Pritchett and Bortel[4] included degenerated facet joints, a loss of lumbar lordosis, and endplate sclerosis with vertebral rotation. Rotational subluxation within the deformity and sagittal plane decompensation are radiographic findings that are associated with significant compromise of health-related quality of life in affected patients.[5]

The etiology of degenerative lumbar scoliosis is multifactorial. The relationship between bone density and degenerative scoliosis has been found to be variable, and there is not a clear causal link to bone mineral density alone.[6] Because Pritchett and Bortel found certain consistent areas of anatomic degeneration, Tribus suggests that an asymmetric degeneration of the anterior disk space or of the posterior facet joints may lead to the rotational and translational deformities associated with degenerative scoliosis.[7] This degenerative cascade, when combined with ligamentum flavum buckling, may explain the more prominent neurogenic symptoms in addition to back or deformity complaints from patients with the disorder.

In adult spinal deformity, there are important correlations between curve and deformity characteristics and patient clinical appearance. Global sagittal plane alignment is the most important radiographic characteristic associated with health status compromise, including pain and functional limitations.[8] Schwab and colleagues[9] proposed a clinical impact classification for adult scoliosis. They demonstrated that radiographic factors associated with disability and surgery include lumbar hypolordosis and intervertebral subluxation.

Radiographic characteristics alone have a poor correlation with the need for operative or nonoperative approaches to deformity. The decision to pursue operative versus nonoperative care is importantly based upon patient self-assessment of health status, and patient and physician combined decision making. Patient self-assessment

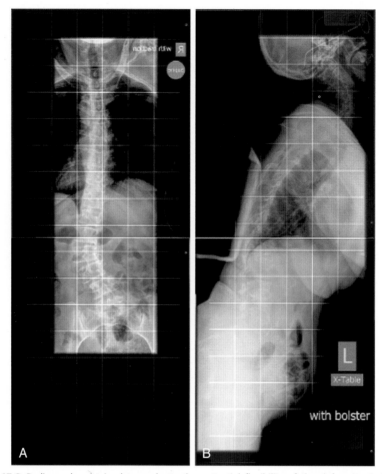

FIGURE 17-2 Radiographs obtained to evaluate the potential flexibility of the deformity, including an anteroposterior traction radiograph (**A**) and a lateral radiograph with a bolster placed under the patient near the apex of the deformity in the sagittal plane (**B**).

of disability is an important determinant of the decision to pursue operative versus nonoperative care for spinal deformity. Glassman and associates[10] demonstrated that patients who were treated with surgery for adult scoliosis had more back and leg pain than patients treated nonoperatively. Patients treated nonoperatively had significantly more comorbid conditions than patients treated operatively. Pekmezci and colleagues[11] demonstrated that functional domain scores, including walking in the Oswestry Disability Index (ODI) and vitality in the Scoliosis Research Society (SRS) instrument, were more important than back or leg pain in distinguishing between operative and nonoperative care in adults with scoliosis.

Bess and co-workers[12] studied factors that differentiated between operative and nonoperative approaches to treatment of deformity in a cohort of 290 adults. They demonstrated that among patients older than age 40, pain and disability were significantly higher in patients who chose operative care rather than nonoperative care. In contrast, among younger patients, curve size and coronal deformity were higher in patients who were treated with surgery rather than nonoperative care, and pain and disability were similar in the operative and nonoperative groups. These findings demonstrate that radiographic considerations may be a more important factor in determining treatment in younger patients, and that health-related quality of life is a more important determinant of treatment course in adults older than age 50.

Spinal deformity and global coronal or sagittal plane imbalance may be related to regional malalignment within the spine or may have extraspinal causes. In the peripheral skeleton, hip and knee flexion contracture may cause global sagittal imbalance and should lead to evaluation of those joints, because osteoarthritis of the hip and knee is common in the older age group. A complaint of altered gait should also lead to evaluation for abnormalities of the cervical spine as a cause of the patient's symptoms. For those who complain primarily of back pain, it is more challenging to determine if the deformity is the source of the pain. Briard and associates[13] found that the convex region of the curve was the area of greatest pain in 75%, with the second most common location being the concave region of the curve. Primary complaints associated with deformity are often related to functional loss from a flat back deformity or a "rib in pelvis" deformity, which can also be accompanied by muscular fatigue and pain due to attempts to compensate for the sagittal and coronal imbalance.

CLINICAL EVALUATION

Evaluation begins with history taking and physical examination, with emphasis on neural evaluation as well as spinal alignment and peripheral joint abnormality. Radiographic evaluation should include full-spine standing radiographs to assess segmental, regional, and global alignment of the spine. The plain radiographs should also be reviewed for other pathologic conditions, because degenerative spondylolisthesis and rotational subluxation may be important causes of stenosis and neural compromise. Bending or traction radiographs will aid in determining the flexibility of the curve. Anteroposterior (AP) and lateral tractions radiographs with or without the patient over a bolster at the apex of the deformity may be useful in preoperative planning for larger curves or rigid deformities that may partially correct during operative positioning.

Advanced imaging, including magnetic resonance imaging (MRI) or computed tomography (CT) myelography, is useful for the evaluation of intraspinal lesions and neural compression. CT myelography may also be valuable in measuring segmental ankylosis and facet joint defects. Evaluation of bone mineral density with a dual energy x-ray absorptiometry (DEXA) scan is particularly important in patients with degenerative scoliosis, because osteoporosis is an important comorbid condition that may affect surgical approaches and fixation strategies. The role of diskography remains controversial in scoliosis. Kostuik[14] has found diskography to be useful in choosing distal fusion levels. However, Grubb and Lipscomb[15] found high rates of concordant pain reproduction and concluded that decision making for surgery was not influenced reliably by diskography results.

An understanding of the natural history of disease progression is important in order for the patient and the physician to participate in informed decision making in adult scoliosis management. Informed choice in the decision to pursue operative or nonoperative care for scoliosis requires information on the outcomes of each option. There is significant variability in clinical and radiographic outcomes depending on treatment, preoperative patient factors, and comorbid conditions. Schwab and associates identified the following as factors that predicted a good outcome from surgery in scoliosis: older age, lower apex of deformity, and greater self-assessment of disability. Patients with high degrees of sagittal imbalance and patients treated with long fusion to the sacrum are most likely to experience perioperative complications.[16] Rates of surgical complications in adult deformity surgery have been reported to be over 70%, and reoperation rates may be greater than 25% at 2 years.[17-20] An understanding of the risks and benefits of operative and nonoperative treatment is important to guide an evidence-based approach to care. Smith and colleagues[21] reported that complication rates were significantly higher in older patients than in younger patients, with complication rates of 17% in patients younger than age 65 and 71% in patients older than age 65. However, older patients experienced significantly greater improvements in pain and disability, which suggests that the risk/benefit ratio may be similar across all ages.

Little evidence exists to demonstrate the long-term effectiveness of nonoperative care of adult scoliosis in improving patient self-assessment of quality of life. Glassman and associates[22] reported that the average yearly cost of nonoperative care of adult scoliosis was more than $10,800 over 2 years, and there was no significant decrease in pain, improvement in function, or reduction in disability in patients treated nonoperatively.

Clinical studies comparing operative and nonoperative care are limited. There is no published prospective randomized comparison of operative and nonoperative care of adult scoliosis. In a study comparing change in quality of life in patients treated operatively or nonoperatively for adult scoliosis, Bridwell and co-workers[23] demonstrated significant improvement in self-assessed quality of life in adults treated operatively but no significant change in quality of life in adults treated nonoperatively. Similarly, Smith and colleagues[24,25] studied operative versus nonoperative care in adults with back pain, leg pain, and scoliosis. These authors demonstrated a significant improvement in ODI and numeric rating scale scores for leg pain and back pain in the operative care group but no significant change in the nonoperative care group. These studies are limited by dissimilarities at baseline between the operative and nonoperative treatment cohorts.

The decision to pursue operative versus nonoperative care in the management of adult scoliosis is as important as the surgical strategy or technique selected in pursuing surgery. An informed choice requires information on the expected outcomes of operative and nonoperative care. Operative care results in greater improvement of self-assessed health-related quality of life in adults with scoliosis compared with nonoperative care. However, a direct comparison of outcomes for patients with similar health status and comorbid conditions at baseline remains to be completed.

SURGICAL OPTIONS

Indications for surgery in adult scoliosis include progression of deformity, neural impairment, and pain or functional limitations that persist despite nonoperative care.[26] There is significant variability in the operative plan for treatment of adult deformity, and the spectrum of surgical approaches may include decompression alone, limited fusion, and fusion of the structural deformity in its entirety. For fusion procedures, approaches may include anterior only, posterior only, and combined anterior and posterior approaches. An evidence-based approach to surgical technique is based on factors such as curve location and stiffness; medical comorbidities, including poor bone quality; and the preferences of the patient and surgeon.

Surgical treatment for the patient described in the Case Presentation must address the following questions: Where is the stenosis that causes the lower extremity pain? Which levels are potentially responsible for the back pain? Is the deformity responsible for some of the patient's disability, and to what extent does it need to be corrected to achieve a satisfactory result for the patient?

Isolated decompression is best performed in a patient with radicular symptoms or symptoms related to spinal stenosis but with minimal back pain. Advanced deformity may be a relative contraindication for isolated decompression, because the destabilization inherent in decompression may worsen the course of the scoliosis in curves already known to be predisposed to progression. Patients should be counseled that back pain symptoms may not improve and may even worsen after isolated decompression. Bridwell[27] presents some guidelines for stratifying surgical treatment based on the amount of deformity in three dimensions as well as the severity of stenosis. Patients with primarily neural symptoms and limited rotational subluxation or spondylolisthesis, as well as patients with ankylosis of motion segments, may be appropriate candidates for decompression alone. The presence of larger bony structures, such as a wide pars interarticularis, and stabilizing osteophytes can help prevent iatrogenic instability. These patients should be followed closely postoperatively for recurrence of neurologic symptoms, iatrogenic instability, and progression of deformity.[28]

A limited fusion may be a useful option to permit decompression of the neural elements, with the decompressed levels stabilized but the extent of the fusion restricted.

Posterior decompression and fusion of a portion of the curve or sometimes even an area below the apex of the curve may be a viable option. The reasons for taking this approach vary, including the need to alleviate iatrogenic instability caused by necessary or aggressive decompression, treatment of arthritic levels responsible for back pain, and avoidance of a larger procedure in a patient who may not tolerate longer time under anesthesia or the metabolic demands of a longer fusion. Once again, as in the case of isolated decompression, the patient must be followed to detect worsening neurologic symptoms and postoperative progression of deformity. In addition, with spinal fusion, adjacent-segment disease may become a concern.

Posterior spinal fusion for deformity correction with decompression of the stenotic levels is often adequate surgical treatment even in the face of significant deformity. It has the advantage of addressing affected levels from a single approach and allowing direct decompression of compressed neural structures. Posteriorly based osteotomies, including Smith-Peterson osteotomies, pedicle subtraction osteotomies, and vertebral column resection, present the opportunity to address coronal and sagittal plane imbalance. For less severe deformity, multiple Smith-Peterson osteotomies may allow enough flexibility in the curve for adequate correction to be accomplished with instrumentation and fusion. The degree of correction of sagittal plane deformity per Smith-Peterson osteotomy is 5 to 8 degrees per level. Pedicle subtraction osteotomies allow greater sagittal correction through a single level and, via asymmetric osteotomy, may allow significant coronal plane correction. Vertebral column resection is the most powerful osteotomy, but carries greater risk to the neural elements. Vertebral column resection may also be less relevant for degenerative scoliosis, in which deformity occurs over several levels, than for a focal deformity, which vertebral column resection is ideally designed to treat.[29]

Anterior approaches are often combined with posterior approaches, and this allows for greater correction of deformity with anterior release. In addition, anterior interbody grafting increases fusion potential. Anterior interbody grafting permits indirect decompression when foraminal height is restored. Performing the anterior stage first and delaying the posterior stage can allow evaluation for resolution of radicular symptoms, which may obviate the need for decompression at the time of posterior instrumentation and fusion.

Since the apex of lumbar degenerative scoliosis is usually in the upper lumbar spine, the lumbosacral junction is not always surgically addressed. In cases in which stenosis is present at the L5-S1 level or long constructs end at L5 or S1, there is the question of whether the L5-S1 disk space can tolerate the increased stress. There is biomechanical and clinical evidence to suggest that when the choice has been made to fuse the L5-S1 joint, augmentation with iliac fixation is beneficial.[30,31] Anterior interbody grafting at the L5-S1 interspace may be necessary simply to improve the fusion rate at this vulnerable level. In this chapter the two approaches to be compared are posterior fusion with lumbosacral junction grafting only (without addressing other levels anteriorly) and a combined anterior and posterior approach.

On the cephalad end there is the question of how high to fuse. Since many curves will have their apex in the upper lumbar spine, fusion constructs that completely address the curve may end at the thoracolumbar junction. Multiple studies have found the potential risk of proximal junctional kyphosis to be 24% to 60%. In general, the fusion should extend proximally to include the entire curve in the coronal plane and cephalad, above the thoracolumbar junction when segmental kyphosis of the thoracolumbar junction is more than 5 degrees.[32-34]

FUNDAMENTAL TECHNIQUE

After discussion of surgical risks and benefits with the patient, she decided to proceed with surgery to address her progressive pain and deformity. The surgical plan was for a posteriorly based fusion with instrumentation from T10 to the pelvis. The possibility of an L2 vertebral column resection was discussed to address deformity in both planes with cephalad instrumentation to T3 to address the kyphotic deformity. After reviewing traction radiographs it was determined

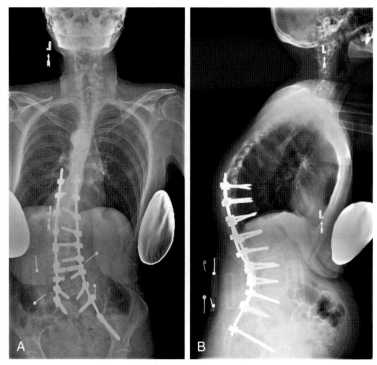

FIGURE 17-3 Postoperative AP (**A**) and lateral (**B**) radiographs after posterior spinal instrumentation and deformity correction.

that multiple Smith-Peterson osteotomies would likely be adequate to achieve deformity correction with cephalad instrumentation to T10. In addition to posterior instrumentation and deformity correction, a staged anterior lumbar interbody fusion for the lumbosacral junction was discussed with the patient.

The primary procedure was a posterior spinal fusion from T10 to S1 with segmental fixation achieved with transpedicular screws at those levels and a right iliac screw using local bone, iliac crest bone graft, and a commercially available bone graft extender. Wide laminectomies were performed from L1 to L5 to help address the patient's lower extremity symptoms and in preparation for the osteotomies. Smith-Peterson osteotomies were performed at T12-L1, L1-2, L2-3, L3-4, and L4-5 (Figure 17-3). At the interstage follow-up appointment, some tenderness to percussion was noted at T9, which raised concern for a compression fracture; this was addressed with a T9 kyphoplasty on the same date as the L5-S1 anteriorly based procedure. Approximately 4 weeks after completion of the first stage, the patient was brought back to the operating room for a planned second stage at which the lumbosacral junction was addressed with anterior lumbar interbody fusion at L4-5 and L5-S1 using prosthetic interbody cages and bone morphogenetic protein-2 (Figure 17-4).

At the 2-month follow-up after the second stage, the patient's pain was significantly better than her preoperative pain level and she was ambulating independently. She did note some mild thigh paresthesias, which were well controlled with medication. Findings of the motor and sensory examination were normal, with significant improvement in observed sagittal and coronal balance. The patient began physical therapy at that point to help her advance her overall conditioning and to continue working on postural stabilization and core strength. At later follow-up she had mild low back discomfort rated as 1 on a visual analog scale of 1 to 10, along with improvement of her thigh paresthesias. Plain radiographs demonstrated the deformity correction. She developed a compression fracture above the upper instrumented vertebra and, as noted earlier, this was treated with a kyphoplasty at the time of her lower lumbar anterior spine fusion. Final radiographs demonstrated a significant residual proximal junctional kyphosis.

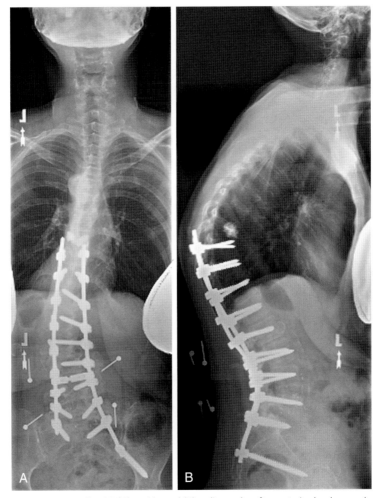

FIGURE 17-4 Postoperative AP (**A**) and lateral (**B**) radiographs after anterior lumbosacral grafting.

DISCUSSION OF BEST EVIDENCE

The surgical management of adult degenerative scoliosis is challenging, and treatment approaches and results are variable. The presence of variability is clear evidence of a lack of an evidence-based approach. A recent review by Bridwell and colleagues[35] examined surgical treatment of adult deformity. None of the 18 reports reviewed in that article provided prospective data, which makes it difficult to evaluate the benefit of surgical treatment of deformity. More recent articles address the potential for surgical intervention to treat back pain and leg pain in the adult patient with spinal deformity. The studies at the highest level of evidence do have prospectively obtained data, but they are still retrospective analyses. These and other studies typically have a heterogenous patient population owing to the limited numbers of patients available for a specific diagnosis, and include patients with de novo scoliosis, adult idiopathic scoliosis, postsurgical deformity, and other conditions. This makes the conclusions of these studies less applicable to patients with lumbar degenerative scoliosis. Data regarding the surgical approach–related complications may be helpful, however, regardless of the initial diagnosis. Another limitation of all of these studies is that the decision regarding surgical approach was always made by the surgeon at his or her discretion, with no explanation of any algorithm or criteria for selecting a dual versus posterior-only approach.

Although the trend in the surgical treatment of lumbar degenerative scoliosis has been to use a posterior-only approach in these cases, this chapter discusses the evidence that supports combined anterior and posterior approaches as well as the complications associated with the dual approach. Traditional indications for the anterior approach included infection (e.g., tuberculosis) and tumor.[36] With tumor surgery, anterior approaches allow en bloc resection of lesions and restoration of anterior column deficiency. Similarly, in trauma patients, the spinal cord can be directly decompressed and anterior support is provided with a structural bone graft or cage reconstruction. In trauma cases use of the anterior approach may also help avoid fusion of multiple adjacent levels as is often necessary in the posterior approach. This potential advantage of the anterior approach is further emphasized by the failures of some of the posterior "fuse short, instrument long" approaches.[37]

Anterior approaches have played a role in treating deformity as well. Adolescent idiopathic scoliosis can be treated via anterior-only, posterior-only, or combined approaches. The important distinction to make between adolescent idiopathic scoliosis and lumbar degenerative scoliosis is that surgical treatment of adolescent idiopathic scoliosis is almost always strictly for deformity. In addition, the curves tend to be much more flexible in the pediatric population. Betz and associates[38] demonstrated that the Cobb angle correction achieved with the anterior approach was similar to that achieved with the posterior approach (approximately 60%). In addition, anterior release and correction permitted greater improvement of preoperative hypokyphosis in the thoracic spine. However, the group undergoing the anterior procedure had higher rates of curve progression, implant breakage, and pseudarthrosis than the group undergoing the posterior procedure.

In a **retrospective study** Berven and co-workers[39] reviewed their institution's results for combined anterior and posterior surgery in patients with deformity, specifically fixed sagittal imbalance. Although the majority of patients had diagnoses of iatrogenic kyphosis or adult idiopathic scoliosis, the analysis of these authors does shed light on some factors to consider when determining whether to use a combined approach in patients with degenerative scoliosis. Many patients with degenerative lumbar scoliosis have hypolordosis, so addressing sagittal balance is essential when correcting the deformity surgically. The cohort in the study by Berven and co-workers was predominantly female and had an average age of 58 years, which is similar to, but slightly younger than, the typical patient with degenerative scoliosis. They evaluated their results clinically by analyzing patient satisfaction using validated surveys, complication rates, and the need for revision surgery (40%), as well as radiographically by examining preoperative, postoperative, and follow-up radiographs. Overall, 82% of patients were satisfied with the results of the surgery. The perioperative complication rate was 32%, and the late complication rate was 40%; wound infection was the most common early complication (4 of 25 patients) and pseudarthrosis was the most common late complication (5 of 25 patients). Other than pseudarthrosis, late reasons for revision were prominent hardware and late infection. Despite the complication rate, 23 of 25 patients stated that they would probably or definitely repeat the surgery. Radiographically, the deformity correction afforded by the combined approach was significant. Preoperative lumbar lordosis improved from an average of −23 degrees to −42 degrees (with positive values implying kyphosis). The average Cobb angle improved from 47 degrees preoperatively to 26 degrees postoperatively. Despite the overall improvement in alignment, the degree of improvement did not correlate well with outcome scores. The authors also found that patients with the greatest preoperative lumbar hypolordosis had the best outcome scores. Specifically, the group that had improvement of lumbar lordosis had better outcomes than those who did not have improvement in regional sagittal balance.

Although the deformity correction afforded by a dual approach may be quite impressive, there is morbidity associated with the additional anesthesia, and more importantly there is morbidity specific to the anterior approach. A patient history of previous abdominal surgery helps alert the spine and approach surgeons of potential difficulty due to adhesions or scar. The most dire consequences arise from mobilizing the aorta and inferior vena cava. Arterial occlusion can lead to limb loss if not addressed promptly. Arterial laceration, although potential devastating, can usually be repaired, whereas laceration of the inferior vena cava is much more challenging to repair. Even smaller vessels that have to be mobilized during the approach, such as the iliolumbar vein and lumbar segmental vessels, can cause significant bleeding if not ligated at the appropriate location. Once the approach procedure is completed, implant placement must be carefully performed to avoid penetration of the spinal canal or prominence deep to the vessels once the latter have been returned to their native locations.

In the immediately postoperative period ileus is quite common, although less so with a retroperitoneal approach. A transperitoneal approach places the hypogastric plexus at greater risk. Injury to this plexus can put men at risk of retrograde ejaculation. Although an ileus may be the most common cause of abdominal discomfort or distention, a retroperitoneal hematoma or lymphocele may also occur and may require a return to the operating room.[40] Heyworth and colleagues[41] reported that a splenic rupture was found on exploratory laparotomy 2 days after an anterior spinal fusion. Patients are also at increased risk of deep vein thrombosis and pulmonary embolism, especially after a right-sided thoracoabdominal procedure.[42] Repeat surgery using abdominal approaches early in the postoperative course may be possible through the original tissue planes, but late surgery may require the use of contralateral retroperitoneal approaches or transabdominal approaches. The literature on revision of lumbar disk arthroplasty warns of some of the risks.[43] Revision surgeries using anterior approaches are potentially life- or limb-threatening operations. Mok and co-workers also found that that staged operations in adult patients with spinal deformity were associated with a higher incidence of infection, although in their study combined anterior-posterior procedures performed on the same day carried infection rates similar to those of posterior-only approaches.[20]

Patients have long-term complaints as well. In a study by Horton and colleagues performed through the SRS, a survey of patients who underwent anterior surgery revealed complaints of incisional pain, umbilical asymmetry, and pseudohernia. The incidence was highest after surgeries using thoracoabdominal approaches, followed by thoracic and then paramedial procedures.[44] Fortunately, most anterior procedures performed to treat adult degenerative scoliosis are paramedial, especially with modern posterior instrumentation.

The posterior approach provides an opportunity to treat deformity and stenosis in a single procedure. Decompression of neural elements, including central, lateral recess, and foraminal, can be performed effectively. The only type of stenosis that may be better decompressed anteriorly is focal kyphosis, for example, from a compression fracture. The process of lateral recess and foraminal decompression naturally leads toward the Smith-Peterson osteotomy and modern posteriorly based interbody fusion techniques. The fusion technique is fairly straightforward with the posterolateral approach and uses segmental instrumentation. A circumferential fusion of the lumbosacral junction may be achieved with a posteriorly based interbody approach. However, deformity correction and restoration of lordosis may be significantly compromised when a posteriorly based interbody approach rather than an anterior and posterior approach is used at the lower lumbar spine.[45,46]

Posteriorly based osteotomies allow gradual correction of deformity with multiple Smith-Peterson osteotomies or greater focal correction with a pedicle subtraction osteotomy. Smith-Peterson osteotomies release an individual level without sacrificing a fixation level and allow 5 to 8 degrees of correction of sagittal balance per level. Pedicle subtraction osteotomies are much more powerful, allowing 10 to 20 degrees of sagittal correction with a single osteotomy. Pedicle subtraction osteotomies also can be performed asymmetrically to help correct coronal imbalance, which of course is important in patients with degenerative scoliosis. The blood loss is more extensive with pedicle subtraction osteotomies, so patients must be monitored carefully by the anesthesia team. These osteotomies are not without risk to the neural elements. Although they are still not risk free with modern neuromonitoring techniques, the addition of electromyography and monitoring of motor evoked potentials to measurement of somatosensory evoked potentials provides much greater sensitivity in detecting neural stretch and compression injuries.[47]

Cho and associates **prospectively** studied outcomes and complication rates for 47 patients undergoing surgery for degenerative scoliosis and **retrospectively** reviewed the radiographic results. The characteristics of the patients in their group were very similar to those of the typical patients this chapter addresses, and a similar surgical approach of posterior decompression and fusion with the aid of pedicle screw instrumentation was used. There was a 68% complication rate, with both early and late complications, and high intraoperative blood loss was an important predictive factor for early complications.[48]

Pateder and co-workers[49] compared results in a heterogenous group of adult scoliosis patients who underwent either posterior-only or combined anterior-posterior surgery to correct their deformity. This was a **retrospective study,** so the need for an anterior approach and the possible use of anterior instrumentation was determined on a case-by-case basis by the senior surgeon in the study. The radiographic correction was comparable for the posterior-only and the combined approaches. Of note, the complication rate was higher (45%) in the combined-approach group when the two procedures were staged, but only 23% to 24% in the single-approach group and in the dual-approach group when both the anterior and posterior procedures were performed on the same day. Similarly, Good and colleagues[50] compared outcomes for posterior-only procedures using osteotomies and transforaminal lumbar interbody fusions with combined anterior-posterior procedures for treatment of adult scoliosis. They found that posterior-only surgery produced better radiographic correction and was associated with shorter surgical time, less blood loss, and shorter hospital length of stay, whereas a trend toward a higher pseudarthrosis rate was seen for anterior-posterior procedures. The complication rate was comparable for the two procedures.

Berven and co-workers[51] reviewed clinical and radiographic outcomes in 38 patients treated surgically for degenerative scoliosis with a minimum of 2 years' follow-up. Thirty patients were treated with posterior-only fusion, four with anterior-only surgery, and four with a combined procedure. All patients with instrumentation above L1 underwent anterior or transforaminal lumbar interbody fusion for structural support of the anterior column. There were clearly some differences between the groups: Patients in the anterior-only group had greater preoperative curves (mean of 54.8 degrees in the anterior-only group vs. 25.6 degrees in the posterior-only group and 36.2 degrees in the combined-approach group) and were younger (mean age of 41.3 years in the anterior-only group vs. 68.3 years in the posterior-only group and 52.5 years in the combined-approach group). The anterior-only group had more lumbar lordosis preoperatively, whereas the posterior-only group had more thoracic kyphosis. Those who underwent fusion of the structural thoracic spine did not require revision, whereas 6 of 33 patients who had fusion below the structural thoracic spine required cephalad revision. Caudually, only 2 of 21 patients who did not have a lumbosacral fusion required revision fusion to the sacrum, whereas none of the 17 patients who initially underwent fusion to the sacrum required revision of distal fixation. Interestingly, the proportion of patients who required revision was similar among those undergoing fusion below the cephalad extent of the coronal curve (3 of 17) and among those undergoing fusion at or above the curve (3 of 15).

Clinical outcomes (evaluated using the Short Form 36 [SF-36] Health Survey and the SRS 30 Patient Questionnaire) were reported in this article and illustrated the variable outcomes in surgical treatment of degenerative scoliosis. Although a majority of patients felt that they had improved with regard to pain and function, 21% felt that their pain was worse, and 34% felt that their function was worse after surgery. Those who had worse function were typically older, and those whose pain was worse tended to have less severe curves and also were older. Patients who underwent an anterior procedure had lower postoperative pain, even after the differences in patient variables were accounted for using multiple regression analysis. As other authors have similarly noted, patients with less preoperative lumbar lordosis were more satisfied with the results of surgery. The investigation by Berven and associates, although presenting a thorough review of results for their patients, highlights some of the limitations in studying patients with degenerative scoliosis, because surgical treatment is difficult to randomize given the need to individualize the management plan to the patient based on the patient's spinal deformity, age, and comorbid conditions.

Kim and co-workers[52] conducted a **retrospective study** of outcomes in 48 patients with lumbar scoliosis, both de novo and adult idiopathic, who were divided into two groups based on treatment. Group I was treated with an anterior release via a thoracoabdominal procedure followed by posterior spinal fusion, whereas group II underwent correction via a posteriorly based procedure with anterior or transforaminal interbody fusion for lumbosacral support. Group II treated with the posteriorly based procedure did have slightly smaller Cobb angles (56 degrees for group II vs. 63 degrees for group I) and more flexible curves (27% for group II vs. 37% for group I on bending radiographs), but the preoperative SRS outcome scores were similar. Postoperative radiographic analysis revealed similar correction in the coronal plane and similar improvement in the sagittal plane. There were more complications in group I, which underwent anterior release first (61%), than in group II, which underwent posteriorly based correction with anterior lumbosacral grafting (20%). Group II had significantly higher postoperative outcome scores (79% for group II vs. 70% for group I), and significant differences favoring group II were also seen in scores on the subscales of pain, self-image, and function with a trend toward differences in satisfaction.

COMMENTARY

The surgical approach to management of adult degenerative scoliosis is characterized by significant variability. There are limited data to guide an evidence-based approach to specific cases, and considerations such as curve characteristics, patient comorbid conditions, and preferences of the patient and surgeon have an important impact on operative strategies.

Posteriorly based approaches to treatment of adult deformity permit a single-stage decompression of neural elements with correction of deformity. Posterior approaches may minimize operative morbidity and limit the need for surgical staging over separate days. Three-column osteotomies, including pedicle subtraction osteotomy and posteriorly based vertebral column resection, may permit significant correction of global sagittal and coronal plane deformity.

The limitations of posteriorly based surgery in the treatment of degenerative scoliosis relate primarily to the lumbosacral junction. In patients with fixed obliquity at the lumbosacral junction and patients with segmental hypolordosis between L4 and S1, a more reliable correction of deformity can be achieved using an anterior approach to the lumbosacral spine. Fusion at the lumbosacral junction is also more reliable when a combined anterior and posterior approach is used. In patients with a structural fractional curve, adopting a limited approach to the lumbosacral junction using a combined anterior and posterior approach may restrict the morbidity of the surgical approach, while providing an effective treatment for well-localized pathologic changes.

REFERENCES

1. Hu SS: Adult scoliosis. In Herkowitz H, editor: *The spine*, ed 5, Philadelphia, 2006, Elsevier, pp 1046–1057.
2. Benner B, Ehni G: Degenerative lumbar scoliosis, *Spine* 4:548–552, 1979.
3. Pritchett JW, Bortel DT: Degenerative symptomatic lumbar scoliosis, *Spine* 18(6):700–703, 1993. This article describes natural course of degenerative lumbar scoliosis and risk factors for progression. Clinical presentation and some nonoperative treatment options were discussed. Radiographs were studied to delineate typical curve cephalad and caudad levels along with concomitant frequency of spondylolisthesis.
4. Grubb SA, Lipscomb HJ, Suh PB: Results of surgical treatment of painful adult scoliosis, *Spine* 19(14):1619–1627, 1994. This article examines idiopathic adult scoliosis and degenerative scoliosis. Degnerative scoliosis patients had improved walking and standing tolerance postoperatively, but no significant change in sitting tolerance. The complication rate and types are well documented. In deciding levels for surgical treatment pain producing pathology was identified, not simply relying on radiographic findings. Coronal and sagittal balance was important in addressing degenerative scoliosis.

5. Schwab F, Farcy JP, Bridwell K, et al: A clinical impact classification of scoliosis in the adult, *Spine* 31(18):2109–2114, 2006.

6. Pappou IP, Girardi FP, Sandhu HS, et al: Discordantly high spinal bone mineral density values in patients with adult lumbar scoliosis, *Spine* 31(14):1614–1620, 2006.

7. Tribus CB: Degenerative lumbar scoliosis: evaluation and management, *J Am Acad Orthop Surg* 11(3):174–183, 2003.

8. Glassman SD, Berven S, Bridwell K, et al: Correlation of radiographic parameters and clinical symptoms in adult scoliosis, *Spine* 30(6):682–688, 2005. **Sagittal balance matters, with positive sagittal balance being correlated with worse function and pain. Coronal balance only matters if greater than 4 cm off midline in previously unoperated patients. Lumbar hypolordosis is also correlated with worse function and pain, independent of global sagittal balance. Upper thoracic kyphosis is well tolerated.**

9. Schwab F, Farcy JP, Bridwell K, et al: A clinical impact classification of scoliosis in the adult, *Spine* 31(18):2109–2114, 2006.

10. Glassman SD, Schwab FJ, Bridwell KH, et al: The selection of operative versus nonoperative treatment in patients with adult scoliosis, *Spine* 32(1):93–97, 2007.

11. Pekmezci M, Berven SH, Hu SS, Deviren V: The factors that play a role in the decision-making process of adult deformity patients, *Spine* 34(8):813–817, 2009. **This article evaluates factors important in proceeding to surgical treatment of adult scoliosis. This article does not analyze patients with degenerative scoliosis separately. The authors found that functional limitation, specifically walking, influenced patients to choose surgery. Pain levels statistically trended towards importance for surgical treatment. Curve magnitude had no impact.**

12. Bess S, Boachie-Adjei O, Burton D, et al: International Spine Study Group: Pain and disability determine treatment modality for older patients with adult scoliosis, while deformity guides treatment for younger patients, *Spine* 34(20):2186–2190, 2009.

13. Briard JL, Jegou D, Cauchoix J: Adult lumbar scoliosis, *Orthop Clin North Am* 19:339–346, 1998.

14. Kostuik JP: Treatment of scoliosis in the adult thoracolumbar spine with special reference to fusion to the sacrum [review], *Orthop Clin North Am.* 19(2):371–381, 1988.

15. Grubb SA, Lipscomb HJ: Diagnostic findings in painful adult scoliosis, *Spine* 17:518–529, 1992.

16. Schwab FJ, Lafage V, Farcy JP, et al: Predicting outcome and complications in the surgical treatment of adult scoliosis, *Spine* 33(20):2243–2247, 2008.

17. Akbarnia BA, Ogilvie JW, Hammerberg KW: Debate: degenerative scoliosis: to operate or not to operate, *Spine* 31(Suppl 19):S195–S201, 2006.

18. Weistroffer JK, Perra JH, Lonstein JE, et al: Complications in long fusions to the sacrum for adult scoliosis: minimum five-year analysis of fifty patients, *Spine* 33(13):1478–1483, 2008.

19. Berven SH, Deviren V, Smith JA, et al: Management of fixed sagittal plane deformity: outcome of combined anterior and posterior surgery, *Spine* 28(15):1710–1715, 2003.

20. Mok JM, Cloyd JM, Bradford DS, et al: Reoperation after primary fusion for adult spinal deformity: rate, reason, and timing, *Spine* 34(8):832–839, 2009.

21. Smith JS, Shaffrey CI, Glassman SD, et al: The Spinal Deformity Study Group. Risk-benefit assessment of surgery for adult scoliosis: an analysis based on patient age, *Spine* 36(10):817–824, 2011.

22. Glassman SD, Carreon LY, Shaffrey CI, et al: The costs and benefits of nonoperative management for adult scoliosis, *Spine* 35(5):578–582, 2010.

23. Bridwell KH, Glassman S, Horton W, et al: Does treatment (nonoperative and operative) improve the two-year quality of life in patients with adult symptomatic lumbar scoliosis: a prospective multicenter evidence-based medicine study, *Spine* 34(20):2171–2178, 2009.

24. Smith JS, Shaffrey CI, Berven S, et al: Spinal Deformity Study Group. Improvement of back pain with operative and nonoperative treatment in adults with scoliosis, *Neurosurgery* 65(1):86–93, 2009. discussion, 93-94.

25. Smith JS, Shaffrey CI, Berven S, et al: Spinal Deformity Study Group. Operative versus nonoperative treatment of leg pain in adults with scoliosis: a retrospective review of a prospective multicenter database with two-year follow-up, *Spine* 34(16):1693–1698, 2009.

26. Bradford DS, Tay BK, Hu SS: Adult scoliosis: surgical indications, operative management, complications, and outcomes, *Spine* 24(24):2617–2629, 1999.

27. Bridwell KH, DeWald RL: Adult scoliosis and related deformities. In Bridwell KH, editor: *The textbook of spinal surgery,* ed 2, vol 1, Philadelphia, 1997, Lippincott-Raven Publishers, pp 777–795.

28. Gupta MC: Degenerative scoliosis: options for surgical management, *Orthop Clin North Am* 34(2): 269–279, 2003.

29. Bridwell KH: Decision making regarding Smith-Petersen vs. pedicle subtraction osteotomy vs. vertebral column resection for spinal deformity [review], *Spine* 31(Suppl 19):S171–S178, 2006.

30. Lebwohl NH, Cunningham BW, Dmitriev A, et al: Biomechanical comparison of lumbosacral fixation techniques in a calf spine model, *Spine* 27:2312–2320, 2002.

31. Kasten MD, Rao LA, Priest B: Long-term results of iliac wing fixation below extensive fusions in ambulatory adult patients with spinal disorders, *J Spinal Disord Tech* 23(7):e37–e42, 2010.

32. Shufflebarger H, Suk SI, Mardjetko S: Debate: determining the upper instrumented vertebra in the management of adult degenerative scoliosis: stopping at T10 versus L1, *Spine* 31(Suppl 19): S185–S194, 2006.

33. Glattes RB, Bridwell KH, Lenke LG, et al: Proximal junctional kyphosis in adult spinal deformity following long instrumented posterior spinal fusion: incidence, outcomes, and risk factor analysis, *Spine* 30(14):1643–1649, 2005.

34. Kim JH, Kim SS, Suk SI: Incidence of proximal adjacent failure in adult lumbar deformity correction based on proximal fusion level, *Asian Spine J* 1(1):19–26, 2007.

35. Bridwell KH, Berven S, Edwards C, et al: The problems and limitations of applying evidence-based medicine to primary surgical treatment of adult spinal deformity, *Spine* 32(Suppl 19):S135–S139, 2007.

36. Hodgson AR, Stock FE, Fang HS, et al: Anterior spinal fusion. The operative approach and pathological findings in 412 patients with Pott's disease of the spine, *Br J Surg* 48:172–178, 1960.

37. McLain RF: The biomechanics of long versus short fixation for thoracolumbar spine fractures, *Spine* 31(Suppl 11):S70–S79, 2006.

38. Betz RR, Harms J, Clements DH 3rd, et al: Comparison of anterior and posterior instrumentation for correction of adolescent thoracic idiopathic scoliosis, *Spine* 24(3):225–239, 1999.

39. Berven SH, Deviren V, Smith JA, et al: Management of fixed sagittal plane deformity: outcome of combined anterior and posterior surgery, *Spine* 28(15):1710–1715, 2003.

40. Patel AA, Spiker WR, Daubs MD, et al: Retroperitoneal lymphocele after anterior spinal surgery, *Spine* 33(18):E648–E652, 2008.

41. Heyworth BE, Schwab JH, Boachie-Adjei OB: Case reports: splenic rupture after anterior thoracolumbar spinal fusion through a thoracoabdominal approach, *Clin Orthop Relat Res* 466(9):2271–2275, 2008.

42. Piasecki DP, Poynton AR, Mintz DN, et al: Thromboembolic disease after combined anterior/posterior reconstruction for adult spinal deformity: a prospective cohort study using magnetic resonance venography, *Spine* 33(6):668–672, 2008.

43. McAfee PC, Geisler FH, Saiedy SS, et al: Revisability of CHARITE artificial disc replacement: analysis of 688 patients enrolled in the U.S. IDE study of the CHARITE Artificial Disc, *Spine* 31(11):1217–1226, 2006.

44. Horton W, et al: Morbidity of the open anterior approach, Paper presented at the Scoliosis Research Society 40th Annual Meeting, 2005.

45. Kwon BK, Berta S, Daffner SD, et al: Radiographic analysis of transforaminal lumbar interbody fusion for the treatment of adult isthmic spondylolisthesis, *J Spinal Disord Tech* 16(5):469–476, 2003.

46. Groth AT, Kuklo TR, Klemme WR, et al: Comparison of sagittal contour and posterior disc height following interbody fusion: threaded cylindrical cages versus structural allograft versus vertical cages, *J Spinal Disord Tech* 18(4):332–336, 2005.

47. Lieberman JA, Lyon R, Feiner J, et al: The efficacy of motor evoked potentials in fixed sagittal imbalance deformity correction surgery, *Spine* 33(13):E414–E424, 2008.

48. Cho KJ, Suk SI, Park SR, et al: Complications in posterior fusion and instrumentation for degenerative lumbar scoliosis, *Spine* 32(20):2232–2237, 2007. **Forty-seven patients were followed for early (less than 3 months postoperatively) and late complications as well as minor and major complications. Age was not a statistically significant risk factor, but $p = 0.053$. Adjacent segment disease was discussed and separated by previous levels of fusion. Other adjacent segment problems such as fractures in addition to stenosis were addressed. Blood loss increased early postoperative problems. Increased number of levels was associated with increased complications. Increased preoperative positive sagittal balance was also associated with increased complications.**

49. Pateder DB, Kebais KM, Cascio BM, et al: Posterior only versus combined anterior and posterior approaches to lumbar scoliosis in adults: a radiographic analysis, *Spine* 32(14):1551–1554, 2007.

50. Good CR, Lenke LG, Bridwell, et al: Can posterior-only surgery provide similar radiographic and clinical results as combined anterior (thoracotomy/thoracoabdominal)/posterior approaches for adult scoliosis? *Spine* 35(2):210–218, 2010.

51. Berven SH, Deviren V, Mitchell B, et al: Operative management of degenerative scoliosis: an evidence-based approach to surgical strategies based on clinical and radiographic outcomes, *Neurosurg Clin N Am* 18(2):261–272, 2007.

52. Kim YB, Lenke LG, Kim YJ, et al: Surgical treatment of adult scoliosis: is anterior apical release and fusion necessary for the lumbar curve? *Spine* 33(10):1125–1132, 2008.

Chapter 18   Sagittal Imbalance: Multiple Smith-Petersen Osteotomies Versus Pedicle Subtraction Osteotomies

Jamal McClendon, Jr., Tyler R. Koski, Stephen L. Ondra, Frank L. Acosta, Jr.

Scoliosis is a complex three-dimensional rotational deformity affecting the spine in the coronal, sagittal, and axial planes. Treatment paradigms should address all three components of this disorder. Surgical treatment of spinal deformities may be accomplished through anterior, posterior, or combined approaches for correction. Fixed thoracic or lumbar deformity is a complex surgical problem that has been addressed by anterior release and posterior correction with fusion.[1] An osteotomy carried through all three columns of the spine offers the advantage of avoiding anterior exposure.[1] The posterior-only approach itself offers many options. Surgical correction through this approach includes various osteotomy techniques. The inferior facetectomy provides limited corrective ability, but the Smith-Petersen osteotomy (SPO), or a modification of this technique, provides comparatively more correction. Techniques with larger corrective potential include the pedicle subtraction osteotomy (PSO), the extended pedicle subtraction osteotomy, and the vertebral column resection (VCR).

In recent years, posterior-only approaches for treatment of deformity have provided the framework for surgical techniques for correction in the sagittal and coronal plane. Segmental fixation with pedicle screws and rods, and the use of osteotomies through a posterior approach, preclude the need for anterior releases or anterior corpectomies.[2] Addressing deformity through a posterior-only approach avoids the morbidity of an anterior approach while obtaining correction equivalent to that achieved using a combined anterior-posterior approach.[2] Before any osteotomy is attempted on the spine for correction of deformity, sufficient surgical experience and a thorough understanding of the anatomy of the spine and regional structures are imperative.[3]

Osteotomies are performed to treat the following conditions: junctional kyphosis, ankylosing spondylitis, posttraumatic kyphosis, postlaminectomy kyphosis, idiopathic kyphoscoliosis, degenerative scoliosis, Scheuermann kyphosis, iatrogenic flat back, neuromuscular kyphosis, and congenital kyphosis. Patients are often classified as having either flexible or fixed deformity. Flexible sagittal deformity implies change in the sagittal vertical axis when gravity is removed as a variable (i.e., the patient is placed in a recumbent position). A flexible coronal deformity is not rigid, so that radiographs taken in the side-bending position demonstrate movement. Patients with a fixed sagittal deformity may have a subjective perception of imbalance.[3,4] They may lean forward, have a stooped posture, develop early fatigue, experience intractable pain, and be unable to maintain a horizontal gaze.[3,4] In cases of flexible sagittal imbalance or mild sagittal deformity, correction can be accomplished through positioning on the surgical table and segmental instrumentation. However, an osteotomy is often needed for correction in cases of rigid or fixed deformity.[3] The goal is to restore sagittal balance so that the patient can stand without flexion at the hips or knees for compensation and to reduce pain with ambulation.

CASE PRESENTATIONS

Case 1

A 48-year-old woman developed progressive pain at the area of a previous lumbar fusion as well as worsening sagittal imbalance.

- PMH: Unremarkable
- PSH: The patient previously underwent an L3-S1 posterior lumbar interbody fusion at another institution. She also had facet arthropathy from T12 to L3.
- Exam: Neurologically normal except positive sagittal balance
- Imaging: Preoperative standing lateral 14 × 36 inch plain films demonstrating positive sagittal balance and lumbar hypolordosis

The patient underwent corrective surgery with removal of her segmental instrumentation from L3 to S1, exploration of her fusion from L3 to S1, placement of segmental instrumentation from T10 to S1, and performance of an L2 PSO for correction of kyphosis (Figures 18-1 and 18-2).

FIGURE 18-1 Preoperative standing lateral scoliosis radiograph. Note the patient's preexisting instrumentation and interbodies.

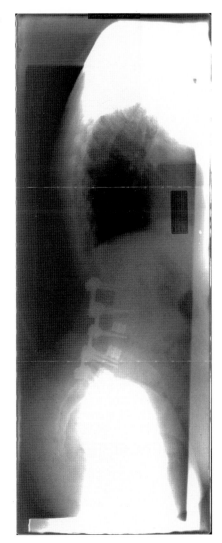

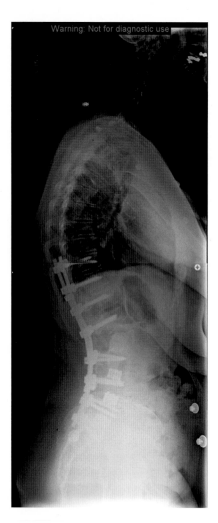

FIGURE 18-2 Postoperative standing lateral scoliosis radiograph. Note the construct extension proximally and the pedicle subtraction osteotomy.

Case 2

A 69-year-old man had progressive lower back pain and bilateral radiculopathy. He has been unable to stand fully erect or ambulate without severe back pain. He has failed conservative management. He also has noted weakness of 4 out of 5 strength in his left dorsiflexion.

- PMH: Unremarkable
- PSH: Unremarkable
- Exam: The patient also had a slight left foot drop.
- Imaging:

The patient underwent surgery that included placement of segmental instrumentation from T10 to S1/ilium, SPOs at T12-L1, L1-2, L2-3, L3-4, L4-5, and L5-6, and transforaminal lumbar interbody fusion at L6 to S1 for correction of kyphosis (Figures 18-3 through 18-6).

SURGICAL OPTIONS

Preoperative workup is important for all patients undergoing osteotomies. Patients may be evaluated preoperatively by an internist, family physician, and/or a cardiologist depending on medical comorbid conditions. Patients often undergo computed tomography (CT) of the spine covering the regions to be included in the intended fusion to evaluate for bone integrity.[1] Thin-cut CT

FIGURE 18-3 Preoperative standing lateral scoliosis radiograph showing gross sagittal alignment. Note the patient's lack of lumbar lordosis.

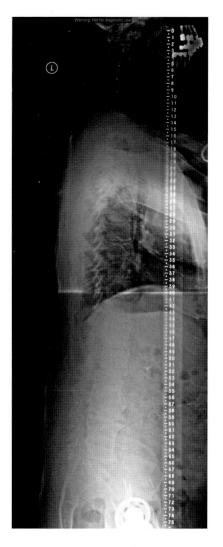

scans with sagittal reconstructions are valuable in accurately identifying anky-losed regions of the spine, both in the anterior and middle columns as well as along the facet joints.[1] Standing long-cassette anteroposterior (AP) and lateral radiographs are obtained for all patients. Also, initial workup includes assess-ment of the flexibility of the spine. Spinal rigidity is assessed based on standing and supine radiographs. For sagittal deformity, this is accomplished by obtain-ing long-cassette AP and lateral radiographs with the patient standing, supine, prone, or supported by a bolster.[5] For coronal deformity, lateral side-bending radiographs are also obtained. If the deformity is fixed and no correction is observed with positional change, or if it is partially fixed with some degree of correction occurring through adjacent mobile segments, then an osteotomy may be appropriate.[5-7]

Patient risk and intraoperative morbidity, including blood loss from surgery, are weighed when deciding what corrective osteotomy will be advantageous for a patient with coronal and/or sagittal imbalance. The larger corrective osteoto-mies, although more powerful, are associated with increased technical demands, longer operative time, greater blood loss, and procedure-related morbidity.[2] The VCR, in particular, carries the greatest risk to the patient in terms of possible neurologic injury, operative time, and potential morbidity, but achieves the most correction in the coronal and sagittal planes.[2] This chapter focuses on the SPO and the PSO.

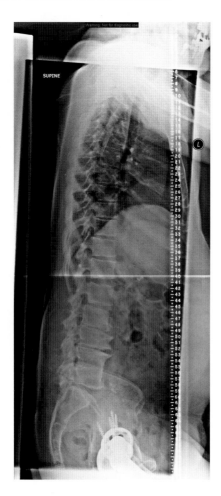

FIGURE 18-4 Preoperative supine lateral scoliosis radiograph. Note that the patient does not have substantial spine flexibility when gravity is removed as a variable.

FUNDAMENTAL TECHNIQUE

Smith-Petersen Osteotomies

In 1945, Smith-Petersen and colleagues[5,8-10] first described the technique of posterior-element osteotomy and posterior compression. It was principally used for treating ankylosing spondylitis. This technique also was used to treat flexion deformities in individuals with rheumatoid arthritis and ankylosed or autofused spines.[2,5,8] They resected the spinous processes, removed the edges of the laminae, resected the ligamentum flavum, and performed oblique osteotomies with an osteotome forward and upward through part of the inferior and superior articular processes (the synostosed articular processes).[11] Correction through rupture of the anterior tension band results in profound anterior lengthening. The middle column or posterior part of the annulus serves as the pivot or fulcrum, and because the wedge is closed posteriorly, the disk space opens anteriorly.[2,3,7,8,12] The SPO involves removal of the posterior ligaments (supraspinous, intraspinous, and ligamentum flavum) and resection of the facets at one or more levels to produce a posterior release, which aids in coronal correction and sagittal plane realignment.[2,5] The osteotomies either hinge or slightly shorten the middle column.[5] Also, producing an anterior gap may make arthrodesis less reliable.[12,13] Rupture of the anterior longitudinal ligament carries the risk of injury to vascular structures anterior to the spine.[2,8] The lengthening of the anterior column can be associated with vascular and neurologic complications.[9,12,14-16] This may be especially true in the elderly or in patients with ankylosing spondylitis, who may have significantly calcified vessels, including the aorta and the vena cava.[6,7] Modifications have been suggested to avoid such complications.[12,17,18]

FIGURE 18-5 Preoperative supine lateral radiograph with the patient over a bolster. Note the curve flexibility seen in the lumbar spine.

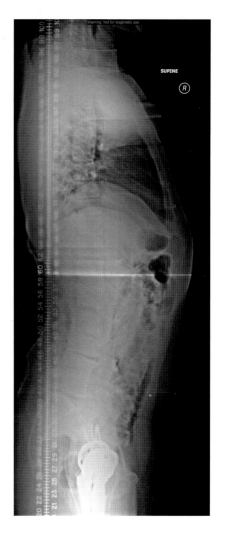

Law[19,20] described a modification of the corrective lumbar osteotomy for ankylosing spondylitis, but found it unnecessary to divide the anterior longitudinal ligament.

Hehne and colleagues[2,17] also described a multisegmented osteotomy that achieved lordosis through resection of a portion of the posterior elements at each level, producing about 10 degrees per segment. The lordosis correction was described as "harmonious." In addition, Ponte and associates[2,21] further elaborated on the use of wide segmental osteotomies and posterior compression along unfused regions of the spine in patients with Scheuermann kyphosis. Ponte[21-23] advocated a posterior-only procedure consisting of posterior column shortening via multiple wide segmental osteotomies and posterior compression with instrumentation and fusion. This modification of the SPO did not require anterior osteoclasis.[3] They were developed for a gentle correction at multiple levels using the same technique.[3] This method gave a more overall correction from the closing of the dorsal osteotomy without fracturing the anterior column.[3,17]

Although the name *Smith-Petersen osteotomy* seems to encompass the original osteotomy technique involving posterior column resection and anterior osteoclasis and also the modification, the technique most commonly used today (modification) is referred to in this chapter. Multiple SPOs have been useful for treating fixed sagittal imbalance in conditions like ankylosing spondylitis and iatrogenic sagittal imbalance.[5,17,24,25] Compression of an SPO after transpedicular fixation can correct kyphosis. An adequate intervertebral disk height and a mobile disk space anteriorly add to the corrective potential.

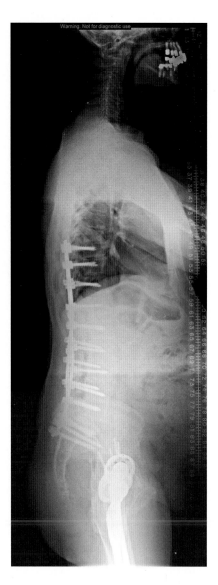

FIGURE 18-6 Postoperative lateral scoliosis radiograph after multiple Smith-Petersen osteotomies and instrumentation from T10 to S1/ilium.

Tips from the Masters 18-1 • Compression can lead to narrowing of the neural foramina, which necessitates a preceding wide facetectomy to prevent nerve root impingement.

However, correction may be challenging if there is a fully ossified anterior longitudinal ligament. PSOs have also been described for the treatment of these conditions.[4,5,11,26,27]

Indications for SPO include ample intervertebral disk height anteriorly and laterally, a mobile disk without ankylosis, and a smooth curve. The SPO requires disk space flexibility to allow for coronal and/or sagittal correction.[6] A long, rounded, smooth kyphosis is often an ideal target for multiple SPOs.[3,5] The classic indication for an SPO is a long, gradual, rounded kyphosis as in Scheuermann kyphosis.[2,3,5] The surgeon may consider another type of osteotomy if there is a thick bridging anterior osteophyte. Although an anterior gap may be present after an SPO, there is no need for an anterior bone graft.[3] Coronal and sagittal imbalance may be addressed with an SPO; it affords gradual correction of kyphotic or scoliotic curves.[2] The degree of kyphotic correction afforded by an SPO has been reported to be in the range of 9.3 to 10.7 degrees per level, with approximately 1 degree per millimeter of bone resected.[2,5,12,22] Technically, these osteotomies can be used at multiple levels within a fusion construct and offer powerful correction globally across a kyphotic segment.[2] However, focal regions of kyphosis may be amenable to use of other osteotomies for correction. If there is a fine bony ridge anteriorly, it can potentially be broken with closed reduction.[5] After closure of an SPO, there is bone on bone of the posterior column centrally and laterally.[5]

At the time of the surgery, patients are appropriately padded and positioned prone on a Jackson table. This permits the patient's abdomen to float freely and allows gravity to assist in pulling the lumbar spine back into lordosis. Lordosis can be achieved by using an open Jackson table so that the abdomen hangs free. This is particularly helpful for nonrigid or flexible sagittal imbalance. Placing additional height on the chest pad helps to achieve further lumbar lordosis on the table. Intraoperatively, you obtain lordosis based on your correction technique. Neurophysiologic monitoring with measurement of somatosensory evoked potentials and transcranial motor evoked potentials is often used for SPOs (and routinely for PSOs). Normotension is always rigorously maintained throughout surgery to ensure adequate spinal cord perfusion. Patients typically have an arterial line and a central venous line in place to allow for blood pressure monitoring and volume resuscitation during surgery. The coagulation profile is closely monitored intraoperatively by the anesthesiologist. The incision is made and subperiosteal dissection is performed to expose the posterior spinal elements. If needed, existing segmental instrumentation is removed, and the old fusion mass is explored if present. Pedicle screws are placed at all levels involved in the fusion. For completion of an SPO, the lamina and facet joints are removed completely using an osteotome, Kerrison rongeur, or high-speed drill in an oblique manner at the desired level. A V-shaped gutter is created.[3] The width of the gutter should be between 10 and 15 mm.[3] Correction is performed by compression of the posterior elements until closure. Compression should be performed gradually over multiple segments at the same time to redistribute the corrective forces over a large area of the spinal column. Rods are set and decortication is performed before wound closure. A cross-table scoliosis radiograph is taken at the end of the procedure to ensure that adequate correction has been obtained.

Pedicle Subtraction Osteotomy

In 1963, Scudese and Calabro described a vertebral wedge osteotomy for the correction of lumbar kyphosis in a patient with ankylosing spondylitis.[3,28] They removed the back part of the upper surface of the body of a lumbar vertebra and wedged the disk space and body with posterior narrowing.[3,28] This led the way to the technique known today as the *pedicle subtraction osteotomy*. The PSO was first described by Thomasen in 1985.[11] This osteotomy has also been referred to as a *transpedicular wedge procedure, closing wedge osteotomy,* and *eggshell osteotomy*.[2,3,11] The technique involves removal of the posterior ligaments and facets—as in an SPO—followed by bilateral pediculectomy and decancellation of a wedge of the vertebral body via a transpedicular corridor.[2] A resection that includes the disk space above the decancellated segment is described as an extended PSO.[2,5] Closure of this osteotomy occurs in wedge fashion, which brings about kyphosis correction through posterior shortening.[2] If performed in an asymmetric fashion, the osteotomy can also lead to significant coronal correction.[2] This closure also creates a large contact area of cancellous bone, which is beneficial for fusion of the vertebral body. The technique also creates a superforamen. Segmental correction by a PSO depends on the level at which the osteotomy is performed.[1]

For a PSO, pedicle screws are placed above and below the level of the osteotomy.

Tips from the Masters 18-2 • A pedicle preparatory hole is created at the level of the PSO, which is useful to maintain orientation during bony removal.

The posterior elements and pedicles are then resected. When there is an existing posterior fusion mass, resection of the fusion mass is performed in accordance with posterior closure goals using osteotomes, rongeurs, and curettes, and all bone is saved for use in later fusion. A temporary rod is often placed to prevent unwanted movement. A laminectomy in excess of the posterior laminar closure goals is performed at the osteotomy level to minimize any dural impingement at the time of PSO closure. In revision cases, exposure of the normal dura is performed at the level adjacent to the previous decompression and a plane is developed between the dura and adjacent scar. This scar tissue is removed from the dura where the osteotomy is intended to prevent the compression that can occur with closure. Thoracic nerve roots are not routinely sacrificed, but can be if needed. The next step is to decancellate the pedicle. Retraction of the thecal sac medially helps in identifying the posterior wall of the vertebral body and the pedicles. After posterior-element and pedicle resection, dissection of the lateral vertebral body wall is carried out bilaterally with Penfield 1 and Kittner dissectors. Lateral vertebral body wall cuts are made with straight osteotomes in a precise wedge based on the desired degree of closure. The apex of the wedge is at the anterior cortical vertebral body wall. This serves as the pivot point. The cancellous bone of the vertebral body is then removed with curettes and rongeurs in a wedge-shaped fashion matching the cuts on the lateral walls. Using angled curettes, the cancellous bone in the body is pushed anteriorly into the body to create a cavity in the vertebra. High-speed drills are used for osteotomy contouring. The final step of bone resection is resection of the posterior vertebral body wall, or the floor of the spinal canal. This is carried out with an impaction technique performed with curettes or with specialized impactors. This pushes the posterior vertebral wall contents anteriorly, completing the osteotomy. PSO closure is performed by gentle compression across temporary rods.

Tips from the Masters 18-3 • Special attention should always be directed to the intraoperative somatosensory evoked potentials at the time of osteotomy closure.

Arthrodesis is performed, and bone graft is used to augment fusion. The wound is then closed in layers. A cross-table scoliosis plain radiograph is obtained to ensure that correction is adequate.

The fascia is closed with vicryl absorbale suture. The dermis and subcutaneous tissue is closed next. Staples are applied to the skin.

Patients may be evaluated using postoperative thin-cut CT scans to assess osteotomy closure and accuracy of implant placement. For all patients, standing AP and lateral 14 × 36 inch scoliosis radiographs are obtained before hospital discharge and every 3 to 6 months thereafter at follow-up appointments. The patient should stand in a natural position without knee flexion or hip hyperextension.[5] Correction at each PSO is often determined by measuring preoperative and postoperative Cobb angles on lateral radiographs across the superior and inferior end plates of the vertebrae at which the osteotomy was performed. The global sagittal balance is evaluated by using a C7 plumb line and noting its relationship to the posterior superior corner of the sacrum.

A thoracic PSO differs from one performed in the lumbar spine in a number of ways.[1] For a thoracic PSO, it is important to resect the rib attachment (2 to 3 cm) to the vertebra so that the body can be approached from a lateral perspective.[1] Thus, the rib heads articulating with the disk spaces above and below the osteotomy need to be released.[1]

Tips from the Masters 18-4 • The thoracic PSO is performed at the level of the spinal cord, and this limits the amount of safe posterior osteotomy closure that can be performed without excessive dural kinking, which may result in spinal cord dysfunction or injury.

This amount has been reported anecdotally to be 20 to 25 mm in the thoracic spine.[1] As noted by Ondra and co-workers[29] and Yang and associates,[30] trigonometric analysis has shown that an osteotomy in the thoracic spine will produce less improvement in global sagittal balance than a similar-sized lumbar PSO. For this reason, patients often require additional osteotomies if a thoracic PSO is needed for global sagittal realignment.[1] Multiple thoracic PSOs also offer the advantage of spreading the cord-level correction over multiple segments and thereby minimizing the risk of focal neurologic injury after correction. Limitations to large correction by thoracic PSOs include shorter vertebral bodies with a triangulated morphology and limited relative sagittal height of the pedicle compared with vertebral bodies.[1]

Complications after multiple osteotomies can include pseudoarthrosis, proximal junctional kyphosis, or instrumentation failure. Postoperative medical complications can include deep vein thrombosis, pulmonary embolism, small bowel ileus or obstruction, myocardial infarction, or stroke. Radiculopathy may be noted following osteotomy closure due to compression of nerve roots as they exit the foramina. Care must be taken to perform wide foraminotomies at the level of the osteotomies. Durotomies are sometimes unavoidable, especially in revision surgery. Careful repair of the cerebrospinal fluid leak is important to prevent pseudoarthrosis. The leak can be repaired primarily, with dural substitutes, or sealants.

Osteotomy closure for a PSO hinges on the anterior column, and typically the anterior cortical wall serves as the fulcrum for closure.[1] In the lumbar spine, there is a broad anterior cortical surface that usually provides a rigid pivot for PSO closure.[1] In the upper thoracic spine, the thin, narrow, and triangulated anterior cortex can be easily disrupted, which can result in a planum fracture of the vertebral body or segmental translation from loss of integrity.[1] This can happen during the osteotomy or during closure. As a PSO is being closed, the spine must be observed for subluxation.[5] In general, when significant correction is needed between T2 and T10, a VCR through a bilateral costo-transversectomy approach is often used, although other osteotomies can still also be performed.[1] A VCR involves opening of the anterior column and closing of the posterior column after complete removal of the three columns with placement of an interbody cage to serve as a pivot.[3] From T11 through L1, multiple osteotomy options are feasible for correction, and the procedure of choice depends on both the correction requirements and the anatomy of the deformity.[1] An extended PSO in which the anterior apex of the wedge-shaped osteotomy is located at the cephalad disk space can be used for correction of thoracolumbar junctional kyphosis and focal junctional deformities.[1] This procedure includes the arthrodesis of the interspace after the cephalad disk is resected.[1] From L2 through L5, a traditional PSO can provide appreciable sagittal correction based on the geometry of the lumbar segments and the trigonometric calculations at this level.[1]

An asymmetric PSO may be used for correction of coronal and sagittal decompensation.[3,5]

Tips from the Masters 18-5 • By placing the wider portion of the osteotomy on the side of the convexity of the curve, coronal correction can be obtained at the same time as sagittal correction.

Bilateral rib osteotomies help in approaching the vertebral body out wide.[5] PSOs are not commonly performed in the distal lumbar spine because fewer fixation points are achievable distally.[5] The best candidates for a PSO are patients with the following conditions: (1) sagittal imbalance of more than 10 cm; (2) sharp, angular kyphosis; (3) fixed sagittal imbalance caused by anterior ankylosis or circumferential fusion between multiple segments.[3,5] A PSO can also be used effectively in most patients with ankylosing spondylitis. The PSO is advantageous because it can produce substantial correction at a single level.[3] It is highly successful at bone union because there is bone contact in three columns, and it can be performed without the use of a supplemental anterior approach with its potentially morbidity. The VCR is recommended in cases in which a substantial amount of correction is needed, which cannot be easily obtained by a PSO.[3] The indications for a VCR include fixed trunk translation, severe scoliosis (often congenital or neuromuscular), spinal tumor, spondyloptosis, rigid spinal deformities or more than 80 degrees in the coronal plane, and asymmetry between the length of the convex column and the length of the concave column of the deformity that precludes the achievement of balance by a simple osteotomy alone.[3,31]

DISCUSSION OF BEST EVIDENCE

A PSO may be used in the thoracic or lumbar spine and is commonly used in the lumbar spine for correction of flat back deformity or fixed kyphotic deformity.[1] It is described as a V-shaped wedge resection (widening from anterior to posterior) of the vertebral body including both pedicles and posterior elements.[5,11,12] The procedure does not create an anterior bony defect.[12] This osteotomy can achieve stable correction at a single segment, potentially reducing the need for an anterior procedure, with an average correction of 30 to 40 degrees.[12,26,32,33] The osteotomy accomplishes bone on bone in the posterior, middle, and anterior columns.[5]

The indications for a PSO overlap with those for multiple SPOs. The PSO is used to achieve major correction over a short segment and correction over levels that have anterior ankylosis or lack anterior flexibility.[2,5] Patients with more than 10 cm of sagittal imbalance would be more likely to benefit from a PSO than an SPO.[2,5,12] A PSO can help with treatment of significant lumbar kyphosis and offer a tremendous degree of correction in the sagittal plane to achieve balance.[2] Ondra and colleagues[2,29] have presented a mathematical model for determining the degree of correction needed through a PSO to achieve sagittal balance. Yang and associates[2,34] compared data for patients undergoing lumbar and thoracic PSOs and found no difference in outcomes between the two groups in terms of scores on the Scoliosis Research Society (SRS) 22 Patient Questionnaire, but complication rates ranged between 10% and 30%. When there is a completely fixed deformity, care must be taken to determine whether there is anterior fixation, as with a bridging osteophyte; in such a case, osteotomies other than an SPO may be indicated.[6]

A PSO addresses focal, angular kyphosis more effectively than an SPO, although not as effectively as a VCR.[2,35,36] The PSO facilitates correction of sagittal imbalance, although it is technically more demanding and is associated with longer operative time, greater blood loss, and higher risk of neurologic complications than the SPO.[2,3,5,12] Dorward and Lenke[2] note that deformities involving a gradual or sweeping kyphosis, mobile disk space, or less than 10 cm of sagittal imbalance may be more amenable to correction with SPOs, whereas those characterized by sharp or focal kyphosis, sagittal imbalance of 10 cm or more, or fixed disk space may benefit from a PSO. A PSO has the advantage of obtaining correction through three columns from a posterior approach.[3] A PSO does not lengthen the anterior column as does an SPO, which thus minimizes stretching of the major vessels and viscera anterior to the spine.[3,12,26] This also maximizes healing potential.[3,26]

Tips from the Masters 18-6 • Patients with anterior column fusion are unlikely to gain significant correction with multiple SPOs, and therefore a PSO is a better option to surgically address a sagittal deformity.

A long, sweeping, rounded, smooth kyphosis, such as Scheuermann kyphosis, is amenable to treatment with multiple SPOs, in part because of its multisegmental nature and because the pathologic changes are in the thoracic spine.[5] SPOs are useful for correction of mild to moderate sagittal imbalances.[5] A short, angular kyphosis such as a posttraumatic kyphosis is more amenable to treatment with a PSO.[5] Depending on the anatomy, ankylosing spondylitis is often treated with a PSO. For some curves, more than one type of osteotomy may be needed, such as multiple SPOs and a PSO. When patients undergo a single PSO, it is often performed in the apical region of the kyphosis or at the epicenter of a junctional deformity.[1] When patients require multiple osteotomies, they are often spread out along the deformity to introduce correction in a harmonious manner. Occasionally multiple PSOs need to be performed for correction. Or a PSO and other osteotomies can be performed. A greater degree of correction is possible at a motion segment with a mobile disk than at a level with a severely degenerated and sclerotic disk space presenting osteotophytes.[6] The Zielke technique involves the performance of multiple SPOs at all levels from T10 to the sacrum.[17]

The PSO is a technique popularized for the surgical treatment of fixed sagittal deformity and can be performed safely in the thoracic and lumbar spine.[1,3-5] The primary advantage of a PSO is that it allows posterior-only correction and obviates the need for an anterior release and its associated morbidity.[1] Focal lumbar lordosis of 30 to 40 degrees can be introduced using this technique.[1,5,27,34,37,38] A PSO in the lumbar spine will accomplish approximately 35 degrees of lordosis, and a PSO in the thoracic spine will accomplish approximately 25 degrees of lordosis.[5] Indications for thoracic PSO include symptomatic severe thoracic kyphosis (more than 80 degrees) that is determined to be rigid based on preoperative radiographs taken with the patient over a bolster.[1] The PSO can be used when other osteotomies associated with potentially less morbidity such as an SPO or inferior facetectomy are not feasible because of a lack of sagittal curve flexibility.[1] A mobile disk is not required to perform a PSO. The

PSO involves removal of all the posterior elements, both pedicles at a particular level, and half of the body with the anterior margin of the body used as a pivot.[3]

COMMENTARY

The SPO and PSO are techniques suited to treat spinal imbalance. Regional kyphosis with overall global balance can be corrected with multiple SPOs. The SPO treats smooth sagittal and coronal curves in both the thoracic and lumbar regions. Three or more SPOs or a PSO is useful for sharp angular kyphosis, regional kyphosis with overall global imbalance, or coronal imbalance. Cho and colleagues[12] reported achieving similar correction using either three SPOs or a single PSO. They also reported accomplishing greater correction in the sagittal plane with a single PSO than with three or more SPOs (5.49 ± 4.5 cm vs. 11.19 ± 7.2 cm, respectively; $P < .01$).[12] However, the C7 plumb line deviation was substantially greater before surgery in the PSO-treated group than in the SPO-treated group.

The PSO allows for bone-on-bone contact throughout all three columns of the spine.[39] The main candidate for a PSO is a patient with some component of fixed sagittal imbalance who needs approximately 30 degrees of additional lordosis.[39] If a patient only needs 10 to 20 degrees of lordosis and the sagittal vertical axis is less than 8 cm from the posterosuperior end plate of S1, then it may be more feasible to perform SPOs. The SPO is indicated for smooth curves, curves featuring mobile disk spaces, and minor sagittal imbalance. Several studies have reported transient neurologic deficits after a PSO.[12] Thus, care should be taken to remove the pedicle edges completely, to undercut the lamina, and to provide generous central canal enlargement.[12,27]

Sagittal plane imbalance is disabling for patients and leads to a poor quality of life.[40] This chapter has described useful tools for restoration of balance. The surgeon must be well versed in executing these various osteotomy techniques. A multidisciplinary approach will decrease perioperative morbidity and complications related to the performance of these osteotomies.

REFERENCES

1. O'Shaughnessy BA, Kuklo TR, Hsieh PC, et al: Thoracic pedicle subtraction osteotomy for fixed sagittal spinal deformity, *Spine* 34(26):2893–2899, 2009. O'Shaughnessy and colleagues evaluated the impact of thoracic pedicle subtraction osteotomies on fixed sagittal plane imbalance. Twenty-five thoracic pedicle subtraction osteomies were performed on 15 patients. Preoperative and postoperative Cobb angles were measured, and degrees of correction were evaluated based on region within the thoracic spine. Surgical and clinical outcomes were presented in detail, with no neurologic complications. This paper also contrasts thoracic and lumbar pedicle subtraction osteotomies, and describes the consideration of a vertebral column resection due to the risk of planum fracture or translation with thoracic pedicle subtraction osteotomy closure.

2. Dorward IG, Lenke LG: Osteotomies in the posterior-only treatment of complex adult spinal deformity: a comparative review, *Neurosurg Focus* 28(3):E4, 2010. Dorward and Lenke describe the indications, technical nuances, and examples of the posterior-only osteotomies (Smith-Petersen, pedicle subtraction, and vertebral column resection). They describe the history and modifications afforded to the Smith-Petersen osteotomy, with a review of the literature. Dorward and Lenke also review the history of the pedicle subtraction osteotomy and discuss the literature on outcomes and complication rates. Finally, the authors review Professor Suk's description of the vertebral column resection, and talk about the significant risk of neurologic injury afforded to the osteotomy technique. An algorithm is provided to aid in the decision making process regarding osteotomy selection. Surgeon judgment and experience is paramount before offering surgery.

3. Kim KT, Park KJ, Lee JH: Osteotomy of the spine to correct the spinal deformity, *Asian Spine J* 3(2):113–123, 2009.

4. Berven SH, Deviren V, Smith JA, et al: Management of fixed sagittal plane deformity: results of the transpedicular wedge resection osteotomy, *Spine* 26(18):2036–2043, 2001.

5. Bridwell KH: Decision making regarding Smith-Petersen vs. pedicle subtraction osteotomy vs. vertebral column resection for spinal deformity, *Spine* 31(Suppl 19):S171–S178, 2006. Bridwell reviews the decision making process regarding when to perform a Smith-Petersen osteotomy, pedicle subtraction osteotomy, or a vertebral column resection. He highlights the nomenclature of the three osteotomy types, and discusses their indications. Bridwell discusses that a long, rounded, smooth kyphosis is amenable to Smith-Petersen osteotomies, and that short, angular kyphosis is correctable with pedicle subtraction osteotomies. He also provides several examples regarding the decision to perform a specific osteotomy type for correction. Bridwell discusses the limitations of the Smith-Petersen osteotomy: it

requires a mobile disk anteriorly and no solid bony bridge. Finally, he provides an algorithm for when to perform a specific osteotomy depending on the type and location of the deformity.

6. La Marca F, Brumblay H: Smith-Petersen osteotomy in thoracolumbar deformity surgery, *Neurosurgery* 63(Suppl 3):163–170, 2008.

7. Wiggins GC, Ondra SL, Shaffrey CI: Management of iatrogenic flat-back syndrome, *Neurosurg Focus* 15(3):E8, 2003.

8. Smith-Petersen MN, Larson CB, Aufranc OE: Osteotomy of the spine for correction of flexion deformity in rheumatoid arthritis, *J Bone Joint Surg Am* 27:1–11, 1945.

9. McMaster MJ: A technique for lumbar spinal osteotomy in ankylosing spondylitis, *J Bone Joint Surg Br* 67(2):204–210, 1985.

10. Kostuik JP, Maurais GR, Richardson WJ, et al: Combined single stage anterior and posterior osteotomy for correction of iatrogenic lumbar kyphosis, *Spine* 13(3):257–266, 1988.

11. Thomasen E: Vertebral osteotomy for correction of kyphosis in ankylosing spondylitis, *Clin Orthop Relat Res* 194:142–152, 1985.

12. Cho KJ, Bridwell KH, Lenke LG, et al: Comparison of Smith-Petersen versus pedicle subtraction osteotomy for the correction of fixed sagittal imbalance, *Spine* 30(18):2030–2037: discussion, 2038, 2005. **Cho and co-workers designed a study comparing the Smith-Petersen osteotomy with the pedicle subtraction osteotomy for correction of fixed sagittal-plane deformity and identified a total of 71 patients. The pedicle subtraction osteotomy group demonstrated statistically significant improvement in sagittal plane correction compared with three or more Smith-Petersen osteotomies. This study also compared operative time and operative blood loss. Clinical and radiographic outcomes are reviewed, and early and late complications are discussed in this manuscript.**

13. Bridwell KH, Lenke LG, Lewis SJ: Treatment of spinal stenosis and fixed sagittal imbalance, *Clin Orthop Relat Res* 384:35–44, 2001.

14. Weatherley C, Jaffray D, Terry A: Vascular complications associated with osteotomy in ankylosing spondylitis: a report of two cases, *Spine* 13(1):43–46, 1988.

15. Adams JC: Technique, dangers and safeguards in osteotomy of the spine, *J Bone Joint Surg Br* 34-B(2):226–232, 1952.

16. Li F, Sagi HC, Liu B, et al: Comparative evaluation of single-level closing-wedge vertebral osteotomies for the correction of fixed kyphotic deformity of the lumbar spine: a cadaveric study, *Spine* 26(21):2385–2391, 2001.

17. Hehne HJ, Zielke K, Bohm H: Polysegmental lumbar osteotomies and transpedicled fixation for correction of long-curved kyphotic deformities in ankylosing spondylitis. Report on 177 cases, *Clin Orthop Relat Res* 258:49–55, 1990.

18. LaChapelle E: Osteotomy of the lumbar spine for correction of kyphosis in a case of ankylosing spondylarthritis, *J Bone Joint Surg Am* 384:851–858, 1946.

19. Law WA: Surgical treatment of the rheumatic diseases, *J Bone Joint Surg Br* 34-B(2):215–225, 1952.

20. Law WA: Osteotomy of the spine, *Clin Orthop Relat Res* 66:70–76, 1969. **A morphometric analysis demonstrated that the lateral mass size decreases from C5 to C7. Also, the T1 pedicle is typically larger than T2. These are important considerations when planning for CTJ instrumentation.**

21. Ponte A, Vero B, Siccardi GL: *Surgical treatment of Scheuermann's hyperkyphosis*, Bologna, Italy, 1984, Aulo Gaggi.

22. Geck MJ, Macagno A, Ponte A, et al: The Ponte procedure: posterior only treatment of Scheuermann's kyphosis using segmental posterior shortening and pedicle screw instrumentation, *J Spinal Disord Tech* 20(8):586–593, 2007.

23. Ponte A: Posterior column shortening for Scheuermann's kyphosis. In Haher TR, Merola AA, editors: *Surgical techniques for the spine*, ed 1, New York, 2003, Thieme Medical Publishers.

24. Lagrone MO, Bradford DS, Moe JH, et al: Treatment of symptomatic flatback after spinal fusion, *J Bone Joint Surg Am* 70(4):569–580, 1988. **This retrospective review evaluated posterior instrumentation across the CTJ for tumor and in parallel hardware evolved from rod-sublaminar to rod/screw systems. This change leads to a reduction in fixation failure from 29% to 0%, establishing the superiority of rod/screw constructs.**

25. Voos K, Boachie-Adjei O, Rawlins BA: Multiple vertebral osteotomies in the treatment of rigid adult spine deformities, *Spine* 26(5):526–533, 2001.

26. Bridwell KH, Lewis SJ, Lenke LG, et al: Pedicle subtraction osteotomy for the treatment of fixed sagittal imbalance, *J Bone Joint Surg Am* 85-A(3):454–463, 2003.

27. Bridwell KH, Lewis SJ, Edwards C, et al: Complications and outcomes of pedicle subtraction osteotomies for fixed sagittal imbalance, *Spine* 28(18):2093–2101, 2003.

28. Scudese VA, Calabro JJ: Vertebral wedge osteotomy. Correction of rheumatoid (ankylosing) spondylitis, *JAMA* 186:627–631, 1963.

29. Ondra SL, Marzouk S, Koski T, et al: Mathematical calculation of pedicle subtraction osteotomy size to allow precision correction of fixed sagittal deformity, *Spine* 31(25):E973–E979, 2006. **Ondra and associates reviewed 15 consecutive patients with fixed sagittal deformity and demonstrated a consistent trigonometric method for predicting the amount of correction needed to achieve a desired outcome using the pedicle subtraction osteotomy. This study also describes the technique of a pedicle subtraction osteotomy. Using this mathematical tool helps surgeons minimize the risk of overcorrection and undercorrection.**

30. Yang BP, Ondra SL: A method for calculating the exact angle required during pedicle subtraction osteotomy for fixed sagittal deformity: comparison with the trigonometric method, *Neurosurgery* 59(4 Suppl 2):ONS458–ONS463: discussion, ONS463, 2006.

31. Bradford DS, Tribus CB: Vertebral column resection for the treatment of rigid coronal decompensation, *Spine* 22(14):1590–1599, 1997.

32. Thiranont N, Netrawichien P: Transpedicular decancellation closed wedge vertebral osteotomy for treatment of fixed flexion deformity of spine in ankylosing spondylitis, *Spine* 18(16):2517–2522, 1993.

33. van Royen BJ, Slot GH: Closing-wedge posterior osteotomy for ankylosing spondylitis. Partial corporectomy and transpedicular fixation in 22 cases, *J Bone Joint Surg Br* 77(1):117–121, 1995.

34. Yang BP, Ondra SL, Chen LA, et al: Clinical and radiographic outcomes of thoracic and lumbar pedicle subtraction osteotomy for fixed sagittal imbalance, *J Neurosurg Spine* 5(1):9–17, 2006.

35. Jaffray D, Becker V, Eisenstein S: Closing wedge osteotomy with transpedicular fixation in ankylosing spondylitis, *Clin Orthop Relat Res* 279:122–126, 1992.

36. Van Royen B, DeGast A: Lumbar osteotomy for correction of thoracolumbar kyphotic deformity in ankylosing spondylitis: a structured review of three methods of treatment, *Ann Rheum Dis.* 58: 399–406, 1999.

37. Kim YJ, Bridwell KH, Lenke LG, et al: Results of lumbar pedicle subtraction osteotomies for fixed sagittal imbalance: a minimum 5-year follow-up study, *Spine* 32(20):2189–2197, 2007.

38. Boachie-Adjei O, Ferguson JA, Pigeon RG, et al: Transpedicular lumbar wedge resection osteotomy for fixed sagittal imbalance: surgical technique and early results, *Spine* 31(4):485–492, 2006.

39. Bridwell KH, Lewis SJ, Rinella A, et al: Pedicle subtraction osteotomy for the treatment of fixed sagittal imbalance. Surgical technique, *J Bone Joint Surg Am* 86-A(Suppl 1):44–50, 2004.

40. Mummaneni PV, Dhall SS, Ondra SL, et al: Pedicle subtraction osteotomy, *Neurosurgery* 63 (Suppl 3):171–176, 2008.

Chapter 19 L1-S1 Fusion: When to Extend to T12 and Pelvis and When to Include L5-S1 Anterior Grafting

Steven Mardjetko

Lumbar spinal fusion is used to treat a wide variety of spinal disorders, including degenerative spinal pathologic processes, degenerative conditions that result in segmental instability, spinal deformities that lead to alterations of normal sagittal and coronal plane alignment, instability due to pathologic bone destruction (tumors and trauma), and acute traumatic lesions. Lumbar fusions are often performed in concert with neural decompression procedures. The development of pedicle-based spinal instrumentation and its widespread use starting in the 1980s has led to significant improvement in fusion rates compared with in situ noninstrumented fusion. These devices make ideal spinal anchors for vertebral segments requiring laminectomy. In addition, pedicle screw instrumentation gives the surgeon segmental control of vertebral position in all three planes.

The determination of fusion levels is based on the underlying pathologic condition, the number and location of levels requiring decompression, and abnormalities in adjacent spinal segments and spinal regions.

Single-level pathologic changes that result in segmental instability, such as spondylolisthesis, can be managed by addressing the single segment. But lesions that involve multiple segments may require more extensive constructs covering multiple spinal segments (Figure 19-1). Degenerative changes of the lumbar spine are often concentrated in the lower three or four segments. Such changes can include disk degeneration, spondylolisthesis, or postlaminectomy instability, among others. Certain pathologic conditions affect the entire lumbar spine. These include lumbar scoliosis and kyphosis. Multisegmental lesions typically require inclusion of all the pathologic segments. Short segmental fusions usually cover one or two segments. Three- to four-segment fusions are usually considered moderate in length. Fusions of five or more levels are defined as long posterior (lumbar) fusions. Fusions extending from L1 to S1 or even further proximally may occasionally be required to adequately address the pathology, provide enough implant fixation to ensure maintenance of spinal construct stability, correct spinal deformity, and address pathologic changes in adjacent segments.

CASE PRESENTATION

A 65-year-old practicing dentist underwent a minimally invasive posterior lumbar interbody fusion (PLIF) procedure at L2 and L3 for radicular pain. The operating surgeon ignored adjacent-segment pathologic changes and did not recognize the severe regional and global sagittal plane imbalance that the patient's history clearly described.

- PMH: Generally healthy and active, with a long history of lumbar pain symptoms and neurogenic claudication associated with forward leaning posture
- PSH: "Minimally invasive" L2-3 PLIF procedure that did not address adjacent segment compressive pathology, or positive sagittal balance
- Exam: Forward-leaning posture secondary to lumbar hypo-lordosis; compensations to maintain vertical truncal position included hip/knee flexion position. Neural exam was normal, but history supported diagnosis of neurogenic claudication.

224

- Imaging: Analysis of the patient's standing anteroposterior (AP) and lateral radiographs revealed severe spinal stenosis at L1-2 and L3-4, with kyphotic disk degeneration at L4-5 and L5-S1. Sagittal vertical axis (SVA) imbalance was +10 cm (Figure 19-2, *A* and *B*).

Further proximal surgery without addressing the lumbar spine alignment would result in a worsening of SVA and flat back syndrome symptoms. The surgical strategy must address the compressive pathology at L1-2 and L3-4, and the multi-level sagittal balance problem. This requires a multi-stage approach.

Stage 1/day 1: The patient underwent posterior laminectomy with prior instrument removal and Smith-Petersen osteotomies from L1 to L4, excluding the solidly fused level L2-3, with insertion of pedicle screws at L1 to S1 and bilateral iliac screws (Figure 19-2, D and E). Surgical time was 4 hours.

Stage 2/day 2: An anterior spinal osteotomy and fusion procedure at L3-L4, L4-L5, and L5-S1 was performed. Titanium mesh and carbon fiber implants were placed and autogenous and allogeneic bone graft and bone morphogenetic protein (BMP; 6 mg per level) were inserted via a retroperitoneal straight anterior approach to address segmental lumbar kyphosis. Surgical time was 3 hours.

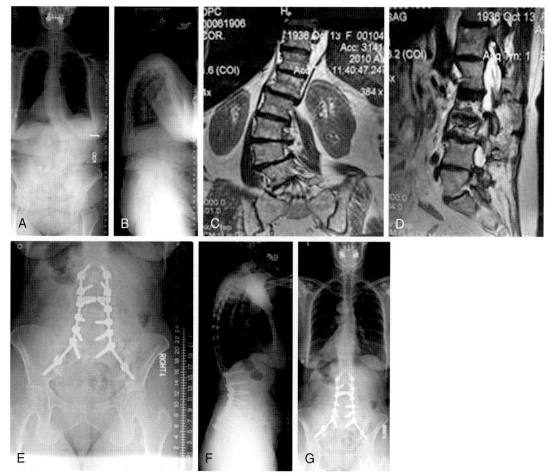

FIGURE 19-1 Coronal plane deformities such as the degenerative scoliosis illustrated in this figure represent multisegmental defects that require extensive instrumented fusion extending from the thoracolumbar junction to the sacropelvis. **A** and **B,** Standing AP and lateral scoliosis radiographs. **C** and **D,** Coronal and sagittal magnetic resonance imaging scans of the lumbar spine revealing degeneration of multiple segments. **E** through **G,** Radiographs taken 2 years after surgery that included L1-S1 fusion with L1 to sacropelvic fixation using bilateral iliac screws.

SURGICAL OPTIONS

Pathologic Conditions That Require Long Fusion and Instrumentation

1. Sagittal plane abnormalities. Sagittal plane imbalances can occur on a segmental, regional, or global level, resulting in serious problems in the individual's ability to maintain an upright posture with an erect and vertical trunk. It has been clearly demonstrated that significant sagittal plane alterations require greater energy expenditure, result in lower quality-of-life scores,[1] and are associated with an increased risk of spinal pain and malalignment (kyphosis)—flat back syndrome (Figure 19-3).[2] Patients with this latter condition frequently complain of a fatiguing spinal pain syndrome affecting the lumbar and thoracic regions, as well as buttock and thigh pain due to the recruitment of the hip extensors and knee extensors to compensate for the forward-leaning posture (Figure 19-4). Patients experience a decrease in walking tolerance, but can perform sitting exercise programs with reasonable facility.

2. Coronal plane deformities. These deformities include many variants of scoliosis. The Scoliosis Research Society classification of adult spinal deformity[3] acknowledges the following coronal plane deformities seen in adults: (1) de novo degenerative scoliosis; (2) adult idiopathic scoliosis, which is seen in a group of patients

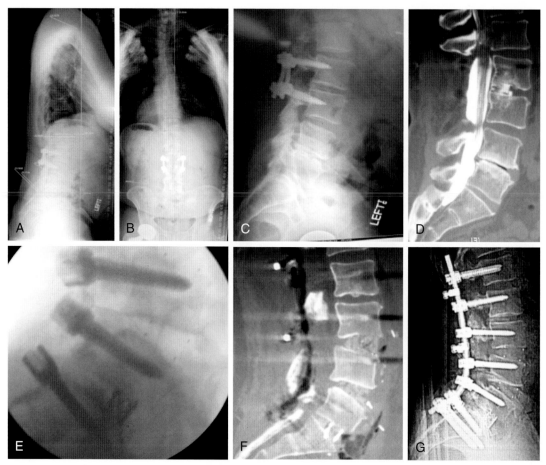

FIGURE 19-2 **A** through **C,** Preoperative AP and lateral radiographs showing instrumentation from previous PLIF procedure at L2 and L3, severe spinal stenosis at L1-2 and L3-4, kyphotic disk degeneration at L4-5 and L5-S1, and sagittal plane imbalance. **D** and **E,** Stage 1: posterior instrument removal and Smith-Petersen osteotomies from L1-2 to L5-S1 with insertion of pedicle screws at L1 to S1 and bilateral iliac screws. Stage 2: anterior osteotomies at L3-4, L4-5, L5-S1 with placement of lordotic cages, bone graft, and BMP to address segmental lumbar kyphosis. **F** through **H,** Stage 3: posterior rod insertion with compression to enhance segmental lumbar lordosis, and posterolateral spinal fusion at L1-S1 with autograft, allograft, DBM, and BMP.

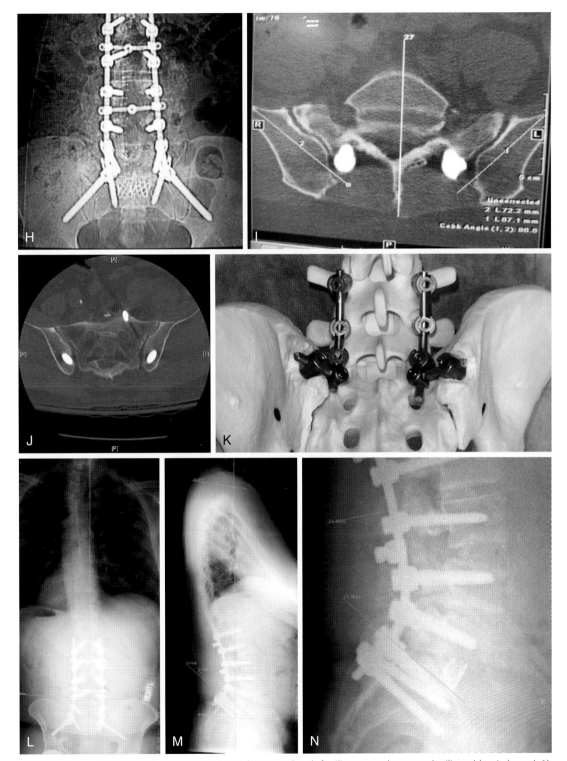

FIGURE 19-2, cont'd I through **K,** Insertion site and proposed path for iliac screws between the iliac tables. **L** through **N,** Standing AP and lateral scoliosis radiographs showing complete restoration of sagittal alignment with the L1-sacropelvis stabilization procedure.

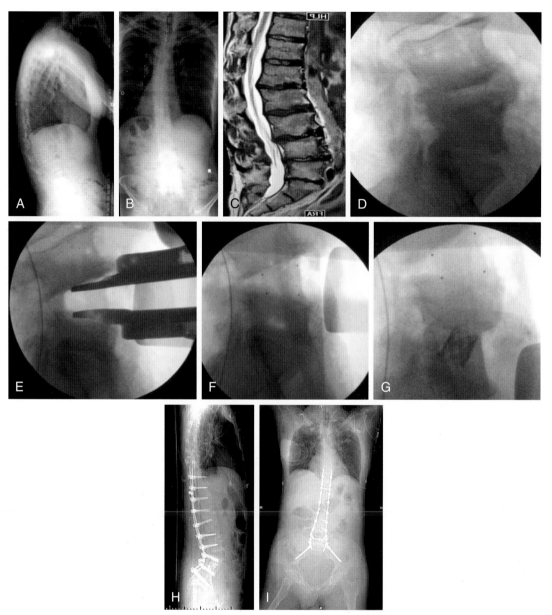

FIGURE 19-3 Sagittal plane abnormalities represent another group of disorders with multisegmental defects. **A** and **B,** Lateral and AP radiographs for a patient with thoracolumbar Scheuermann disease who had severe lumbar pain and flat back symptoms, a common presentation of this type of defect. **C** and **D,** Sagittal MRI and radiographic images demonstrating the patient's rigid sagittal plane deformity. Osteotomy procedures are often required to realign the involved spinal regions back to physiologic range. **E** though **G,** Intraoperative images during the first stage of surgery for this patient, which included anterior osteotomies with placement of large lordotic cages. At L4-5 a carbon fiber implant was used and at L5-S1 titanium mesh cages were inserted. **H** and **I,** Lateral and AP radiographs taken after the second stage of surgery during which posterior Smith-Petersen osteotomies were performed followed by posterior spinal fusion and instrumentation from T10 to L5-S1 with bilateral iliac screw fixation. The upper instrumented vertebra of T10 was chosen based on the presence of reasonable sagittal thoracic alignment and reasonable disk health in the lower thoracic spine.

who had adolescent scoliosis in whom the lumbar curve demonstrates degenerative progression; (3) degenerative lumbar kyphosis, a condition that is seen more commonly in Asian countries but is increasingly being recognized in the United States; and (4) primary lumbosacral scoliosis, which results in severe coronal plane decompensation. Lower lumbar disk degeneration is the proximate cause of the latter, but this deformity may be associated with a preexisting congenital lumbosacral obliquity.[4]

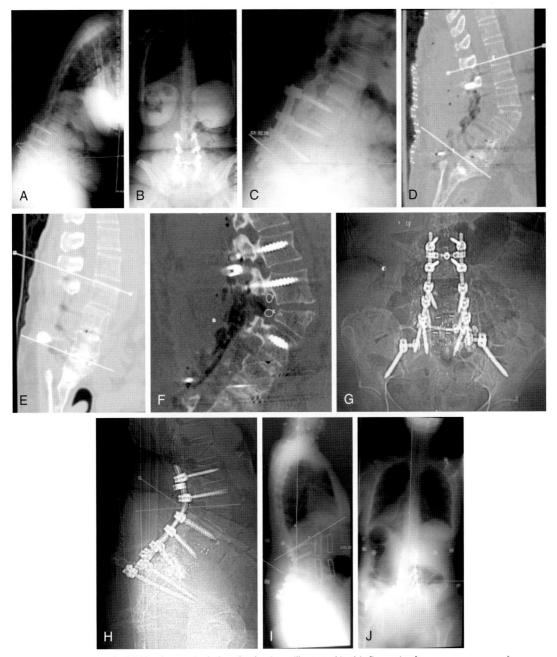

FIGURE 19-4 Iatrogenic rigid lumbar sagittal plane kyphosis, as illustrated in this figure, is often a consequence of sequential fusions of the lumbar spine without adequate attention to the lumbar segmental sagittal alignment. Symptoms of adjacent-segment spinal stenosis and instability combined with symptoms of flat back syndrome are typical. **A** through **D,** Lateral and AP radiographs and sagittal CT scan revealing a very flat TLIF of L3 to S1 of 16 degrees coupled with a pelvic incidence of 80 degrees. A pelvic incidence of 80 degrees requires at least 50 degrees of lumbar lordosis to maintain sagittal alignment. **E** through **H,** Sagittal CT image and lateral and AP radiographs taken after corrective surgery that involved decompression and stabilization from L1 to the sacropelvis with iliac screws combined with an L3 Tomesen pedicle subtraction osteotomy popularized by Bridwell. This three-column osteotomy was performed from a posterior approach at L3 and resulted in a 30- to 40-degree correction at a single level. **I** and **J,** Postoperative standing lateral and AP radiographs, demonstrating that the preoperative SVA of +26 cm has been corrected to +3 cm.

    3. Combined sagittal and coronal plane deformities
    4. Fixed sagittal or coronal plane deformities owing to the following:
       a. Degenerative ankylosis
       b. Spondyloarthropathy with ankylosis
       c. Previous fusion procedures

5. Multilevel lumbar spinal instability, which can involve three or more levels
   a. Multilevel spondylolisthesis, usually combined with degenerative retrolisthesis or deformity
   b. Postlaminectomy instability

Biomechanical Differences between Short (Two or Fewer) and Long (Five or More) Spinal Constructs

The biomechanical demands on spinal implants, the bone-implant interface, and the adjacent spinal segments are affected by the number of lumbar segments included in the construct. Biomechanical and anatomic differences exist between the lumbosacropelvic junction, the midlumbar spine, and the thoracolumbar junction. These differences can explain the variation in fusion and pseudarthrosis rates and in implant failure rates reported for these different regions. Mechanical failures in the early postoperative period are most often due to a failure of the bone-implant interface. Although the adjacent segment is not actually considered part of the construct, it is exposed to increased forces that intensify as the length of the construct increases. This can lead to adjacent-segment failures such as vertebral body fracture or posterior ligament failure. Pseudarthrosis rates are directly related to the number of segments stabilized, and pseudarthrosis most commonly occurs at the lumbosacral junction. This can result in late instrument failure, usually around 6 months after surgery.

The surgical decision depends on the extent of the pathologic changes, the spinal alignment on standing spinal radiographs, and the findings on dynamic radiographs, which may include left- and right-bending radiographs, flexion-extension lateral radiographs, and traction radiographs. Careful attention to the patient's hip and knee joints is warranted to assess for concomitant appendicular abnormalities that may impact the clinical and radiographic outcome and be a source of pain.

The clinical and radiographic analysis is augmented by neuroimaging studies. These should include magnetic resonance imaging (MRI) scans of the thoracic and lumbar spine and, if necessary, dynamic gravity-loaded myelography followed by computed tomographic (CT) scanning. The myelography may reveal pathologic changes not picked up on a supine MRI. The CT scan gives the surgeon a clear view of the posterior elements and the health of the facet joints. CT without myelography may also be useful for the latter purposes.

Not uncommonly, the pathologic changes are multisegmental but the primary abnormality involves the lumbosacral junction, and one may be able to concentrate on the lumbosacral defects without needing to address the more proximal pathologic elements. This situation is commonly seen in patients with a combination of L4-L5 degenerative spondylolisthesis and degenerative lumbar scoliosis. If the neural compressive syndromes are related to lumbosacral pathologic changes, one may address the lumbosacral segments primarily. (See case 1.)

It is not uncommon to see significant degeneration and coronal and/or sagittal deformity extend through the entire lumbar spine.

Tips from the Masters 19-1 • Carefully analyze the standing lateral scoliosis radiograph to determine the desired sagittal plane alignment.

In these cases all the pathologic areas must be included in the surgical plan. (See case 1.)

The management of multisegmental disease requires an intimate understanding of the sagittal alignment of the adult spine. In single-level lesions, which requires a one-level fusion, the other spinal segments can accommodate for a hypolordotic fused segment via adjacent-segment hyperextension. Although this has been implicated as a cause of precocious demise of the adjacent segment, most often the overall effect in the sagittal plane is minimal.

In long fusions no compensation is possible, so physiologic sagittal alignment must be achieved at the time of surgery. Glassman, Schwab and others have shown that sagittal plane alignment is the primary determinant of the patient's clinical outcome.[1,3]

Evaluation of the sagittal plane starts with the clinical evaluation, and if necessary radiographic evaluation, of the hip-knee-ankle alignment. One should then evaluate the pelvic index.[5]

The pelvic index in adults describes a constant anatomic relationship of the sacrum and pelvis to the hip joints, and helps to determine the amount of lumbar lordosis that is necessary to maintain an appropriate sagittal balance. Generally, a SVA that is within ±4 cm of the posterior superior sacral corner is considered normal. Significant positive values are often associated with symptoms of flat back syndrome.[2] The clinical presentation of a forward-leaning posture has been correlated with increased energy expenditure and significantly increased spinal extensor, gluteal, and quadriceps muscle activity during standing and walking. Individuals with increased pelvic incidence require greater degrees of lumbar lordosis to maintain appropriate sagittal alignment. Other factors that enter into the sagittal balance formula include the thoracic kyphosis and cervical spine position. Pelvic incidence is the sum of the pelvic tilt and the sacral slope. Generally, the lumbar lordosis should be 20 degrees greater than the thoracic kyphosis. These guidelines can help the surgeon determine the minimum amount of lumbar lordosis that should be obtained, if possible, at the time of surgery.

To correct coronal or sagittal plane deformities, or to address translational instabilities, surgeons depend on spinal release procedures, including posterior, anterior, and three-column spinal osteotomies, to restore alignment. These techniques, combined with the rigid three-dimensional control afforded by pedicle screw systems, allow the surgeon to achieve coronal, sagittal, and translational correction.

Lumbopelvic Fixation

Practical experience has taught surgeons that sacral pedicle screw fixation alone cannot stabilize the lumbosacral junction in long fusion constructs (encompassing five or more levels), and multiple studies have demonstrated the inadequacy of sacral fixation in these circumstances. Early sacral screw–bone interface failure results in loss of sagittal alignment and increases the risk of lumbosacral pseudarthrosis. Iliac fixation to control the lumbopelvis was initially conceived for the treatment of children with neuromuscular spinal deformity and used the Galveston post in a modification of Luque rod fixation to the ilium-pelvis. They used a unique three-dimensional rod bend and inserted a 5- to 10-cm segment of rod between the iliac tables, starting at the posterior superior iliac spine and then directing it to the anterior inferior iliac spine. The rod remains completely within the ilium and is located in strong supra-acetabular bone, approximately 1 cm proximal to the sciatic notch. Modifications to the Cotrell-Dubousset system also resulted in the development of iliac screws as well as an iliosacral screw that crossed the sacroiliac joint. McCord and Asher performed a biomechanical evaluation of this pelvic fixation.[6] They defined the concept of the pivot point and noted the importance of extending iliac screws anterior to this point. This iliac fixation was found to be biomechanically superior to any combination of sacral fixation, with or without structural anterior interbody lumbosacral grafting.

Tips from the Masters 19-2 • Utilize iliac screw fixation to ensure sacro-pelvic stability.

Bridwell and Lebwohl's follow-up biomechanical studies demonstrated clearly the superior biomechanical effects of the iliac screws and supported the combination of structural anterior interbody grafting with bilateral iliac screw placement as the most secure method of stabilizing the lumbopelvic junction.[7,8] Today, many spinal surgeons augment the bicortical sacral screws with iliac screws when dealing with spinal lesions that demand a long fusion extending from the thoracolumbar junction to the sacrum.

Anterior Column Reconstruction

The next surgical decision that must be tackled is to determine the need for anterior column reconstruction. Advantages of anterior column reconstruction are that it allows achievement of circumferential fusion with thorough diskectomy and grafting techniques, correction of fixed sagittal and coronal segmental misalignment, and reconstruction of anterior column support function with structural implants. Disadvantages include the need for a second surgical intervention, the longer hospitalization required, and the risk of exposure-related complications such as hernias, sympathetic and parasympathetic chain injury, abdominal wall paresis, and vascular and visceral injuries.

Anterior column reconstruction can be achieved via standard anterior lumbar approaches that include direct anterior retroperitoneal access for the L3-L4 to L5-S1 levels, standard left or right retroperitoneal flank exposures that allow access from L1-L2 to L5-S1, and more extensile thoracolumbar transdiaphragmatic exposures that allow exposure from T3 to S1.

Tips from the Masters 19-3 • Utilize anterior interbody fusion techniques when necessary to optimize sagittal alignment and ensure anterior column fusion.

Over the past 5 years minimally invasive lateral flank exposures that traverse the psoas muscle have been developed and have specific utility at L2-L3, L3-L4, and L4-L5 if neural anatomy allows. But deformity correction is limited to these segments, and by the inability to achieve a substantial anterior release, so the segmental spinal deformity must be positionally correctable.

Restoring anterior column support function requires placement of structural interbody grafts or implants that provide adequate end-plate support and enhance osseous healing across the disk space. Historically, these structural grafts were obtained from autogenous sources such as the ilium, ribs, and fibula. Although this worked well to achieve the goals for the spine there were issues with donor site pain and complications. This led to the evolution of allograft structural bone graft options, usually configured as tricortical iliac wedges and femoral rings. Initially, these were used as fresh frozen grafts, but concern for disease transmission led to the development of processes that could "sterilize" the implants, with variable diminution of biomechanical characteristics and biologic healing potential. This has led to the creation of anterior interbody structural devices that can provide structural support and cover a majority of the vertebral body end plate. These cages are packed with bone graft that can serve as conduits for interbody fusion. Because of their ease of use and modularity these hybrid devices for anterior column reconstruction are now favored by most spinal deformity surgeons. Materials most commonly used include polyetheretherketone (PEEK), PEEK with carbon fibers, and titanium mesh cages. Cylindrical screw-shaped cages lost popularity as standalone devices, but have had a resurgence for specialty use in interbody fusion procedures via the lateral approach, in which they are placed coronally across the disk space. Recent developments in cage design include cages that affix to the vertebral bodies with screws and vertically expandable cages. Although these are clever innovations, they do not offer a significant advantage in multilevel thoracolumbar deformity correction.

Posterior Lumbar Interbody Fusion/Transforaminal Lumbar Interbody Fusion Technique

An additional option for reconstruction of the anterior column is the use of a PLIF or transforaminal lumbar interbody fusion (TLIF) technique from the posterior approach (Figure 19-2). Certain criteria must be met to use this technique. For one, the surgeon must be able to achieve the sagittal and coronal plane realignment goals from this approach. Limitations include the need to remove large claw osteophytes and contracted anterior longitudinal ligaments or anterior column ankylosis. PLIF/TLIF techniques can be applied up to the conus medullaris, but become increasingly challenging to implement when the disk spaces are narrow. Previous surgery can also create a great deal of scar in the spinal canal and limit the amount of neural retraction, which may be required to safely perform these procedures. Generally, all of these levels are amenable to posterior Smith-Petersen osteotomies, which improves the window for cage-graft insertion. Temporary segmental distraction through the pedicle screws allows improved posterior disk space access. Once the disk space is accessed, a variety of intradiskal instruments allow sequential distraction of the disk space. This can be done to correct coronal or sagittal misalignment. Once the segmental correction is made, anterior column support needs to be restored to maintain the desired alignment. This requires placement of structural interbody implants that are inserted from the posterolateral window into the disk space. Interbody fusion with bone graft, augmented with BMP if desired, is then performed. A variety of these devices are available, and they come in a wide range of shapes, sizes, and materials. One preferred option is oval carbon fiber or PEEK implants placed in coronal orientation from a unilateral approach into midbody position in the disk space. Titanium mesh cages, ranging from 10 to 16 mm in diameter and available in a wide range of heights from 8 to 20 mm, may be placed via unilateral or bilateral annulotomies. Coronal realignment can be achieved by adjusting left and right cage heights to level disk spaces. Sagittal realignment can be improved by placing the cage in the anterior third to midbody position. These modular implants allow surgeons to insert two or three implants, improving end-plate coverage and anterior column support. Titanium mesh cages also have the added benefit of limiting sheer forces across the disk space. This is most important at spondylolisthetic L4-L5 and L5-S1 levels.

Spinal Osteotomy Procedures to Correct Spinal Deformity

Spinal osteotomy procedures increase segmental mobility and are used to achieve correction in all types of spinal deformity. Osteotomies are usually defined by the location where the vertebral column is cut.

Posterior osteotomies are generally done from a posterior approach. These involve excision of a portion or the entirety of the facet joints on one or both sides at each level. Often these osteotomies are named for the surgeons who used them to address a specific pathologic condition. The Smith-Petersen osteotomy is done by performing a complete excision of the superior and inferior facet in conjunction with ligamentum flavum excision and hemilaminotomy or laminectomy. It was developed to improve segmental lordosis in kyphotic lumbar defects. Ponte used the same osteotomy for correction of thoracic kyphosis in Scheuermann disease.[9] These posteriorly based osteotomies depend on a mobile disk space to achieve correction in any plane. They are ineffective in conditions in which the anterior column is stiff or rigid.

For abnormalities associated with anterior column stiffness, rigidity, or ankylosis, anterior spinal osteotomy procedures must be used. These can be done by an anterior, lateral, or posterior approach.

Tips from the Masters 19-4 • Utilize technical advances such as anterior and posterior osteotomies to achieve the desired sagittal alignment.

The anterior osteotomy is performed via a standard anterior approach and involves cutting through the anterior column. This is usually done through the disk space level and is often combined with posterior osteotomies to maximize correction. In certain pathologic conditions complete removal of a vertebral body is often performed in conjunction with decompression of the thecal sac. This may be necessary to address neurologic and deformity concerns. It is often required for posttraumatic spinal deformity. For maximal corrective potential the procedure can be expanded into a vertebrectomy, done by excision of the anterior vertebral body and posterior elements at corresponding levels. This disconnects the spine and allows the surgeon complete control in correcting the deformity. This generally requires a two-exposure procedure, with the stages performed sequentially or simultaneously.

The posterior vertebral column resection procedure has recently been popularized to achieve three-column osteotomy and shortening through a single approach. It is highly effective in managing severe and rigid thoracic and thoracolumbar spinal deformity, but is not typically used in the lumbar spine except when dealing with spinal neoplasms.

To address rigid lumbar kyphotic and scoliotic deformities, a posterior-approach three-column osteotomy done by excising a wedge of bone based on the pedicles and carried through the middle column to the anterior column was popularized in the United States as the pedicle subtraction osteotomy (PSO) by Bridwell and others.[10] This osteotomy is very useful for dealing with rigid kyphotic spinal deformity in the lumbar spine. Common pathologic conditions treated by this method include iatrogenic flat back syndrome, ankylosing spinal conditions, and posttraumatic spinal deformity. In their original 2003 study of 66 patients who underwent PSO, Bridwell and colleagues reported a mean SVA correction from +16 cm to +4 cm. Complications included pseudarthrosis in two patients and transient neural deficits in five patients.[10]

The PSO typically yields approximately 30 degrees of correction at a single level. Although this does not re-create the normal segmental alignment, it does correct sagittal plane imbalance and does address the symptoms of flat back syndrome. PSO with asymmetric coronal plane cuts can be used to address combined coronal plane and sagittal plane imbalances, simultaneously correcting both planes.

Selection of the Distal Instrumented Vertebra: L5 Versus Sacropelvis

In the treatment of multilevel spinal lesions, it is not uncommon to consider extending the fusion construct to the sacrum. Although the L5-S1 segment is spared when the spinal lesion can be treated with short segment fusion constructs (L2 to L5), the biomechanical demands on L5-S1 with long fusions extending to the thoracolumbar junction are great and result in unpredictable and precocious failures of this segment.[8]

Tips from the Masters 19-5 • In the vast majority of adult spinal deformity work, fusion to the sacro-pelvis is indicated.

Recently published comparative studies suggest that patients who had fusions stopping at L5 had poorer clinical and radiographic outcomes than those who had fusions to the lumbopelvis. The high rates and unpredictable nature of failure of open L5-S1 segments under long fusions has resulted in changes in spinal deformity practice, with most surgeons carrying fusions that extend to the thoracolumbar junction distally to the sacropelvis. The preferred method of fixation is bilateral S1 pedicle screw fixation augmented by iliac screws placed in the Galveston position. The most common argument against extending to the sacropelvis had been the risk of increased lumbosacral pseudarthrosis. With current fusion and fixation techniques, including iliac screws, fusion augmentation with BMPs, and strategic use of anterior column reconstruction via anterior lumbar interbody fusion or PLIF/TLIF, this complication can be minimized and addressed when recognized.

Selection of the Proximal Instrumented Vertebra

Selection of the proximal end vertebra in multisegmental lumbar fusion is much more complicated than selection of the distal end vertebra and requires analysis of a number of important factors to ensure clinical and radiographic success and to maximize the survival of the spinal segment adjacent to the proximal instrumented vertebra (PIV).

Some important considerations in determining a PIV for long lumbar fusion constructs are the following:

1. Are the sagittal alignment of the segment adjacent to the PIV, the alignment of the adjacent spinal region, and global sagittal alignment (SVA) normal?
2. Is the PIV deviated by coronal plane spinal deformity? Can the PIV be brought to within 4 cm of the coronal spinal axis?
3. Is the PIV in neutral axial rotation?
4. Does the adjacent segment demonstrate healthy facet joints and a healthy intervertebral disk?
5. Is the adjacent segment stable on flexion-extension radiographs?

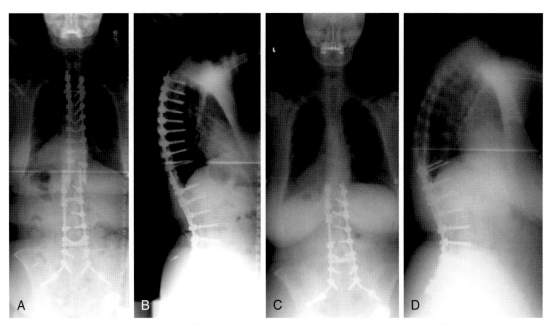

FIGURE 19-5 AP and lateral radiographs illustrating adjacent segment failure via acute "chance" flexion-distraction fracture through the pedicles of the UIV with acute kyphotic deformity. Treated with posterior osteotomy and extension of instrumentation to T3.

In 2007, Suk reported longer adjacent-segment survival time in long lumbar fusions that were carried to T9 or T10 in the lower thoracic spine. He concluded that ending fusions on these rib-bearing vertebrae afforded the next adjacent segment protection from premature breakdown.[11]

Tips from the Masters 19-6 • Proximal end vertebra choice depends on global and regional sagittal concerns, coronal plane alignment, and the relative health of the adjacent spinal segments.

If the conditions are not ideal for stopping at T11, T12, or L1, it is probably safest to extend up to T9 or T10 to maximize survival of the adjacent segment.

Current opinion suggests that certain factors are important when choosing the PIV. These include adequate pedicle dimensions, which vary based on spinal level; healthy adjacent spinal segment with little or no degeneration; normal sagittal segmental alignment; and no rotational or translational malalignment.

Acceptable Regional and Global Sagittal and Coronal Balance

Assuming the aforementioned conditions are met, specific anatomic and biomechanical determinants may be important in the survival of the adjacent spinal segments. Theoretically, stopping at or proximal to T10 may be protective to the adjacent segments because of the enhanced stability provided by the rib cage. Stopping at the relatively mobile lower thoracic (T11-T12) and upper lumbar (L1-L2) spine may predispose to precocious degeneration of the adjacent segments. The surgeon must weigh the pros and cons of extending the fusion across the thoracolumbar junction, including the risk of precocious adjacent-segment failure (Figure 19-5). Prospective longitudinal studies with long-term follow-up should provide information on relative survival based on the selected PIV level. The surgeon should be aware that age-related changes in the proximal unfused spine and adjacent-segment degeneration will uniformly occur with longer follow-up. The patient and family also should be made aware that the likelihood of revision will increase with longer follow-up.

PIV and adjacent-segment failure can take many forms. Acute failures often relate to (1) acute anterior wedge compression fractures at the PIV, the adjacent segment, or even more proximal segments, and/or (2) chance fractures through the proximal pedicle screw trajectory, posterior facet joint fractures, and/or dislocations. Long-term problems include precocious degeneration of the adjacent segment, which can present as a proximal root syndrome or myelopathy secondary to disk herniation, and spinal stenosis with or without segmental instability. Sagittal plane alterations may include development and progression of adjacent-segment kyphosis or proximal thoracic kyphosis. Both can be secondary to age-related degeneration and the natural tendency to develop thoracic kyphosis over time.

Regardless of the pathologic condition that requires fusion of the entire lumbar spine, and regardless of which segment the surgeon ultimately chooses as the PIV, there will remain a risk of short- or long-term failure by a variety of mechanisms at the adjacent segment.

Stage 3/day 2: Immediately following the anterior surgery the patient was repositioned for insertion of posterior rods, application of sequential compression to enhance segmental lumbar lordosis, and completion of posterolateral spinal fusion at L1-S1 with autograft, allograft, demineralized bone matrix, and BMP (6 mg per level). Surgical time was 2 hours. Bone grafts were taken from the iliac crest bilaterally, and an extraarticular iliosacrolumbar fusion was performed (Figure 19-2, F though K). One year after surgery, standing scoliosis radiographs and a CT scan (Figure 19-2, L through N) showed solid anterior column healing and posterolateral fusion. The patient returned to dentistry full time.

COMMENTARY

The management of multisegmental spinal lesions that require fusion of the entire lumbar spine can be a daunting task for any spine surgeon. Deciding how best to address the spinal abnormality requires a careful preoperative planning algorithmic approach. Practical experience has shown that placement of sacral screws alone cannot protect the lumbosacral junction during the healing process. Iliac screw fixation appears to have solved this biomechanical dilemma. The use of anterior column support and anterior spinal fusion procedures offers a great opportunity for the surgeon to fully restore disk space height and lumbar segmental lordosis and thereby positively affect the sagittal balance, which is perhaps the most important factor in achieving good clinical outcomes. Fusion rates are enhanced at the level most prone to pseudarthrosis, L5-S1. Alternatively, the PLIF/TLIF procedure can be used when the pathologic features and anatomy allow.

Spinal osteotomies are important surgical techniques that allow the surgeon to correct sagittal and coronal plane deformity. Management of multisegmental lumbar lesions requires the surgeon to be skilled and facile in applying these techniques.

Selection of the PIV continues to challenge even the most experienced spinal deformity surgeon. Criteria for determining the PIV were presented earlier, but the final answer is not yet available. The controversy between extending to the lower thoracic spine versus stopping at the thoracolumbar junction is centered on whether or not survival of the adjacent segment is significantly improved when instrumentation is extended three or four segments higher than the defect demands. Regardless of where the surgeon stops, careful scrutiny of the adjacent segment is required to recognize adjacent-segment failure over time.

REFERENCES

1. Glassman SD, Berven S, Bridwell K, et al: Correlation of radiographic parameters and clinical symptoms in adult scoliosis, *Spine* 30(6):682–688, 2005. The 298 patients studied include 172 with no prior surgery and 126 who had undergone prior spine fusion. Positive sagittal balance was the most reliable predictor of clinical symptoms in both patient groups. Thoracolumbar and lumbar curves generated less favorable scores than thoracic curves in both patient groups. Significant coronal imbalance of greater than 4 cm was associated with deterioration in pain and function scores for unoperated patients but not in patients with previous surgery. This study suggests that restoration of a more normal sagittal balance is the critical goal for any reconstructive spine surgery. The study suggests that magnitude of coronal deformity and extent of coronal correction are less critical parameters.

2. Lagrone MO, Bradford DS, Moe JH, et al: Treatment of symptomatic flatback after spinal fusion, *J Bone Joint Surg Am* 70(4):569–580, 1988. Fifty-five patients who had loss of lumbar lordosis after spinal fusion and subsequently had corrective osteotomies were studied. When they were first seen, 52 patients (95%) were unable to stand erect and 49 (89%) had back pain. The previous use of distraction instrumentation with a hook placed at the level of the lower lumbar spine or the sacrum was the factor that was most frequently identified as leading to the development of the flatback syndrome. Sixty-six extension osteotomies were performed in these 55 patients; of these, 19 (35%) had an associated anterior spinal fusion, and 33 (60%) had one or more complications, including pseudarthrosis, a dural tear, failure of hardware, neurapraxia, and urinary tract infection. The results of the operation were evaluated at follow-up by review of clinical records, radiographs, and questionnaires. At an average follow-up of 6 years (range, 2-14 years), most patients felt they had benefited from the corrective osteotomies. However, 26 patients (47%) continued to lean forward and 20 patients (36%) continued to have moderate or severe back pain. The failure to restore sagittal plane balance led to a higher rate of pseudarthrosis, which was associated with recurrent deformity. Anterior spinal fusion combined with posterior osteotomy resulted in greater maintenance of correction. The prevention of flatback syndrome is important, since its treatment is difficult. When a spinal fusion must be extended to the level of the lower lumbar spine or the sacrum, the use of distraction instrumentation should be avoided in order to prevent this deformity.

3. Schwab F, el-Fegoun AB, Gamez L, et al: A lumbar classification for scoliosis in the adult patient: preliminary approach, *Spine* 30:1670–1673, 2005.

4. Brown KM, Ludwig SC, Gelb DE: Radiographic predictors of outcome after long fusion to L5 in adult scoliosis, *J Spinal Disord Tech* 17(5):358–366, 2004.

5. Roussouly P, Gollogly S, Berthonnaud E, et al: Classification of the normal variation in the sagittal alignment of the human lumbar spine and pelvis in the standing position, *Spine* 30(3):346–353, 2005.

6. McCord DH, Cunningham BW, Shono Y, et al: Biomechanical analysis of lumbosacral fixation, *Spine* 17(Suppl 8):S235–S243, 1992. Flexion testing was performed until failure on 66 lumbosacral bovine spinal segments comparing 10 different lumbosacral instrumentation techniques. Maximum flexion moment at failure, flexural stiffness, and maximum angulation of the lumbosacral joint at failure were determined as well as strain measurements across the anterior aspect of the lumbosacral intervertebral disk using an extensometer. The maximum moment at failure was significantly greater for the only two devices that extended fixation into the ilium anterior to the projected image of the middle osteoligamentous column: ISOLA Galveston and ISOLA iliac screws (F = 12.2, P < 0.001). The maximum stiffness at failure reinforced these findings (F = 23.7, P < 0.001). A second subset of stability showed the advantages of S2 pedicle fixation by increasing the flexural lever arm (Cotrel-Dubousset butterfly plate, and Cotrel-Dubousset Chopin block, P < 0.05). This exhaustive in vitro biomechanical study introduces the concept of a pivot point at the lumbosacral joint at the intersection of the middle osteoligamentous column (sagittal plane) and the lumbosacral intervertebral disk (transverse plane). A spinal surgeon can increase the stability of lumbosacral instrumentation by extending fixation through the anterior sacral cortex (Steffee plate group with pedicle screws that medially converge in a triangular fashion). A means of enhancing this fixation was to achieve more inferior purchase by extending the fixation down to the S2 pedicle (Cotrel-Dubousset Chopin and Cotrel-Dubousset butterfly groups). However, the best fixation was achieved by obtaining purchase between the iliac cortices down into the superior acetabular bone.

7. Lebwohl NH, Cunningham BW, Dmitriev A, et al: Biomechanical comparison of lumbosacral fixation techniques in a calf spine model, *Spine* 27(21):2312–2320, 2002.

8. Bridwell KH: Utilization of iliac screws and structural interbody grafting for revision spondylolisthesis surgery, *Spine* 30(Suppl 6):S88–S96, 2005. Past studies and experience have suggested that there is a relatively high rate of sacral screw failure both in long constructs to the sacrum in the adult population and also with treatment of both high-grade and adult spondylolisthesis at L5-S1. It has been noted that anterior column support at L5-S1 and additional fixation points in the sacropelvic unit provide some protection to the sacral screws. For many of these cases of both high-grade dysplastic spondylolisthesis and low-grade adult isthmic spondylolisthesis, a reasonable combination of anterior column support and/or iliac screw fixation may be logical to reduce the incidence of failure and need for revision. The biggest concern with using iliac screw fixation is that these screws are prominent in a percentage of patients and the ultimate impact on the sacroiliac joint is not fully investigated. However, at our institution with 5- to 10-year follow-up, the impact on the sacroiliac joint has been minimal.

9. Geck MJ, Macagno A, Ponte A, Shufflebarger HL: The Ponte procedure: posterior only treatment of Scheuermann's kyphosis using segmental posterior shortening and pedicle screw instrumentation, *J Spinal Disord Tech* 20(8):586–593, 2007.

10. Bridwell KH, Lewis SJ, Edwards C, et al: Complications and outcomes of pedicle subtraction osteotomies for fixed sagittal imbalance, *Spine* 28(18):2093–2101, 2003.

11. Suk SI, Kim JH, Kim WJ, et al: Posterior vertebral column resection for severe spinal deformities, *Spine* 27(21):2374–2382, 2002.

Chapter 20   High-Grade Spondylolisthesis: Reduction and Fusion Versus In Situ Fusion

Matthew B. Maserati, Christopher I. Shaffrey, Adam S. Kanter

High-grade lumbosacral spondylolisthesis is rare and likely a distinct entity from low-grade spondylolisthesis. Although the etiology of the condition is not completely understood, it is likely the result of a congenitally dysplastic lumbosacral segment with incompetent posterior elements that cannot withstand typical forces associated with maintenance of an upright posture. Unlike low-grade slips, whose manifestations are typically limited to painful segmental instability or neural compromise at the affected level, high-grade slips invariably provoke secondary changes in the regional pelvic anatomy and thus produce global sagittal deformity. It is this global deformity that makes the surgical management of high-grade spondylolisthesis so complex and so challenging.

Although slip reduction was contemplated as early as 1921, the procedure was undeniably associated with an unacceptably high rate of neurologic injury, and most experts agreed that in situ fusion was safer and produced acceptable results. Still, some surgeons continued to pursue reduction, believing that correction of the underlying deformity was supported by sound mechanical principles and—in the right hands—could be safely accomplished. With the advent of modern transpedicular instrumentation, what had once seemed unsafe became possible, and the debate was rekindled between proponents of reduction and advocates of in situ fusion. Unfortunately, no randomized, controlled trials exist to definitively answer the question of which approach is superior. Nevertheless, a close examination of the evidence is warranted and will allow the modern spine surgeon to formulate a cogent approach to the treatment of the patient with high-grade spondylolisthesis.

CASE PRESENTATION

A 22-year-old woman came for treatment of low back pain that had persisted for the past 8 years; was worse when she was sitting, standing, or walking; and had progressed over the previous year. Nonsteroidal antiinflammatory drugs and physical therapy were initially helpful but no longer provided relief from the pain. In addition, her pain had recently begun to radiate into the buttocks and legs in a nondermatomal distribution.

- PMH: Unremarkable
- PSH: Unremarkable
- Exam: On physical examination, the patient was a well-appearing young woman who, when standing erect, showed a subtle sagittal deformity in which the trunk was thrust forward relative to the hips. Motor strength was full throughout, and no sensory deficit was detected. Hamstring tightness was present bilaterally. Deep tendon reflexes were normal throughout. The lumbar paraspinous muscles were moderately tender to manual palpation. The patient reported no bowel or bladder dysfunction.

- Imaging: Plain spinal radiographs were obtained, including 36-inch standing posteroanterior and lateral radiographs and flexion-extension views of the lumbar spine. These demonstrated Grade IV lumbosacral spondylolisthesis with the following characteristic findings: retroversion of the pelvis, dysplasia of the posterior elements of L5, including bilateral pars interarticularis defects, rounding of the sacral dome, trapezoidal shape of the L5 vertebral body, and positive sagittal balance. Magnetic resonance imaging of the lumbar spine was obtained to evaluate neural element involvement and confirmed severe, bilateral L5 and S1 neural foraminal narrowing (Figure 20-1).

SURGICAL OPTIONS

Among the many decisions to be made when planning a surgery for high-grade spondylolisthesis is whether to reduce the deformity or simply perform fusion in situ[1-3] (Table 20-1). If reduction is to be performed, will complete anatomic realignment be attempted, or is partial reduction of the slip angle sufficient (Tips from the Masters 20-1)? It has become widely accepted that when reduction is to be attempted, wide decompression is essential to minimize the risk of iatrogenic neurologic deficit. Instrumentation, on the other hand, is for most surgeons a must—although in rare cases (such as with severe osteoporosis or renal osteodystrophy) a noninstrumented fusion might be considered, followed by postoperative immobilization in a brace or cast. How, and which levels, to instrument must then be determined.

Tips from the Masters 20-1 • Partial reduction (particularly of slip *angle*) offers significant biomechanical advantages, whereas complete (anatomic) reduction is rarely necessary.

Traditional pedicle screw-rod constructs remain the gold standard, but additional options exist, particularly for fixation of the lumbosacral joint; for example, transvertebral screws directed through the S1 pedicle, across the L5-S1 disk space, and into the body of L5 provide excellent fixation across multiple cortices when significant reduction is not desired or achievable, or when significant dysplasia of the L5 pedicles precludes adequate fixation (Tips from the Masters 20-2).

FIGURE 20-1 Preoperative sagittal T2-weighted magnetic resonance imaging scan demonstrating Grade IV lumbosacral spondylolisthesis.

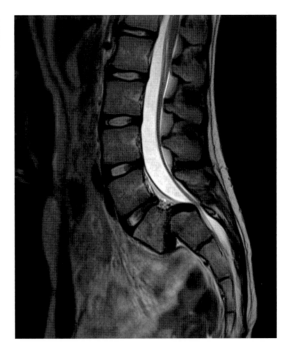

TABLE 20-1 Surgical Options When Addressing High-Grade Spondylolisthesis

1. ± Reduction
   a. Partial vs. complete (anatomic) reduction
   b. Correction of kyphosis alone vs. reduction of slip percentage
2. ± Instrumentation
   a. Pedicle screws vs. transvertebral/transdiskal screws
   b. Navigation (live or virtual fluoroscopy, computed tomography)
3. ± Decompression
   a. Loose posterior (dysplastic) elements of L5
   b. Sacral dome resection (osteotomy)
4. Approach
   a. Interbody device or graft vs. transvertebral cage or dowel
   b. Anterior vs. posterior/posterolateral vs. combined approach
   c. Single stage vs. multiple stages
5. ± Extension of instrumentation/fusion to "normal" levels
   a. Caudal (e.g., S2, ilium) fixation
   b. Rostral (e.g., L4) fixation
6. ± Postoperative immobilization
   a. Bed rest
   b. Lumbosacral orthosis
   c. Casting

Tips from the Masters 20-2 • Strong consideration should be given to incorporating supplemental fixation such as iliac screws, S2 pedicle screws, and/or L4 pedicle screws to protect the construct from the powerful shear forces acting at the lumbosacral junction, especially if anatomic reduction is not performed.

Next, the surgeon must decide whether to perform a decompression, which can simply consist of the removal of the loose posterior elements of L5 or may involve wide removal of the pars interarticularis; in addition, osteotomy (Tips from the Masters 20-3) of the sacral dome may in some cases facilitate reduction and increase the safety of the procedure. Options for arthrodesis include posterior (if decompression is not performed), posterolateral, anterior, or a combination of posterior-posterolateral and anterior (Tips from the Masters 20-4). Anterior interbody arthrodesis may be accomplished through an anterior (transperitoneal) approach, or via a transforaminal or posterior approach. Typically, interbody arthrodesis is accomplished using an interbody device (e.g., titanium or carbon fiber cage) or structural bone graft. Alternatively, a metal cage or fibular dowel may be inserted—with either a posterior or anterior trajectory—across the lumbosacral junction.

Tips from the Masters 20-3 • Wide decompression of the neural elements with particular attention to compressive dysmorphic elements (e.g., fibrocartilaginous pars, sacral dome), in addition to judicious distractive reduction under direct visualization of the neural elements, is essential to avoid iatrogenic neural injury.

Tips from the Masters 20-4 • Interbody fusion, whether performed from an anterior or posterior approach, is essential to the long-term success of the final construct.

Surgical staging must additionally be considered, particularly in regard to the patient's ability to tolerate the extended time under anesthesia required by a combined anterior-posterior procedure. Finally, the surgeon must decide whether to extend the arthrodesis and instrumentation beyond the lumbosacral segment.

FIGURE 20-2 Postoperative lateral radiograph demonstrating partial slip reduction and instrumented fusion of L4 to S1 with interbody graft at L5-S1.

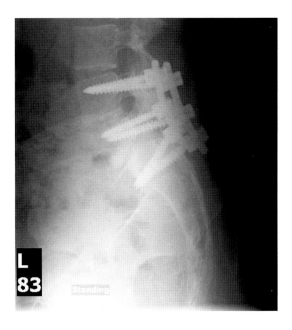

Incorporation of L4 is typical, but the addition of S2 pedicle screws or iliac screws is gaining acceptance for improved construct strength.

Given the severity of the patient's symptoms, her failure to obtain lasting relief from conservative measures, and her dramatic lumbosacral deformity, she elected to proceed with surgery. She subsequently underwent a single-stage procedure using a posterior midline approach for wide decompression of L5 and pedicle screw fixation at L4, L5, and S1, followed by partial reduction of her lumbosacral slip, lumbosacral interbody fusion, and bilateral L4-S1 inter–transverse process (and interalar) fusion (Tips from the Masters 20-5). There were no intraoperative or postoperative complications and she was able to ambulate without the need for a brace on the second postoperative day. She was discharged home on the third postoperative day and, at latest follow-up, remains pain-free without any need for oral analgesic medicines (Tips from the Masters 20-6). Plain lumbar radiographs obtained postoperatively revealed successful partial slip reduction (Figure 20-2).

Tips from the Masters 20-5 • Consider transsacral, transvertebral fibular dowel and/or screws when anatomic reduction is not performed.

Tips from the Masters 20-6 • Consider using the Gaines method when reduction of spondyloptosis is deemed necessary.

FUNDAMENTAL TECHNIQUE

The patient is positioned on a radiolucent Jackson table to decompress the abdomen (and thereby decrease intraoperative bleeding) and enable flexion of the pelvis and extension of the lumbar spine via positioning of the anterior superior iliac spine pads. Following wide lateral decompression and exposure of the neural elements, including sacral dome osteotomy when necessary, the reduction maneuver is executed using pedicle screw fixation with extended tab reduction screws from L4 to S1 followed by distraction under direct visualization of the exiting nerve roots. Care is taken not to distract excessively to avoid screw loosening, nerve stretch injury, and iatrogenic instability at adjacent levels. Upon completion of reduction, the nerves are palpated to ensure that they are not under tension, and direct nerve root stimulation is performed.

The recommendation is that continuous neurophysiologic monitoring be performed routinely, including measurement of somatosensory and motor evoked potentials and electromyography, and reduction is terminated if any abnormality is detected with the maneuver. Posterolateral instrumented fusion from L4 to S1 is performed and augmented in essentially all cases by interbody fusion. Use of the anterior approach to the lumbosacral interspace is often impractical, given the limited access to the disk space when slip percentage and angle are severe, and thus the anterior fusion is in almost all cases executed via the transforaminal approach. To reiterate, the many benefits afforded by interbody fusion include (1) availability of increased surface area for fusion, (2) compressive load sharing to increase the stability of posterior instrumentation, (3) indirect neural decompression of the neural foramen via increased intervertebral height, and (4) restoration of segmental lordosis. Iliac fixation is commonly included, particularly when anatomic reduction is not achieved. In cases of spondyloptosis, one of three options is selected, depending on the particular anatomy and clinical presentation: (1) fusion in situ from L4 to the sacrum using fibular dowel grafts, (2) posterior reduction and fusion with iliac fixation, or (3) the Gaines procedure of anterior-posterior L5 spondylectomy and placement of L4 onto the sacrum, supplemented by iliac fixation.

Patients are in most cases mobilized by the second postoperative day. Occasionally, a thoracolumbosacral orthosis (including thigh extensions) is provided to adequately control the pelvis for 3 or 4 months or until radiographic fusion is confirmed.

DISCUSSION OF BEST EVIDENCE

Due in large part to the rarity of high-grade lumbosacral spondylolisthesis, no prospective studies exist comparing reduction with fusion in situ. The best evidence available to date is limited to retrospective case series with a small number providing a comparison of surgical strategies. Of the several dozen retrospective series reported, more than one third predate modern techniques of transpedicular instrumentation, which makes any conclusions from these publications of limited relevance to contemporary surgical practices.

Further confounding the interpretation of this body of literature is the fact that many series suffer from profound heterogeneity: Study populations frequently included both skeletally mature and immature patients, combined new cases and salvage procedures, and comprised a mixture of patients with spondyloptosis and Grade III/IV slips (many experts posit that spondyloptosis requires a fundamentally different approach). The surgical approach was seldom uniform, with many studies describing a mixture of anterior, posterior, and combined approaches, inconsistent decompression, variable fusion methods, and widely varying degrees of reduction. Finally, the length and quality of follow-up frequently varied significantly both within a given study and between series. Perhaps most problematic of all is the inconstant use of validated outcome measures; moreover, those studies that do use metrics such as the Oswestry Disability Index (ODI) and the Scoliosis Research Society (SRS) questionnaire only rarely report preoperative scores.

In an attempt to draw meaningful conclusions from this heterogeneous body of literature, the available studies have been stratified into three tiers according to the quality of the evidence presented. After exclusion of historical studies that did not use transpedicular instrumentation, each study was evaluated with respect to size, length of follow-up, and use of a validated outcome measure. High-quality studies were of at least moderate size (10+ patients), had at least 2 years of follow-up in all cases, and used a validated outcome measure; intermediate-quality studies were deficient in meeting only one of these criteria; low-quality studies were deficient in meeting two of these criteria.

High-Quality Studies

Of the 19 eligible studies, 3 case series and 1 retrospective comparative study were identified as "high quality" (Table 20-2).

TABLE 20-2   High-Quality Studies

Ruf et al.[4]

- Retrospective series (27 patients, aged 9-29 years)
- Anatomic reduction, decompression, and instrumented circumferential fusion of L5 to S1 (18 PLIF, 9 ALIF); 14 patients had temporary L4 fixation (electively removed at 3 months); spondyloptosis was treated using the Gaines method
- Follow-up 24-80 months (mean, 45 months)
- 1 case of permanent neurologic deficit (L5 sensory) (3.7%); 5 cases of transient L5 motor weakness; 1 reoperation to decompress L5 roots
- No cases of nonunion or device failure, no loss of correction
- Outcome (SRS-30 mean scores, data available for 24 patients): pain 21.9/25,* function/activity 20.5/25, self-image 25.2/30, mental health 19.5/25, satisfaction 9/10
- Weaknesses: SRS-30 data not obtained preoperatively; surgical techniques somewhat heterogeneous; mix of Grade III/IV and Grade V slips; mix of both skeletally mature and immature patients

Sasso et al.[5]

- Retrospective series (25 patients, aged 10-50 years)
- Reduction of slip angle only, decompression, and L4-S1 instrumented fusion using transvertebral fibular dowel (posterior-only approach in 8, with instrumented posterolateral L4-S1 fusion and posterior L5-S1 dowel; anterior-posterior approach in 17, with L4-L5 ALIF and anterior L5-S1 dowel followed by instrumented posterolateral L4-S1 fusion)
- Follow-up 30-71 months (mean, 39 months)
- No cases of permanent neurologic deficit
- No cases of nonunion or loss of correction
- Outcome: 24 of 25 patients were either extremely or somewhat satisfied (SRS score); mean score on visual analog pain scale improved from 8.2 preoperatively to 3.4 postoperatively
- Weaknesses: very heterogeneous surgical approach; mix of Grade III/IV and Grade V slips; mix of skeletally mature and immature patients

Hanson et al.[6]

- Retrospective series (17 patients, aged 13-56 years; 10 primary and 7 revision cases)
- Decompression, partial reduction, and instrumented posterolateral fusion, followed by anterior placement of transvertebral fibular dowel in 15; 2 patients had decompression, in situ noninstrumented posterolateral fusion, and posteriorly inserted transvertebral fibular dowel; instrumentation was from L4 to S1 in 11, L4 to ilium in 1, L5 to ilium in 1, L3 to ilium in 1, and T5 to ilium in 1
- Follow-up 2-8 years (mean, 4.6 years)
- No cases of permanent neurologic deficit
- 2 cases of nonunion (22%), including 1 fractured fibular dowel; no cases of loss of correction
- Outcome: mean ODI was 11.4%, mean SRS score was 37.3/45 (mean SRS satisfaction subscore was 14.1/15)
- Weaknesses: heterogeneous surgical technique; mix of skeletally mature and immature patients; mix of primary and revision surgeries; ODI and SRS data not obtained preoperatively

Poussa et al.[7]

- Retrospective comparative series (22 patients, aged 10.7-18.5 years)
- 11 patients had decompression, reduction, instrumented posterolateral fusion of L5 to S1 (in 2) or L4 to S1 (in 9) and L5-S1 ALIF; 11 patients had decompression (in 7), in situ L5-S1 ALIF, and *noninstrumented* posterolateral fusion of L5 to S1 (in 4) or L4 to S1 (in 7)
- Follow-up 11.6-18.7 years (mean, 14.8 years)
- 1 case of permanent L5 injury (9.1%) in reduction group; no permanent injuries in in situ group (2 L5 injuries resolved after reoperation)
- 2 cases of nonunion (18%) in reduction group; no cases of nonunion in in situ group
- 1 patient in reduction group had significant (>10%) loss of correction
- Outcome: mean ODI and SRS scores better for in situ group than for reduction group (ODI 1.6% vs. 7.2%, $P = .0096$; SRS 103.9 vs. 90, $P = .046$)
- Weaknesses: somewhat heterogeneous surgical technique within each cohort; mix of Grade III/IV and Grade V slips; mix of skeletally mature and immature patients; ODI and SRS data not obtained preoperatively

ALIF, Anterior lumbar interbody fusion; *ODI,* Oswestry Disability Index; *PLIF,* posterior lumbar interbody fusion; *SRS,* Scoliosis Research Society; *SRS-30,* Scoliosis Patient Questionnaire: Version 30 (Scoliosis Research Society).
*Values following virgule indicate maximum possible score.

Following spondylolisthesis reduction in 27 patients, Ruf and colleagues[4] concluded that anatomic reduction and circumferential instrumented fusion from L5 to S1 is feasible and safe, and thus superior to in situ fusion because it accomplishes the ultimate goal of surgery for high-grade spondylolisthesis—restoration of sagittal balance with minimal functional restriction. They note that neurologic injury may largely be avoided by using four key techniques: (1) wide, lateral exposure of the nerve roots; (2) removal of potentially compressive disk material or bony sacral ledge; (3) avoidance of excessive distraction, which is permitted by sufficient resection of the sacral dome and use of small interbody cages; and (4) adequate correction of the sacral retroversion, which thereby relieves tension on the nerve roots.

Sasso and associates[5] reported their results of partial reduction (of slip angle only) in 25 patients and concluded that complete (anatomic) reduction of severe slips is not essential and that partial kyphosis correction followed by fusion from L4 to S1 is safe and results in high satisfaction scores.

Hanson and co-workers[6] reported positive results after partial reduction and circumferential instrumented fusion using a transvertebral fibular dowel in 15 patients. They concluded that partial reduction was safe and effective, noting that use of anterior grafts is critical to the success of the operation.

Poussa and colleagues[7] authored the only comparative series in this group of studies. They reported lengthy follow-up (average, 14.8 years) after in situ fusion or reduction for treatment of high-grade spondylolisthesis. They noted a higher rate of permanent neurologic deficit in the reduction group (9.1% vs. 0%) and found that, although partial correction of slip percentage was achieved and sagittal alignment was improved in the reduction group, outcome (as measured by the SRS questionnaire and ODI) was superior in the in situ fusion group. They concluded that good clinical results are achieved mainly because the slip is stabilized and the neural elements decompressed, and that in situ fusion should therefore be considered the surgical treatment of choice for high-grade spondylolisthesis.

In summary, four studies met the criteria for "highest quality." Three of the four are case series in which patients were treated with reduction, and these report positive results: high patient satisfaction and function scores (as measured by the SRS questionnaire, ODI, and visual analog scale [VAS]), low rates of permanent neurologic deficit (0% to 3.7%; weighted average, 1.5%), and no loss of correction. The sole comparative study in the group demonstrated inferior results after reduction. This study, however, suffered from significant variability in surgical technique, and although permanent neurologic injury was reported only in the reduction group (one patient), two patients in the in situ group required reoperation to decrease the graft height after emerging from the initial surgery with bilateral peroneal palsies. Furthermore, the poor results after reduction reported by the authors are not consistent with the results reported in the other three studies.

In conclusion, these studies suggest that partial reduction, when accomplished in conjunction with wide neural element decompression and circumferential instrumented arthrodesis, is safe, effective, and durable with low rates of neurologic injury (0% to 9.1%; weighted average, 2.6%), high patient satisfaction, high fusion rates, and infrequent loss of correction at more than 3 years of follow-up.

Intermediate-Quality Studies

Eleven studies, consisting of eight case series and three retrospective comparative series, met the criteria for "intermediate quality" (Table 20-3).

All but one of these 11 series reported favorable results after reduction. Muschik and associates,[8] in the largest comparative series in the literature, reported a higher rate of permanent neurologic deficit in the reduction group than in the in situ fusion group (3.3% vs. 0%, respectively), and despite achieving statistically significant improvement in slip percentage and slip angle in the reduction group, found no difference between the groups in overall satisfaction or number of patients free of symptoms. However, the rate of pseudarthrosis was greater in the in situ group

TABLE 20-3   Intermediate-Quality Studies

Muschik et al.[8]

- Retrospective comparative series (59 children, aged 9-19 years; *high-grade slip defined as offset of >30%*)
- 29 children were treated with anterior in situ L5-S1 fusion from 1980 to 1986; 30 children were treated with posterior reduction, instrumented posterior L5-S1 fusion, and L5-S1 ALIF after 1986; no decompression was performed
- Follow-up 56-160 months (mean, 125 months) for in situ group, 24-90 months (mean, 67 months) for reduction group
- 1 case of permanent neurologic deficit (bilateral foot drop) in reduction group (3.3%)
- Nonunion greater for in situ group (24% vs. 7%; *P* < .02)
- No statistically significant loss of correction seen in reduction group
- Outcome: number of patients free of symptoms increased in both groups equally
- Weaknesses: no validated outcome measure; chronologic bias in surgical technique; only reduction group underwent posterior surgery; length of follow-up differed dramatically; unclear how many patients actually had high-grade slip; decompression not performed, even for reduction

Sailhan et al.[9]

- Retrospective series (44 patients, aged 10-50 years)
- Reduction and fusion without decompression: anterior only (ALIF) in 2, posterior only (instrumented posterior fusion of L4 to S1) in 21, and anterior-posterior (instrumented posterior fusion of L4 to S1 followed by ALIF) in 21
- Follow-up 13 months-13 years (mean, 3.75 years; only 41 of 44 patients had at least 2 years of follow-up)
- 2 cases of permanent L5 injury (4.5%)
- 11.4% nonunion (4 of 21 [19%] in anterior-posterior group vs. 1 of 21 [5%] in posterior-only group)
- Outcome: 28 patients (63.6%) had "good" outcome, 10 patients (22.7%) had "fair" outcome, and 6 patients (13.6%) had "poor" outcome; 2 patients who initially had "poor" outcome underwent reoperation and were subsequently reclassified as having "fair" outcome for overall rate of 91% for good-fair results; 13 patients (31%) had persistent low back pain at last follow-up
- Weaknesses: no validated outcome measure; decompression not performed; heterogeneous surgical technique, with only half undergoing anterior fusion (which was performed 1 week after the posterior stage); higher rate of nonunion associated with circumferential arthrodesis, compared with posterior-only fusion, is inconsistent with a large body of evidence showing increased fusion rates with the incorporation of anterior column fusion and calls into question the surgical technique and/or assessment methods used

Molinari et al.[10]

- Retrospective comparative series (32 patients, aged 9-20 years)
- 11 patients had in situ noninstrumented posterior fusion followed by immobilization in a hyperextension cast for 4-7 months; 7 patients had reduction (except in 1 patient), decompression, and instrumented posterolateral fusion of L4 to ilium or L5 to ilium (in 1 patient), followed by immobilization with bed rest—and in some cases casting as well—for 4 months; 14 patients, plus 5 from the other groups undergoing revision, had reduction, decompression, instrumented posterolateral fusion (L4 to ilium or, in 3 patients, L5 to ilium) and anterior fusion (3 through a posterior-only approach, 16 through a separate anterior approach), followed by bed rest—and in some cases casting as well—for 4 months
- Follow-up 2-10 years (mean, 3.1 years)
- 1 case of permanent foot drop (4.5%) in a patient who underwent reduction
- 45% nonunion in in situ group, 29% nonunion in reduction and posterolateral fusion group, 0% nonunion in reduction and circumferential fusion group
- Outcome measure combined questions from AAOS and SRS questionnaires; scores did not differ significantly between groups *as long as fusion was achieved,* although there was a tendency toward better scores in the reduction and circumferential fusion group
- Weaknesses: no validated outcome measure; very heterogeneous surgical methods

Gaines[11]

- Retrospective case series (30 patients, aged 12-50 years; 26 primary and 4 revision cases)
- All patients underwent Gaines procedure of L5 vertebrectomy from an anterior approach, followed by placement of L4 onto the sacrum and instrumented posterolateral fusion from L4 to the sacrum; first 3 patients had fixation with Harrington compression rods, whereas remaining 27 patients had fixation with pedicle screw-rod constructs; all patients were immobilized with bed rest for 4-6 weeks
- Follow-up 1-25 years (mean, 15 years; 28 of 30 patients had at least 2 years of follow-up)
- 3 cases of permanent neurologic injury: foot drop in 2 patients and retrograde ejaculation in 1 patient; 24 of 30 patients experienced at least transient neurologic deficit
- 6.7% nonunion with screw breakage (fusion was achieved after reoperation)
- No cases of loss of correction

Continued

TABLE 20-3 Intermediate-Quality Studies—cont'd

- Outcome: all patients had resolution of their preoperative back and leg pain, experienced improved functional capacity and regained work and leisure time capacity, and would recommend the procedure to others; no patient was taking narcotic analgesics at last follow-up
- Weaknesses: no validated outcome measure; combined skeletally mature and immature patients; combined primary and revision cases

DeWald et al.[12]

- Retrospective comparative series (21 patients, 20 operated, aged 21-68 years; included 5 revision cases)
- 16 patients had partial kyphosis correction with posterior decompression, instrumented posterolateral fusion of L4 to S1 (in 10), L3 to S1 (in 1), or L5 to S1 (in 5), and interbody fusion (ALIF in 7, PLIF in 9); 4 patients had fusion in situ with instrumented posterior fusion of L4 to S1 (in 2) or L3 to S1 (in 2), and interbody fusion (anterior strut in 3, transvertebral screws without fusion in 1)
- Follow-up 1-14 years (mean, 6.6 years; 14 of 16 patients had at least 2 years of follow-up)
- 3 cases of permanent neurologic injury: L5 palsies in 2 patients, worsening of preoperative cauda equina syndrome in 1 patient
- No cases of nonunion or instrumentation failure; loss of correction not mentioned
- Outcome: 11 had "excellent" outcome, defined as minimal to no pain, occasional NSAID use; 7 had "good" outcome, defined as significant improvement in pain but continued requirement for occasional pain medications; 1 had "fair" outcome, defined as good pain relief with occasional to intermittent narcotic use; 1 patient had "poor" outcome, defined as worsening of neurologic function or pain; outcome for in situ group was excellent in 3 and good in 1; outcome after complete reduction was excellent in 1 and fair in 1
- Weaknesses: no validated outcome measure; heterogeneous surgical methods; combined primary and revision surgeries; combined skeletally mature and immature patients; combined spondyloptosis and Grade III/IV spondylolisthesis

Shufflebarger & Geck[13]

- Retrospective case series (18 patients, aged 10-16 years)
- All patients had decompression, reduction, and instrumented circumferential arthrodesis of L5 to S1
- Follow-up 2.3-5.0 years (mean, 3.3 years)
- No cases of neurologic complication
- No cases of nonunion; 2 cases of structural failure without instrumentation failure: 1 patient experienced loss of correction (slip angle progressed from 4 degrees postoperatively to 20 degrees at latest follow-up) but achieved solid fusion nonetheless, and 1 patient developed S1-S2 kyphosis without recurrence of symptoms and the condition was stabilized with a TLSO
- Outcome: patient/parent survey revealed that all patients thought their activity level much improved, and every patient would undergo the procedure again
- Weaknesses: no validated outcome measure

Hu et al.[14]

- Retrospective case series (16 patients, aged 11-42 years; 9 primary and 7 revision cases)
- All patients had decompression, reduction, and instrumented posterolateral fusion of L4 to S1, in 4 cases followed by anterior fusion with fibular dowel (including 1 case performed for delayed union after 10 months)
- Follow-up 1.6-5.4 years (mean, 3.8 years; 15 of 16 patients had at least 2 years of follow-up)
- 1 case of permanent L5 injury (6.25%); 1 case of lumbar plexus palsy that resolved after reoperation
- 1 case of nonunion (6.25%) and 4 failures of fixation; all patients underwent reoperation and fusion was confirmed at last follow-up; 1 case was associated with loss of correction
- Outcome: 10 "excellent," defined as no pain, no need for medication, and no activity restrictions; 5 "good," defined as mild pain, occasional NSAID use, or minor activity restriction; and 1 "fair," defined as moderate to severe pain, need for narcotic medications, or significant activity restriction
- Weaknesses: no validated outcome instrument; mixed primary and revision surgeries; mixed skeletally mature and immature patients; mixed spondyloptosis and Grade III/IV spondylolisthesis; somewhat variable surgical technique

Bartolozzi et al.[15]

- Retrospective case series (15 patients, aged 11-37 years; included 1 revision case)
- All patients had posterior decompression, distractive reduction, instrumented posterolateral fusion of L4 to S1 (in 13) or L5 to S1 (in 2), with L4-L5 posterior lumbar interbody fusion (except for 2 patients) and L5-S1 anterior fusion without diskectomy using a posteriorly placed transsacral titanium cage filled with autograft bone
- Follow-up 12-58 months (mean, 31.4 months; 10 of 15 patients had at least 2 years of follow-up)
- 1 case of permanent L5 injury (6.7%)
- No cases of nonunion, instrumentation failure, or loss of correction

TABLE 20-3 Intermediate-Quality Studies—cont'd

- Outcome: all patients except 1 (who experienced injury to the iliac vein and required laparotomy for repair) were reasonably or extremely satisfied with the result, with mean scores of 4.26/5* for satisfaction, 4.52/5 for pain, 3.84/5 for self-image, 3.87/5 for function/activity, and 4/5 for mental health (modified SRS outcomes instrument)
- Weaknesses: short follow-up; no preoperative SRS data; mixed skeletally mature and immature patients

Smith et al.[16]

- Retrospective case series (9 patients, aged 8-51 years; included 2 revision cases)
- All patients had decompression, partial reduction, and instrumented (L4-S1) circumferential fusion of L5 to S1 using a posteriorly placed transsacral fibular dowel (2 patients did not initially have instrumentation but underwent reoperation after developing pseudarthrosis and fracture of the fibular graft)
- Follow-up 2-3 years (mean, 3.5 years)
- No cases of permanent neurologic deficit
- No cases of nonunion (except in 2 patients who subsequently had fusion after revision with instrumentation); no cases of instrumentation failure or loss of correction
- Outcome: all patients were either extremely or somewhat satisfied with the result, with mean scores of 4.6/5 for satisfaction, 3.7/5 for mental health, 3.6/5 for function, 3.6/5 for self-image, and 3.5/5 for pain (modified SRS outcomes instrument); the 2 patients with multiple previous surgeries reported significantly lower scores for pain, function, and self-image
- Weaknesses: mixed skeletally mature and immature patients; mixed spondyloptosis and Grade III/IV spondylolisthesis; mixed primary and revision cases

Boachie-Adjei et al.[17]

- Retrospective case series (6 patients, aged 13-29 years)
- All patients had posterior decompression, partial reduction, and instrumented (L4-S1 in 5, L3-S1 in 1) circumferential fusion of L5 to S1; 5 patients had supplemental fixation with S2 alar screws; all patients were immobilized in a TLSO for at least 3 months postoperatively
- Follow-up 2-5 years (mean, 3.5 years)
- No cases of neurologic deficit
- No cases of nonunion, instrumentation failure, or loss of correction
- Outcome: all patients had resolution of preoperative radicular pain and numbness, 4 of 6 had resolution of back pain; mean score was 4.3/5 for pain, 4.5/5 for self-image, 4.2/5 for function, and 4.5/5 for overall satisfaction (modified SRS outcomes instrument)
- Weaknesses: small series; no preoperative SRS data; mixed skeletally mature and immature patients; mixed spondyloptosis and Grade IV spondylolisthesis

Mehdian et al.[18]

- Case report (14-year-old boy with Grade III spondylolisthesis)
- Described three-stage procedure (single setting): (1) posterior decompression and diskectomy; (2) transperitoneal anterior release of the annulus fibrosus; (3) posterior reduction, instrumented posterolateral fusion of L4 to S1, and posterior interbody fusion of L5 to S1
- Follow-up 3 years
- No neurologic deficit
- Solid fusion without instrumentation failure or loss of correction
- Outcome: patient "delighted" with cosmetic result, resolution of back and leg pain; VAS score of 1 for back pain, 0 for buttock and calf pain; ODI 6%
- Weaknesses: single case; VAS/ODI scores not obtained preoperatively

AAOS, American Academy of Orthopaedic Surgeons; *ALIF,* anterior lumbar interbody fusion; *NSAID,* nonsteroidal antiinflammatory drug; *ODI,* Oswestry Disability Index; *PLIF,* posterior lumbar interbody fusion; *SRS,* Scoliosis Research Society; *TLSO,* thoracolumbosacral orthosis; *VAS,* visual analog scale.
*Values following virgule indicate maximum possible score.

(24% vs. 7%: *P* < .02), relief from symptoms was statistically less in those with pseudarthrosis, and there was a tendency toward greater satisfaction with the cosmetic result in the reduction group.

This series suffers from a number of problems, however. First, severe spondylolisthesis was defined as a slip of more than 30%, yet determination of which patients actually possessed a high-grade slip was not possible from the data presented. Second, the two techniques were not used concurrently, with all in situ fusions performed before 1986 and all reduction procedures performed after 1986, which resulted in a significant follow-up discrepancy between the two groups (mean of 125 months for the in situ group vs. 67 months for the reduction group). Finally, decompression was not performed, even for those undergoing reduction, which suggests that the permanent injuries encountered in the reduction group might have been avoided.

Sailhan and co-workers[9] performed reduction of high-grade spondylolisthesis in 44 patients. Despite encountering two cases of permanent neurologic deficit (4.5% of patients) and a 31% incidence of persistent low back pain at last follow-up (which they theorize was due to reduction without decompression), the authors concluded that reduction was safe and produced good clinical results.

Molinari and colleagues,[10] in a heterogeneous study comparing (1) in situ non-instrumented posterior fusion, (2) reduction with decompression and instrumented posterolateral fusion, and (3) reduction with decompression and instrumented circumferential fusion, found a tendency toward improved outcome (as measured by a questionnaire combining elements of the American Academy of Orthopaedic Surgeons and SRS versions) in the reduction and circumferential fusion group, although statistical significance was not demonstrated. They further noted that in situ fusion is inadvisable in the subgroup of patients with severe dysplasia of the posterior elements of L5, due to an unacceptably high rate of pseudarthrosis.

Gaines,[11] who pioneered the method of anatomic reduction of spondyloptosis that bears his name, reported his personal experience in the treatment of 30 patients with spondyloptosis over 25 years. He reported a 10% rate of permanent neurologic deficit and a 6.7% nonunion rate at a mean follow-up of 15 years, and concluded that his method of L5 vertebral body resection followed by reduction of L4 onto the sacrum is safe and produces positive, long-lasting clinical results.

DeWald and associates[12] treated 20 patients with high-grade spondylolisthesis, 16 of whom had at least partial reduction, and concluded that in situ fusion is adequate except in those patients with "significant" sagittal malalignment, for whom partial kyphosis correction may be safely achieved and should decrease the rate of pseudarthrosis.

Shufflebarger and Geck[13] reported positive results after reduction with decompression and instrumented circumferential fusion of L5 to S1 in 18 patients. They concluded that reduction is essential to create a permissive biomechanical environment for successful fusion and positive clinical results, and advocated the use of pelvic fixation for protection of sacral screws.

Hu and colleagues[14] obtained good results in their series of 16 patients treated with decompression, reduction, and instrumented posterolateral fusion from L4 to S1, followed in 4 patients by an anterior L5-S1 fusion with fibular strut. The authors concluded that reduction is safe and effective, and emphasized that physical appearance is often critical, especially for spondyloptosis patients, and is not addressed by in situ fusion.

Bartolozzi and associates[15] reported high satisfaction scores (measured using the SRS questionnaire) with a low rate of permanent neurologic injury, 100% fusion rate, and no loss of correction in 15 patients who underwent posterior decompression, partial reduction, and transsacral interbody fusion using a titanium cage. The authors presage the comments of Shufflebarger and co-workers in noting that only those procedures that address the lumbosacral deformity will permit restoration of sagittal balance through derotation of the sacrum and reduction of the compensatory lumbar hyperlordosis.

Smith and colleagues[16] reported good results (as measured by the modified SRS outcomes instrument) in nine patients after decompression, partial reduction, and instrumented (L4 to S1) circumferential fusion of L5 and S1 using a transsacral fibular strut. Although the series was small, follow-up was at least 2 years in all cases (mean, 27 months) and the outcome measure was validated. Based on these results, the authors recommend partial reduction of high-grade spondylolisthesis in both adults and children with a sagittal plane imbalance of more than 5 cm or cosmetic deformity resulting from sagittal imbalance.

Boachie-Adjei and associates[17] reported favorable results in a series of six patients followed for at least 2 years after partial reduction and circumferential instrumented fusion, including no cases of permanent deficit, a 100% fusion rate, and high scores on the modified SRS outcomes instrument. The authors advocate partial reduction (primarily of slip angle) of severe spondylolisthesis, noting that in these patients, the high sheer stresses at the lumbosacral junction necessitate at least partial reduction to enable placement of the fusion mass under adequate compression. Failure to effect some degree of reduction, they posit, will predispose any fusion to delayed failure (i.e., slip progression despite solid fusion, which has been reported in some series in up to 26% of cases) and also perpetuate the global sagittal imbalance and cosmetic deformity resulting from compensatory lumbar hyperlordosis and thoracic hypokyphosis.

Mehdian and co-workers[18] reported excellent results in a 14-year-old boy with Grade III spondylolisthesis who underwent a three-stage procedure without complication (posterior decompression, transperitoneal anterior release, and posterior reduction and circumferential instrumented arthrodesis of L4 to S1). At 3-year follow-up, the patient had solid fusion, no loss of correction, no back pain (as measured by VAS), and a score of 6% on the ODI. The authors note that the procedure they describe is technically demanding, may not always produce such positive results, and is therefore not applicable to all patients with severe lumbosacral spondylolisthesis.

In summary, the 11 intermediate-quality studies almost uniformly reported good results after partial reduction, with low rates of permanent neurologic deficit (0% to 6.7%; weighted average, 5.9%), nonunion, instrumentation failure, and loss of correction, and a high degree of patient satisfaction. Although three series included fewer than 10 patients, five were relatively large, with 20 or more patients. Follow-up extended, for the most part, to at least 2 years postoperatively. Four of the 11 series used a validated outcome measure. The authors of all eight case series concluded that partial reduction is safe and effective, whereas the authors of only one of the three retrospective comparative studies concluded that partial reduction is warranted. However, the two dissenting views emerged from comparative studies that suffered from significant shortcomings (Muschik and colleagues[8] and DeWald and associates,[12] see earlier).

Low-Quality Studies

Four studies, all of which reported the authors' experience with reduction, were determined to be of "low quality" (Table 20-4).

Ani and co-workers[19] reported favorable results after reduction, although long-term follow-up was available for only 50% of patients, the patients' ages were not specified, and whether decompression was performed was unclear.

Dick and Schnebel[20] concluded from the results in their series of 15 patients undergoing reduction that, although positive results were achieved in all cases, the technical challenges of the procedure and the 20% incidence of permanent neurologic injury should preclude its use in all but a select group of patients with debilitating symptoms associated with severe deformity.

Fabris and associates[21] reported complete resolution of symptoms in 12 patients undergoing reduction, without any cases of nonunion, instrument failure, or loss of correction, although long-term follow-up was largely lacking.

Finally, Boos and co-workers[22] reported positive results after reduction in 10 patients, emphasizing that if reduction is to be performed, circumferential fusion is essential to avoid the unacceptably high rate of nonunion seen in their series.

In summary, although their myriad shortcomings preclude one from deriving any meaningful conclusions, these four studies report results similar to those of other, higher-quality studies. Furthermore, the authors of these four reports echo the sentiments shared by most of the other authors regarding the use of reduction in high-grade spondylolisthesis: reduction, although technically challenging and not indicated in all cases, may be safely performed with favorable results provided certain key guidelines are followed.

Summary of the Evidence

The aforementioned 19 series provide ample evidence of the safety and efficacy of reduction of high-grade spondylolisthesis. Although significant variability exists both within and among these studies, it is clear that reduction (at least partial and

TABLE 20-4   Low-Quality Studies

Ani et al.[19]

- Retrospective case series (41 patients, ages not specified; included 17 revision cases)
- All patients (except 1, see later) had posterior reduction and instrumented (L4-S1) circumferential fusion of L5 to S1; Gaines procedure was performed for all cases of spondyloptosis and for cases of some Grade IV spondylolisthesis; not clear whether decompression was performed
- Follow-up (reported only for 20 patients with >24 months follow-up): 24-70 months (mean, 40 months)
- 1 case of permanent L5 palsy; 1 case of lumbar stretch palsy that resolved after reoperation to decrease graft height
- Nonunion with loss of correction occurred only in the initial 3 patients, who did not undergo interbody fusion up front; 2 underwent reoperation and developed solid fusion with preserved correction; 1 patient later experienced fusion essentially in situ
- Outcome: all of the 20 patients followed for >24 months reported "good" to "excellent" satisfaction with the result (10-question assay of pain and function)
- Weaknesses: follow-up data not reported for 50% of patients; outcome measure not validated; combined spondyloptosis and Grade III/IV spondylolisthesis; combined primary and revision cases; heterogeneous surgical methods; age range not specified

Dick et al.[20]

- Retrospective case series (15 patients, aged 14-41 years)
- Posterior reduction and instrumented fusion of L5 to S1 (in 13) or L4 to S1 (in 2), followed by anterior release and interbody fusion of L5 to S1 (in 14); 4 patients underwent decompression
- Follow-up 4-52 months (mean, 24 months; 6 patients had follow-up of >24 months)
- 3 cases of permanent L5 injury (2 in patients who underwent substantial slip correction, and 1 that was likely due to screw misplacement)
- 2 cases of (presumed) nonunion in patients with loss of correction; solid fusion was confirmed in 13 patients at the time of elective hardware removal; screw breakage occurred in 2 patients, 1 of whom had not had upfront anterior fusion and underwent reoperation
- Outcome: all patients had complete relief of pain and improvement in posture and would choose to have the operation again
- Weaknesses: no validated outcome measure; short follow-up; combined skeletally mature and immature patients; somewhat heterogeneous surgical methods

Fabris et al.[21]

- Retrospective case series (12 patients, aged 13-18 years)
- Posterior decompression, reduction (using temporary distraction device extending from L1 to the sacral ala), and circumferential instrumented fusion of L5 to S1
- Follow-up 6-36 months (mean, 16 months; number with follow-up of >24 months not specified)
- No cases of permanent neurologic deficit
- No cases of nonunion, instrumentation failure, or loss of correction
- Outcome: all patients were asymptomatic at last follow-up
- Weaknesses: outcome measure not validated; short follow-up

Boos et al.[22]

- Retrospective case series (10 patients, aged 9-50 years)
- Posterior decompression, reduction, and instrumented posterolateral fusion at L4 to S1 (in 9 patients) or L5 to S1 (in 1 patient); L5-S1 interbody fusion was performed for spondyloptosis (ALIF in 3, PLIF in 1); reduction was performed intraoperatively in 6 patients, and preoperatively in 4 patients (with a temporary AO external spine fixator in 3 patients and with a Cotrel frame in 1 patient)
- Follow-up 43-75 months (mean, 56 months)
- 1 case of permanent L5 injury
- 5 patients with nonunions with loss of reduction (none of whom had upfront anterior fusion, and all of whom eventually achieved fusion, 4 after reoperation with circumferential fusion); no cases of hardware failure
- Outcome: all patients subjectively rated their final result as "good" (1 patient) or "excellent" (9 patients)
- Weaknesses: outcome measure not validated; combined skeletally mature and immature patients; heterogeneous surgical methods; combined spondyloptosis and Grade III/IV spondylolisthesis

ALIF, Anterior lumbar interbody fusion; *PLIF,* posterior lumbar interbody fusion.

particularly of slip angle) is achievable with minimal morbidity provided that (1) great care is taken to widely decompress the neural elements, (2) distraction is neither rapid nor excessive, and (3) meticulous circumferential (instrumented) arthrodesis is performed.

The consensus appears to be that reduction offers overwhelming biomechanical advantages and that procedures that do not incorporate some degree of correction will inevitably provide an inferior result due to persistent physical deformity or construct failure. Expert opinion notwithstanding, the question of which is clinically superior—reduction or in situ fusion—cannot be decided until a well-designed prospective cohort study is performed and long-term follow-up data are obtained.

COMMENTARY

Although nonoperative management is the mainstay of treatment for low-grade spondylolisthesis, high-grade slips frequently require surgery due to refractory pain, progressive deformity, neurologic impairment, or a combination of these. Although reduction of high-grade slips was proposed as early as 1921 (Scherb and colleagues[23]) the accepted approach as advocated by Meyerding[24] and others was for many decades posterior in situ fusion (typically from L4 to S1), with proponents citing satisfactory results and a lower rate of complications. Attempts at reduction continued, however, with varying degrees of success, notably by Capener[25] in 1932 (using traction), Jenkins[26] in 1936 (using traction followed by interbody fusion), and Harrington[27] in 1971 (using open reduction and internal fixation). Nevertheless, reports of iatrogenic cauda equina syndrome and L5 nerve root injuries continued to discourage widespread use of these techniques. As recently as 1976, Nachemson and Wiltse[28] stated without equivocation that in situ fusion worked so well that reduction was rarely warranted, citing an increased risk of neurologic complications, longer operative time, and greater blood loss with reduction.

Over the past quarter century, tremendous advances have been made in surgical techniques, particularly in the realm of spinal instrumentation, with the result that reduction can now be accomplished more safely and effectively than ever before. Historically, the cosmetic deformity of high-grade spondylolisthesis has been underappreciated or felt to be of secondary importance to those who experience significant pain. In contemporary surgical practice, the complex deformity often associated with high-grade spondylolisthesis and its secondary effects on pelvic version and global sagittal balance impel a reconsideration of the role of reduction.

Although an in-depth discussion of the pathoanatomy of spondylolisthesis is beyond the scope of this chapter, a serviceable comprehension of the forces at work is essential to understand the rationale for reduction. First, high-grade slips are fundamentally different from low-grade slips in that (1) there is invariably a dysplastic component, with implications for the feasibility of fixation and posterolateral fusion; and (2) the slip angle becomes a greater source of deformity than the degree of forward translation.[29] Second, the local deformity of the high-grade slip invariably induces compensatory changes in the regional pelvic anatomy—changes that are propagated up the spinal column, ultimately producing a global postural deformity.[30-32] As L5 slips anteriorly and then inferiorly on the sacrum, the mass gravity line (and with it the trunk and head) is drawn forward, forcing the patient into positive sagittal balance. Two attempts to restore balance ensue: (1) tonic activation of the paraspinous (e.g., erector spinae) muscles, and (2) progressive retroversion of the pelvis. Pelvic retroversion induces lumbar hyperlordosis, which is followed in turn by loss of thoracic kyphosis. The hips adapt first by externally rotating (which permits greater hip extension) until the pelvis is maximally retroverted, and then by flexing (along with the knees), producing a stereotypical crouched posture.[33]

These postural changes represent the end stage of severe lumbosacral spondylolisthesis and are typically accompanied by clinical sequelae of low back pain (presumably due to chronic paraspinous muscle activation and/or segmental instability), tight hamstrings, postural deformity, and in some cases radiculopathy or even cauda equina syndrome. Although proponents of in situ fusion have argued that good results are predictably obtained simply through the elimination of abnormal segmental motion, reduction offers several benefits over in situ fusion. First, in situ fusion has been consistently associated with higher rates of nonunion, up to 44% in some series, presumably due to the continued presence of powerful sheer forces acting at the lumbosacral junction and also to decreased available surface area for fusion.[22] The troublesome phenomenon of slip progression despite solid fusion, which has been reported after in situ fusion in up to 26% of cases, is further testament to the perils of leaving the kyphotic deformity of severe lumbosacral spondylolisthesis uncorrected.[34] Finally, although some patients may not express dissatisfaction with their appearance due to the mildness of the deformity or the severity of their back pain or leg complaints, there are many patients for whom cosmetic concerns remain paramount. For this subset of patients, surgery that does not incorporate some element of reduction will inevitably produce an inferior result.

The principal argument against reduction has historically hinged on the associated unacceptably high rate of neurologic deficit. It must be emphasized that iatrogenic neurologic deficit is *not* a constant finding after reduction and that when neurologic deficits do occur, they are typically transient, with rates of *permanent* neurologic deficit after reduction averaging 5% and rarely exceeding 10%. Moreover, deficits have also been reported after in situ fusion.[35] In 1988, the SRS morbidity and mortality report indicated no difference in the rates of neurologic deficit after reduction and in situ fusion in this patient population. The existence of several series in which patients underwent reduction without neurologic complication offers proof that, through adherence to the principles of wide decompression and judicious correction, reduction of high-grade lumbosacral spondylolisthesis can be achieved safely.

Recommended practice when performing surgery for high-grade spondylolisthesis is to include at least partial reduction of the lumbosacral deformity. In situ fusion is preferred only in the rare patient with Grade III or IV lumbosacral spondylolisthesis who (1) presents with back pain in the absence of radicular complaints, neurologic deficit, or cosmetic deformity; (2) has adequate neural foraminal space; and (3) has acceptable overall sagittal balance and good sagittal alignment of the proximal instrumented vertebra.

REFERENCES

1. Bridwell KH: Surgical treatment of high-grade spondylolisthesis, *Neurosurg Clin N Am* 17:331–338, vii, 2006.
2. Hu SS, Tribus CB, Diab M, et al: Spondylolisthesis and spondylolysis, *Instr Course Lect* 57:431–445, 2008.
3. Marchetti PB, Bartolozzi P: Classification of spondylolisthesis as a guideline for treatment. In Bridwell KD, DeWald RL, editors: *The textbook of spinal surgery*, ed 2, Philadelphia, 1997, Lippincott-Raven Publishers, pp 1211–1254.
4. Ruf M, Koch H, Melcher RP, Harms J: Anatomic reduction and monosegmental fusion in high-grade developmental spondylolisthesis, *Spine* 31:269–274, 2006. **Harms—another master in the field of deformity surgery—and colleagues report positive results after complete (anatomic) reduction, decompression, and instrumented circumferential fusion in 27 patients with a minimum follow-up of 2 years (mean, 3.75 years). A low rate of permanent neurologic deficit (one patient), high satisfaction scores (as measured by the SRS-30 questionnaire), and no cases of nonunion, device failure, or loss of correction led the authors to conclude that anatomic reduction and circumferential instrumented fusion is feasible and safe and thus is superior to in situ fusion. They emphasize that the ultimate goal of surgery for high-grade spondylolisthesis is restoration of sagittal balance with minimal functional restriction.**
5. Sasso RC, Shively KD, Reilly TM: Transvertebral transsacral strut grafting for high-grade isthmic spondylolisthesis L5-S1 with fibular allograft, *J Spinal Disord Tech* 21:328–333, 2008. **From results for their series of 25 patients who underwent partial reduction (of slip angle only), decompression, and circumferential instrumented fusion with transvertebral fibular dowel, the authors conclude that complete (anatomic) reduction of severe slips is not essential and that partial correction of kyphosis followed by fusion from L4 to S1 is safe and results in high satisfaction scores. At a follow-up of 2+ years (mean, 3 years), there were no cases of permanent neurologic deficit and no cases of nonunion or loss of correction, and VAS-measured pain scores improved by almost 5 points from the preoperative values.**
6. Hanson DS, Bridwell KH, Rhee JM, et al: Dowel fibular strut grafts for high-grade dysplastic isthmic spondylolisthesis, *Spine* 27:1982–1988, 2002. **In this retrospective case series, the authors—who are widely acknowledged to be masters in the field of deformity surgery—report positive results after decompression, partial slip reduction, and circumferential instrumented fusion using a transvertebral fibular dowel in 17 patients. At a follow-up of 2+ years (mean, 4.5 years), there were no cases of neurologic deficit, no loss of correction, and two cases of nonunion. The authors conclude that partial reduction is safe and effective, and emphasize the importance of anterior grafts.**

7. Poussa M, Remes V, Lamberg T, et al: Treatment of severe spondylolisthesis in adolescence with reduction or fusion in situ: long-term clinical, radiologic, and functional outcome, *Spine* 31:583–590; discussion, 591-582, 2006. **In the only high-quality study comparing reduction with in situ fusion, Poussa and associates report a higher rate of permanent neurologic deficit and worse outcome after reduction. Follow-up was longer than 10 years (mean, 15 years) in all 22 patients, but the surgical technique was variable, and 2 patients in the in situ group required reoperation for an L5 injury (they were therefore not counted as having a permanent neurologic deficit). The authors conclude that good clinical results are achieved mainly because the slip is stabilized and the neural elements decompressed, and that in situ fusion should therefore be considered the surgical treatment of choice for high-grade spondylolisthesis.**

8. Muschik M, Zippel H, Perka C: Surgical management of severe spondylolisthesis in children and adolescents. Anterior fusion in situ versus anterior spondylodesis with posterior transpedicular instrumentation and reduction, *Spine* 22:2036–2042; discussion, 2043, 1997.

9. Sailhan F, Gollogly S, Roussouly P: The radiographic results and neurologic complications of instrumented reduction and fusion of high-grade spondylolisthesis without decompression of the neural elements: a retrospective review of 44 patients, *Spine* 31:161–169; discussion, 170, 2006.

10. Molinari RW, Bridwell KH, Lenke LG, et al: Complications in the surgical treatment of pediatric high-grade, isthmic dysplastic spondylolisthesis. A comparison of three surgical approaches, *Spine* 24:1701–1711, 1999.

11. Gaines RW: L5 vertebrectomy for the surgical treatment of spondyloptosis: thirty cases in 25 years, *Spine* 30:S66–S70, 2005.

12. DeWald CJ, Vartabedian JE, Rodts MF, et al: Evaluation and management of high-grade spondylolisthesis in adults, *Spine* 30:S49–S59, 2005.

13. Shufflebarger HL, Geck MJ: High-grade isthmic dysplastic spondylolisthesis: monosegmental surgical treatment, *Spine* 30:S42–S48, 2005.

14. Hu SS, Bradford DS, Transfeldt EE, et al: Reduction of high-grade spondylolisthesis using Edwards instrumentation, *Spine* 21:367–371, 1996.

15. Bartolozzi P, Sandri A, Cassini M, et al: One-stage posterior decompression-stabilization and trans-sacral interbody fusion after partial reduction for severe L5-S1 spondylolisthesis, *Spine* 28:1135–1141, 2003.

16. Smith JA, Deviren V, Berven S, et al: Clinical outcome of trans-sacral interbody fusion after partial reduction for high-grade L5-S1 spondylolisthesis, *Spine* 26:2227–2234, 2001.

17. Boachie-Adjei O, Do T, Rawlins BA: Partial lumbosacral kyphosis reduction, decompression, and posterior lumbosacral transfixation in high-grade isthmic spondylolisthesis: clinical and radiographic results in six patients, *Spine* 27:E161–E168, 2002.

18. Mehdian SM, Arun R, Jones A, et al: Reduction of severe adolescent isthmic spondylolisthesis: a new technique, *Spine* 30:E579–E584, 2005.

19. Ani N, Keppler L, Biscup RS, et al: Reduction of high-grade slips (grades III-V) with VSP instrumentation. Report of a series of 41 cases, *Spine* 16:S302–S310, 1991.

20. Dick WT, Schnebel B: Severe spondylolisthesis. Reduction and internal fixation, *Clin Orthop Relat Res* 232:70–79, 1988.

21. Fabris DA, Costantini S, Nena U: Surgical treatment of severe L5-S1 spondylolisthesis in children and adolescents. Results of intraoperative reduction, posterior interbody fusion, and segmental pedicle fixation, *Spine* 21:728–733, 1996.

22. Boos N, Marchesi D, Zuber K, et al: Treatment of severe spondylolisthesis by reduction and pedicular fixation. A 4-6-year follow-up study, *Spine* 18:1655–1661, 1993.

23. Scherb R: Zur indication und technik der albec de quervain operation, *Schweiz Med Wochenschar* 20:763, 1921.

24. Meyerding HW: Spondylolisthesis, *Surg Gynecol Obstet* 54:371–377, 1932.

25. Capener N: Spondylolisthesis, *Br J Surg* 19:374, 1932.

26. Jenkins JA: Spondylolisthesis, *Br J Surg* 24:80–85, 1936.

27. Harrington PR, Dickson JH: Spinal instrumentation in the treatment of severe progressive spondylolisthesis, *Clin Orthop Relat Res* 117:157–163, 1976.

28. Nachemson A, Wiltse LL: Editorial: spondylolisthesis, *Clin Orthop Relat Res* 117:2–3, 1976.

29. Lenke LG, Bridwell KH: Evaluation and surgical treatment of high-grade isthmic dysplastic spondylolisthesis, *Instr Course Lect* 52:525–532, 2003.

30. Acosta FL Jr, Ames CP, Chou D: Operative management of adult high-grade lumbosacral spondylolisthesis, *Neurosurg Clin N Am* 18:249–254, 2007.

31. Hresko MT, Labelle H, Roussouly P, et al: Classification of high-grade spondylolistheses based on pelvic version and spine balance: possible rationale for reduction, *Spine* 32:2208–2213, 2007.

32. Legaye J, Duval-Beaupere G, Hecquet J, et al: Pelvic incidence: a fundamental pelvic parameter for three-dimensional regulation of spinal sagittal curves, *Eur Spine J* 7:99–103, 1998.

33. Harms J: *Severe spondylolisthesis: pathology, diagnosis, therapy*, Darmstadt, Germany, 2002, Steinkopff Verlag.

34. Boxall D, Bradford DS, Winter RB, et al: Management of severe spondylolisthesis in children and adolescents, *J Bone Joint Surg Am* 61:479–495, 1979.

35. Schoenecker PL, Cole HO, Herring JA, et al: Cauda equina syndrome after in situ arthrodesis for severe spondylolisthesis at the lumbosacral junction, *J Bone Joint Surg Am* 72:369–377, 1990.

Index

Page numbers followed by *f* indicate figures; *t*, tables, *b*, boxes.

Thoracolumbar vertebral metastasis *(Continued)*
  laminectomy or radiation therapy for, 183
  lateral extracavitary transpedicular approach to,
      185–186
    best evidence discussion of, 191–192
    commentary on, 193
  optimal surgical treatment of, 183
  preoperative angiography in, 186
  surgical options for, 185–186
    best evidence discussion of, 188–193
  ventral and dorsal approach combination to,
      185
    best evidence discussion of, 189–191
    commentary on, 193
  vertebral body reconstruction in, 192–193
Titanium mesh support cages, 232
Tong traction reduction technique, 164–166
  best evidence discussion of, 166–169
  commentary on, 169
  contraindications to, 164–165, 165b
  magnetic resonance imaging prior to, 165b, 168
  neurologic examination at traction weight
      addition, 165, 165b
Total (cervical) disk replacement (TDR), 1
  best evidence discussion of, 5–11
  biomechanical data on, 10
  commentary on, 11
  complications of, 10
  FDA approved prostheses for, 7
    randomized controlled trial results, 7–10
  indications and contraindications to, 4, 4t, 6–7
  multilevel, 10–11
  postoperative course in, 5, 6f
  technique of, 4–5
    adequate foraminal decompression, 5b
    diskectomy performed-endplate preparation,
        4b
    implant sizing and placement, 5b
    midline identification and appropriate
        implant placement, 4b
  two-level, 10
Total (lumbar) disk replacement (TDR), 78
  and adjacent level disease, literature review and
      studies, 87–88
  commentary on, 89
  complications of, clinical trial results, 88
  contraindications to, 78, 78b
  financial considerations of, 88
  versus fusion, clinical trials, 87
  postoperative radiography of, 79f
  technique of, 78–85
    completed approach to disk space, 81f
    diskectomy and end plate preparation, 82,
        82b–83b, 82f
    incision and access strategy, 77b, 79–80, 80f
    midline identification and level confirmation,
        81–82, 82b

Total (lumbar) disk replacement (TDR)
    (Continued)
  patient positioning, 78–80
  prosthetic device placement, 84, 84t, 85f
  restoration of disk height, 82–83, 83f
  retroperitoneal dissection for mini-open
      approach, 80, 81f
  trial implant insertion, 83–84, 84f, 84t
Transarticular screw fixation, in type II odontoid
      fracture, 137–138
  anatomic precautions in, 137–138, 138f
  technique of, 139–140
Transcervical endoscopic odontoidectomy,
      117–118, 117b–118b, 118f
Transfacet approach, to thoracic disk herniation,
      41–42
  indications for, 43b
Transforaminal lumbar interbody fusion (TLIF),
      77–78, 77f, 232–233
Transitional area surgery, fusion or nonfusion,
      180–181. *See also* Cervicothoracic junction
      laminectomy; L1-S1 fusion; Lumbosacral
      spondylolisthesis
Transoral-transpharyngeal decompression, and
      posterior stabilization
  morbidity associated with, 122
  procedure for, 116–117, 117b

V
Vertebral body reconstruction, after surgery for
      metastatic tumors, 192–193
Vertebral column resection, 201, 233
Vertebral metastases, ventral and dorsal approach
      or lateral extracavitary transpedicular
      approach, 183–195
  case presentation of, 184b, 184f–185f
  dorsal surgical approach, advantages and
      disadvantages, 185–186
  laminectomy or radiation therapy, 183
  lateral extracavitary transpedicular approach,
      185–186
    best evidence discussion of, 191–192
    commentary on, 193
  optimal surgical treatment, 183
  preoperative angiography in, 186
  surgical options for, 185–186
    best evidence discussion of, 188–193
  ventral and dorsal approach combination,
      185
    best evidence discussion of, 189–191
    commentary on, 193
  vertebral body reconstruction in, 192–193

Z
Z-plasty technique, 59, 59f